COMPANION TO
PAKISTANI CUISINE

Edited by
Shanaz Ramzi

Foreword by
Humayun Gauhar

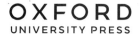

OXFORD
UNIVERSITY PRESS

OXFORD
UNIVERSITY PRESS

Oxford University Press is a department of the University of Oxford.
It furthers the University's objective of excellence in research, scholarship,
and education by publishing worldwide. Oxford is a registered trade mark of
Oxford University Press in the UK and in certain other countries

Published in Pakistan by
Oxford University Press
No. 38, Sector 15, Korangi Industrial Area,
PO Box 8214, Karachi-74900, Pakistan

ISBN 978-969-7343-09-6

Typeset in Minion Pro
Printed on 80gsm Offset Paper

Printed by Delta Dot Technologies (Pvt.) Ltd., Karachi

COMPANION TO
PAKISTANI CUISINE

Dedicated to the memory of

ZUBAIDA TARIQ, IRFAN HUSAIN, *and* MICHAEL JANSEN

Contents

Foreword

I am honoured to write the foreword for Shanaz Ramzi's book, *Companion to Pakistani Cuisine*. Her first book, *Food Prints: An Epicurean Voyage through Pakistan* (OUP, 2012), is a journey through the history of food in Pakistan and how and where it evolved and includes a valuable collection of recipes of various dishes. But this one is different. It does not feature recipes but is a veritable encyclopaedia of cuisine in Pakistan and its evolution. It is the first such encyclopaedia on Pakistani cuisine ever published. That makes it very interesting indeed and a painstaking piece of work covering all culinary related headwords and more. If some foods originated along the Grand Trunk Road, others in the homes of the poor. That is why I have always said that Pakistan's is a poverty-based cuisine. This book should be of great value to culinary students as well as anyone wanting information on Pakistan's food, its communities, provinces, utensils, techniques, popular ingredients, aromatics as well as legends attached to certain food.

Here is a legend: the rich always used to take the choicest cuts of the meat from an animal and discard mostly the offal. The poor would take the trotters of a goat or cow, its tripe, its tail, its liver, kidneys, and brain and cook them with a great deal of spices which made the product very tasty. So much so that the rich developed a fondness for a lot of such dishes especially the trotters, liver, kidneys, brain and so forth and included them in their menus. This is how evolution takes place.

There is another legend: did we take *shahi tukra* from the English bread and butter pudding or vice versa? There is no incontrovertible proof of either that I have heard of. There will be many who tell you that *shahi tukra* originated in the kitchens of the Mughals while others will tell you that local chefs got the idea while making bread and butter pudding for their British colonizers. Whatever you want to believe is also part of the legend.

In Pakistan's culinary evolution, special occasions like marriages, food related to the two Eids, and even food served at funerals have played a significant role.

I should add that a lot of Pakistani delicacies originated in the kitchens of the *rajas*, *nawabs*, and other local princelings and they were very good indeed. Their old recipes are written in another lingo—in *mashas* and *tolas*. Today, they are not that easy for us to follow. There is a story that *shami kebabs* were invented by the chefs of a *maharaja* who had lost his teeth and could only eat soft food. You will find many such legends and special occasion foods mentioned in this book.

Even within Pakistan there is diversity in cooking techniques and palate. The cuisines of the Pakhtun and the Baloch are totally meat-based and without spices except salt. Whereas the cuisine of the people of Karachi is probably the spiciest and most varied in Pakistan, people consider Lahore as the cuisine capital of Pakistani food. But to me, it is the cuisine of Gujranwala some forty miles from Lahore which is the best. Considering that Gujranwala is famous for its wrestlers, it's not surprising.

Meat cooked in whole spices has its own story. Leather workers from Chakwal and Chiniot used to take the cured hides to Calcutta (now Kolkata) which took four days by train. So, they would cook whole spiced meat or *kharay masalay ka gosht* in an earthen pot and take it with them on the journey with the pot acting as a kind of a refrigerator and the meat would last for four days. It came to be known variously as *kattay masalay ka gosht, kharay masalay ka gosht,* and *Calcutta ka gosht.* There are many such stories that await telling.

As such, if you really want to know a country, its peoples and history, you should research its culinary traditions and you will learn a lot. Pakistani food has at its roots Turkish, Persian, Central Asian, Arabic, Goan, Bengali, and of course, English and Chinese cuisines. Over time, Americans have also influenced Pakistan a great deal so that burgers and the like have also been included in Pakistani cuisine.

It is always an exercise in discovery when one starts studying cuisine in a scientific way. This book should be a great companion to books on recipes, methodologies of cooking, cooking in a certain culture, and so much more. You can learn a lot about utensils, cooking pots and cooking mediums. For example, the belief here is that food cooked in an earthen pot over a wood fire will boast flavours that will be otherwise missing if cooked in a modern utensil over a regular stove.

The many riveting essays by renowned writers on various interesting food-related subjects enrich this book further. There is also an article on the iconic eateries of Pakistan which should be of great interest for foodies and travellers to Pakistan.

While there is influence of Indian cuisine on Pakistani—as the Muslim migrant communities from India naturally brought their cuisines with them to Pakistan—there is a lot of influence of Pakistani cuisine on Indian because they have now taken to eating more and more meat.

HUMAYUN GAUHAR

Humayun Gauhar is a renowned writer, editor, and columnist of Pakistan. Currently he is the editor-in-chief of *Blue Chip*, a monthly magazine that specializes in economics, business strategy, and politics. He was a lead op-ed columnist of *The Nation*, Pakistan till the end of 2009. Now he writes a weekly column for *Pakistan Today*. Gauhar's weekly articles also appear in a number of Pakistan's Urdu/English newspapers and on international websites. He also writes occasionally for *The Sunday Times*, London, and is a regular television commentator and analyst on Pakistani and international affairs. In the 1980s, while living in London, Gauhar published around a dozen magazines, including the flagships, *South* and *Third World Quarterly*. Gauhar is known as the ghost-writer of former President General Pervez Musharraf's internationally bestselling autobiography, *In the Line of Fire*, which has been translated into 30 languages, including Italian. Last, but not least, Gauhar enjoys cooking Pakistani cuisine and has done two cooking shows on television.

Introduction

In 2012 when my first book, *Food Prints: An Epicurean Voyage through Pakistan*, was published by Oxford University Press (OUP) Pakistan, at its launch event the then Managing Director of OUP asked me if I would be interested in doing a second title with them, this time a companion—*Companion to Pakistani Cuisine*—to be precise. I immediately said yes—for two reasons: I have always felt that Pakistan has taken a back seat in promoting its diverse and rich cuisine that has evolved through centuries of invasions by armies, and inflows of trade and immigrants into the region; the blending of their food with indigenous recipes, has developed one of the most delectable and varied cuisines in the world. When people talk about exotic cuisines they think 'Indian'—they have no concept that, thanks to our shared history and geography, Indian cuisine is in many ways Pakistani too, and, in fact, thanks to Pakistanis' proclivity for meat, our cuisine is a lot more delightful and varied than that of our neighbouring country. A chance to let the world know all that Pakistan's magnificent cuisine has to offer through this one and only *Companion* was too tempting to pass.

The other reason for me to jump at the opportunity of doing this collection was that I felt that since it would be more or less an extension of my previous book, I would be at an advantage, and would be able to complete it fairly quickly. Suffice it to say, that was far from the case. It took me seven years to write *Food Prints*, and even longer to edit and contribute to the *Companion*. I had not bargained for how difficult it was going to be to identify people who could write on food-related entries, and worse, submit them by their given deadlines.

Admittedly, it may have been much easier if I could have just written the whole book myself instead of having to chase contributors, but then there would have been no diversity in style. There is no denying that the *Companion* benefits greatly from the entries by the many experts that have contributed to it, and I am deeply grateful to each of them for their valuable input and for sparing the time to enrich this book.

Having said that, I must admit that I did land up tackling a large number of entries myself—thanks to Covid-19 that provided a lot of spare time under lockdown—and so managed to finally complete all the pending entries. There is always a silver lining to every cloud and this surely proved to be one for me!

While I am deeply indebted to all the contributors, I would like to particularly record my gratitude to the late Irfan Husain, and Anjali Malik who sent in their timely contributions without expecting any remuneration. I am also deeply grateful to Husain Haroon for sparing his valuable time to go through the entries, and then meeting me to share his thoughts on them.

Most headwords have been explained as briefly as possible, but there are a handful that have been covered in essay form, as I felt that they merited greater detail. I am sure readers will find those entries as enjoyable as they are informative.

I hope this book serves not just as a reference book for those looking to find out about a particular Pakistani dish, ingredient, utensil, or community's culinary preferences, but as a go-to book to read at leisure just to discover more about Pakistan, its people, their culture, and their cuisine. Having said that, I must add that I have learned from experience, that, despite my best efforts, there will, very likely be undetected errors in the book, or some entries that may have been inadvertently overlooked. I would be glad to be told of them, preferably with compassion! Errors/omissions will be rectified in the next edition.

HAPPY READING!

SHANAZ RAMZI

Contributors

Editor

Shanaz Ramzi. Currently, Chief Executive Officer of StarLinks PR and Events and President TravelinPk, Shanaz Ramzi has been working as a freelance journalist since 1994. A prolific writer, she has written on a variety of subjects for various publications, both local and international, and is the author of *Food Prints: An Epicurean Voyage through Pakistan* (OUP, 2012), and *Food Tales* (2021). A regular contributor to the magazine sections of the English daily *Dawn* and the erstwhile monthly magazine *Newsline*, Ramzi has been twice nominated for the Gender in Journalism Award by UNESCO. Her essays have been published in the book titled *Pakistan's Radioactive Decade: An Informal Cultural History of the 1970s* (OUP, 2019). She has also edited various publications including *Humsay, Masala TV Food Mag*, Pakistan's widely circulated food magazine, *Mise en Place, Glam,* and the World Gourmand Peace Award-winning book *Zaiqay Frontier Ke: Dera Ismail Khan Ke Bhule Bisre Pakwan.*

Contributors

Note: All entries in this *Companion* which are without a byline are by Shanaz Ramzi.

Sunita Achria. Born and raised in Bombay, Sunita Achria moved to Karachi in 1977 and while raising three children, dabbled in fashion, going on to run her own fashion business with partners. An inherent multi-tasker, alongside her sartorial enterprises, Sunita also dabbled in her other passion: food. Inspired by her mother, who she saw preparing exotic Indian dishes in her childhood and teen years, Sunita began experimenting with assorted cuisines. The success of her culinary ventures, judging by the response of friends invited to soirees at her home, finally resulted in a restaurant: The Patio. The cuisine at the restaurant reflects Sunita's culinary vision. It is an eclectic mix of food from around the globe—tried and tested dishes, and an unusual one-of-a-kind fare.

Kausar Ahmed. A chef, culinary educator, recipe and content developer, and food and prop stylist specialising in South Asian cuisine, Kausar Ahmed is based in Seattle. She launched her debut cookbook *The Karachi Kitchen in North America* in November 2017. The book consists of traditional and contemporary Pakistani recipes from Karachi, where she was born and grew up. It is a curated piece featuring her favourite recipes from childhood and, later, motherhood.

Naheed Ansari. A renowned name in the field of food management in Pakistan, Naheed Ansari holds over thirty-five years of experience in cooking, food presentation, and home decor. She has appeared on several channels such as Pakistan Television (PTV), Indus TV, Indus Plus, Ary Digital/Ary Zauq, Samaa TV, Health TV, Geo TV and Masala TV and has several TV programmes under her belt. She has become an icon of good taste and fabulous cooking for women in Pakistan. Her experience in cooking and presentation has made her immensely popular among fans at home and overseas.

Irfan Husain. The late Pakistani newspaper columnist and civil servant residing in the UK, Irfan Husain wrote weekly columns for *Dawn* newspaper. Although Husain has written on a wide range of subjects for newspapers in Pakistan and elsewhere since 1970, his food-related articles probably garnered the most readership as he was quite the foodie and loved to cook and experiment with his food. He died on 16 December 2020.

Michael Jansen. The late Prof. Jansen studied architecture and building history until 1974. In 1976, he studied South Asian archaeology at Delhi University and the Archaeological Survey of India. In 1979, he received his doctorate from Aachen on his thesis 'Architecture of the Harappa Culture.' From 1978 to 1987, he was, in collaboration with Gunter Urban, project leader of the DFG research project 'Mohenjo-Daro'. His main research interests include the Indus culture (Mohenjo-Daro), colonial architecture in South Asia, and archaeology and architecture in Southeast Arabia. He died in July 2022.

Yasmeen Lari. Co-founder and CEO of Heritage Foundation, and founder chair of INBAU Pakistan, Yasmeen Lari is an architect, architectural historian, heritage conservationist and philanthropist. Recipient of several national and international awards, her works have been exhibited widely. She has devised barefoot social architecture for attaining social and ecological justice and one of her latest projects, the Pakistan *Chulah*, has not only bagged her an international award and recognition but is also being emulated in other countries.

Lal Majid. Owner and master chocolatier at Lal's Chocolates, Lal Majid trained for years in schools and kitchens from Karachi to Canada, working all hours to learn the tricks of her trade. Now at the pinnacle of her career, she has a shop and chocolate café in Karachi, two shops in Lahore, done a cooking show on Masala TV—*All About Chocolates*—and authored a Gourmand Award-winning chocolate cookbook titled *Deliciously Yours*, published by Markings.

Anjali Malik. A retired Associate Professor at the University of Delhi, India, and having specialised in Ancient Indian History, Anjali Malik has a teaching experience of more than four decades. She has participated and presented papers in many national and international seminars. Her book, *Merchants and Merchandise in Northern India AD 600–1000*, published in 1998 was well received and is considered an authoritative work on this subject. Her papers on society and economy of ancient India have also been published in various journals. Her interest in the history of food began when she edited and wrote two chapters on the cuisine of 'Frontier' for her mother Shrimati Pushpa Kumari Bagai's bilingual book (in Hindi and Urdu), titled *Zaiqay Frontier Ke: Dera Ismail Khan Ke Bhule Bisre Vyanjan*, published in 2015 in Pakistan. The book was launched by Anjali Malik at the Jaipur Literature Festival, Bhutan Literature Festival, Rekhta Festival in Delhi, and the Faiz International Festival in Lahore during 2015 and 2016. It went on to win the World Gourmand Cookbook Award for 'Harmony Through Food: Indo-Pak Cookbook' at Yantai, China, in 2015. The book is about the delectable cuisine of North West Frontier Province (now Khyber Pakhtunkhwa) from where the Bagai Family migrated after the Partition of the country.

Sibtain Naqvi. An independent researcher, Sibtain Naqvi, focuses on institutional and cultural history. A frequent contributor to Pakistan's English newspapers, Naqvi's research has been presented in Oxford, Cambridge, Columbia, and other institutions. His essays have been published by Oxford University Press in *Pakistan's Radioactive Decade*. He has been heavily cited in *Through the Eyes of Tiger Cubs: Views of Asia's Next Generation* published by Time Magazine, Asia Business Council, and the Lee Kuan Yew School of Public Policy at National University of Singapore. He has authored *Unravelling Gordian Knots: The Works and Worlds of Dr. Ishrat Husain*; *Chronicling Excellence: A History of IBA*; *Cobwebbed World of Sadequain: A Retrospective*; *Ghalib: Call of Angel*; *Sadequain: Drawings 1970*; *Surah-e-Rehman: Calligraphy*; and *Rubaiyaat-e-Kuliyaat-Sadequain*.

Asif Noorani. Belonging to a bilingual (Urdu and English) family, Asif Noorani was born in what was Bombay in 1942. He migrated to Pakistan in 1950 with his parents and two younger brothers. He has written three books and contributed to quite a few including the one on Karachi, published by Oxford University Press, Pakistan. He also edited *Eastern Film*, Pakistan's most widely circulated English magazine to date, way back in the 1960s, and *Star Weekend*, the popular colour magazine that was distributed with the daily *Star* in the 1990s. He is a freelance journalist and contributes to daily *Dawn*. He writes on art, literature, culture, and, somewhat rarely, on cuisine. He loves *desi* food, particularly *nihari*, *paya*, and fried fish. As far as his talent for cooking is concerned, it doesn't exceed beyond pouring boiling water in a cup furnished with a tea bag.

Nayyer Rubab. Researcher, author, translator and storywriter for children, Nayyer Rubab has produced programmes for radio and TV, with experience of more than thirty years in advertising, and electronic and print media. She has developed content of thousands of hours on different subjects for HUM TV and PTV Ramazan transmission, and is also doing a weekly radio programme. She has translated four books published by Faiz Foundation, while the fifth is underway.

Deborah Santamaria. Known as Debbie, Deborah Santamaria was born and raised in Karachi where she was the secretary, and then president of Goinkars Own Academy (GOA), established in 2000 to help solidify the existence of their mother tongue Konkani, and the Goan culture in an Islamic country. Goinkars Own Academy was among the twenty-five Konkani associations from around the world to be presented with an award by President of India, Smt. Pratibha Devisingh Patil, for its contribution to the growth and preservation of Konkani in the region. Besides taking part in church activities, Debbie has been on the executive committee of various organisations such as Catholic Women's Guild (CWG), The Distinguished Secretaries Society of Pakistan (DSSP), and Karachi Goan Association (KGA). She moved to the USA in 2016 and in 2020 she created a Food blog, Debs Kitchen, where she shares her love for cooking with the world in an attempt to promote Goan cultural cuisine along with cherishing cuisines that other worlds have to offer.

Zarnak Sidhwa. A household name practically throughout Pakistan and one of the most popular television chefs on Masala TV, Zarnak Sidhwa has been sharing recipes and cooking tips with Pakistani audiences for 11 years now on her exclusive show, *Food Diaries*.

Shaha Tariq. After a long association with the education industry working at various leadership positions, Shaha has now moved her skillset of content development and marketing to Nutshell Group where she heads Content. She is appreciated for her innovative strategies that have helped turn struggling institutions into success stories. She is a certified trainer from the University of Cambridge and has been part of training teams for various educational and multinational institutions. She

has also contributed to Heritage Foundation's literacy and development projects. Her series on children's literacy is used by the literacy centres in Khairpur. She scripted a digital short (film) in 2021 which crossed a two-million viewership mark.

Zubaida Tariq. The late Zubaida Tariq Ilyas, commonly known as Zubaida Aapa, was a Pakistani chef, herbalist, and cooking expert. She was the first celebrity cook of Pakistan, who appeared on numerous TV shows, and was also known for her household tips and culinary advice. She died on 4 January 2018, aged 72.

Bisma Tirmizi. A former *Dawn* staffer and currently a freelance journalist, Bisma Tirmizi is also an author at Rupa Publications India and Aleph Book Company. She frequently writes a food-related column for *Dawn*'s magazine *EOS*, published on Sundays.

Summaya Usmani. A Pakistan-born cookery writer, blogger and teacher based in Scotland, Summaya Usmani is the published writer of two award-winning and award-nominated cookbooks and continues to write for many international food and culture publications. She is currently working on a non-fiction and fiction book, with food as a common theme.

Aab gosht. One of the dishes included in the Kashmiri *Wazwan* (traditional feast) today, *aab gosht* is a wholesome meat dish originating in Persia—*aab* means water in Persian. Mixed with the flavours of fennel, cardamom, cumin, cinnamon, and black pepper which are placed in a muslin bag and cooked on low heat all night, it makes for a unique lamb chops dish that is cooked in its stock with yoghurt, small onions and tomatoes. A slow-cooking dish, it is easy to cook, very nourishing and full of taste.

NAYYER RUBAB

Aaloo chaap. A delicious, Khoja-community version of potato cakes with ground meat filling, the cutlets could be of any size, though traditionally they are big and round, and served as a side dish at a meal. They could also be served on their own as a snack, accompanied by ketchup or chutney. Potatoes are boiled and mashed, a little amount is spread on the palm, the filling is placed inside, and then another layer of mashed potato is placed over it. The cooked minced meat could be beef or chicken, with onion and fresh coriander generally added into it, along with seasoning of choice. The cutlets are then dipped into a beaten egg and coated with breadcrumbs before being deep fried in oil.

SHAHA TARIQ

Aaloo gosht. Known as *aaloo gosht* or *gosht ka salan* in most communities and as *aaloo salan* among the Dilliwallay, this is a mutton and potato curry cooked in basic spices. It is perhaps the most widely consumed curry dish in the country and is regarded as comfort food. A savoury and aromatic dish with light spiciness, its meat is very tender, while the gravy is a little soupy with balanced spices.

According to legend, this erstwhile royal dish became a common man's household dish when Haji Karimuddin, son of Mohammad Aziz (a cook in the royal Mughal kitchen, whose ancestors used to cook for Babar, the first Mughal emperor), set up a roadside stall selling just two dishes—*aaloo gosht* and *daal* (lentils) for the coronation celebration of King George V. He served both the dishes with *roomali roti*.

Later, as a matter of tradition, people in UP began to cook *aaloo gosht* in combination with *daal maash* (white lentils) and served it with *roti* (roasted or baked flat bread) or plain rice. There are various methods of cooking *aaloo gosht*, the most common being to fry the lamb/mutton with onion, tomato, and spices, and then simmer with potato over medium heat.

NAYYER RUBAB

Aam ka rus aur puri. A summer favourite when mangoes are in season, *aam ka rus* is usually made in two styles. One is served hot; mango pulp is cooked in oil infused with cloves and cardamom, with a cup of flour added to give it consistency. Water and sugar are also added. It is served piping hot after meals as a dessert.

The other style is more Gujarati in tradition and is made with fresh, ripe mangoes. *Saunth* (dry ginger powder) is added for flavour to freshly diced and blended mangoes, along with milk and sugar. It is served chilled with hot *puri* (fried, puffed version of *chapati* (roasted flat bread), though smaller in size, and generally made with refined flour).

A Rajasthani variation of *aam ka rus* also exists which incorporates saffron instead of dry ginger. *Aam ka rus* is a popular breakfast item in summer when mangoes are in season.

SHAHA TARIQ

Aash. A popular dish in Iranian, Azerbaijani, Caucasian, and Turkish cuisine, and also prepared by the Parsis living in Pakistan, *aash* immediately conjures an image of a big pot of thick hot soup cooked by grandmothers in winter. Typically consisting of various beans, legumes, fresh herbs, vegetables, broth, yoghurt, spices, meat and oil, the term *aash* has such great significance in Persian culture that *aash paz khoneh* means kitchen in Persian and *aash paz* means cook.

Aash is commonly served in low-income groups, especially at large gatherings, as the dish is very nutritious, easy to serve, and cost-effective as well.

There are more than 50 varieties of *aash*, depending on the occasion. *Aash-e-reshteh* (*reshteh* meaning spaghetti/noodles) is the standard soup or meal as it is very filling. In the Parsi community, it is normally made on a happy occasion, especially the day after the wedding in the bride's maternal home when both the bride and the groom are called over to the bride's parents' house.

NAYYER RUBAB

Abresham. A traditional Sindhi herbal drink originating from Thatta valley, this sherbet is allegedly the creation of Hakeem (traditional medicine physician) Mohammad Vasil Dars who lived in Thatta. The formula was very sacred and only known to Hakeem sahib. When Hakeem sahib was on his death bed, he passed on the formula of *abresham* to his young son. The factory is still in Thatta, and the drink is made with the extract of very rare flowers and herbs, used in Unani (Greco-Arab) medicine. The concentrate is mixed with water or milk, and sugar just before serving. As per the claim, it quickly gives strength to the heart and brain. It is cool in composition and therefore mostly consumed in Ramazan and summers. *Abresham* is red in colour, and hence is popularly known as *Sindh ka lal sherbet* (Sindh's red sherbet). It tastes best when consumed chilled.

NAYYER RUBAB

Accompaniment. Sometimes referred to as a side dish, accompaniment is a food item that accompanies the entrée or main course at a meal, served as a smaller portion, or something that supplements or complements the dish.

Traditionally, Pakistani accompaniments are derived from three broad cultures—the Middle Eastern, the Central Asian, and the South Asian. Historical influences of serving accompaniments go back to the Mughal era. Significant influence emerged in the 16th century, when the Mongol Empire began ruling the area and introduced a style of cooking called Mughlai.

Accompaniments, such as raw salads, chutneys, pickles (*achars*), *kachumbers* (a tangy onion-based salad), and *raitas* are commonly used with the main courses in Pakistan. When indulging in traditional Pakistani dishes with spices that linger in the mouth long after one has finished eating, a great way to cool off the hot flavours is by tempering side dishes like the *raita*, a traditional yoghurt dip. Some popular Pakistani dishes such as *nihari* and *haleem* are served with a variety of accompaniments which could include fried onions, lemon, coriander, mint leaves, chopped green chillies, and finely julienned ginger.

Mangoes (in season) are also consumed as accompaniments to the main meal in many households that can afford to serve fruits. Beverages, such as milk, tea, juice, green tea and *lassi* (buttermilk) are also regarded as accompaniments.

Modern day accompaniments are inspired by continental and Western influences and include a variety of French fries, baked potatoes, soups, salads, butter, and sweet and savoury sauces, whereas the health conscious even opt for steamed vegetables.

Accompaniments may or may not be a part of the regular meal but the likelihood of their presence becomes higher over the weekends and on special occasions.

KAUSAR AHMED

Achar. The English term for *achar*, commonly thought to be of a Persian or Arabic origin, is pickle. However, Georg Rumphius in AD 1750 states that the word *achar* is derived from terms like *axi* or *achi* used for chilli. There are other theories too about the origin of the word. According to Hobson-Jobson (1903; see Yule and Burnell, 1979), the term is used across the subcontinent for all acid and salt relishes. Pickling is an age-old technique used to preserve food and, judging from some archaeological evidence, was invented in the subcontinent. Traditionally, certain varieties of fresh fruits and vegetables were mixed in oil and spices so as to increase their shelf-life and to be enjoyed out of season. Now, even meats such as mutton, fish, and chicken, are pickled and eaten with food as accompaniments. Pickles make the food spicy and tangy.

To make *achar*, fruits and vegetables are cut into bite-size pieces, while small size vegetables could be kept whole. They are then spread on a clean sheet in the sun for some time so that the surface moisture is evaporated. Once they are dry, they are mixed with various spices and oil, and put in glass or porcelain jars that have been thoroughly cleaned and dried as there must be no trace of moisture in them. These *achar*-filled jars are then kept in the sun for a few days for the pickle to age and the flavours of all the spices to blend in. Oil, salt, brine or vinegar and spices act as preservatives, preventing fungi and also giving a quintessential sourness to pickles, not to mention increasing the nutritional value of the basic ingredients, which, as they ferment, introduce vitamin B, in the form of good bacteria. This, in turn, inhibits the growth of harmful microbes in the human digestive system. The vitamin C content of pickles also tends to be very high which is an additional health benefit.

Some pickles such as of lemon, lime, and raw mango, can last for many years. Traditionally, mustard oil is used for making *achar* because it has a pungent taste but sesame oil is also used for making pickles. The main spices used are fenugreek seeds, nigella seeds, mustard seeds, fennel, salt, chilli powder, asafoetida, *garam masala* (mixed spices) and turmeric.

There are many recipes for making *achar*. Spices are mixed according to individual tastes. Some *achars* are spicy while others are sweet and sour. To make sweet and sour pickles, jaggery is added along with spices. Generally, carrot, turnip, and cauliflower are mixed together to make sweet and sour pickle.

The most common fruits and vegetables used in making *achar* are raw mango, lemon, lotus stem, onion, potato, pumpkin, radish, chilli, garlic, ginger, aloe vera, carrot, turnip, and cauliflower. Sometimes vegetables are combined to make pickles. If five types of vegetables are combined, it is called *panchranga achar* and if seven are used then it is termed *satranga achar*.

Achars are a common accompaniment to Pakistani meals. Whether the staple is *roti/parathay*, or rice, and the main course *daal* or curry, *achars* add a zing to the meal and are always welcome. They also help digest food easily.

Once exclusively made at home, pickles are now commercially produced in factories and are generally bought by households, especially in the cities, where few people have the patience or the inclination to go through the tedious procedure of making them at home.

ANJALI MALIK

Achari murgh. Literally, pickled chicken, this dish derives its name from the ground roasted spices and whole spices used in its cooking, that are commonly incorporated in pickles. A rare Awadhi cuisine of Uttar Pradesh (UP), although Hyderabad Deccan also claims its origin, it is now very popular among Pakistanis all over the world, having been introduced to Pakistan by the immigrant community moving from India at the time of Partition.

The key ingredients used in equal proportion are onion seeds, fenugreek seeds, fennel seeds, cumin seeds, and nigella seeds (collectively known as *panch phoran*) but the taste may differ depending on whether one is adding tamarind paste, tomatoes or yoghurt to the dish, and onions. Cooked in mustard oil, *achari murgh* is generally served with *naan/paratha/roti* as it tends to be dry but is sometimes also served with plain rice.

Variations of the above could be made using mutton instead of chicken, and vegetarian versions incorporating cottage cheese to make *achari paneer* or vegetables to make *achari sabzi*.

NAYYER RUBAB

Achcho borh. A variation of the Balochi dish *rosh* (white lamb curry) which was introduced from Persia, *achcho borh* is a popular dish in Sindh. *Achcho* means white in Sindhi, and *borh* means curry. A white curry made with sautéed mutton or chicken (*gosht jo achcho borh/ murghi jo achcho borh*), it does not incorporate the otherwise ubiquitous turmeric, red chilli powder/flakes, or tomatoes that lend colour to most curries.

The basic ingredients in this curry, aside from the meat are salt, yoghurt, crushed black pepper, a little bit of coriander powder, ground onions, almonds and *sabut garam masala* (whole mixed spices). It tastes best when cooked covered, over slow fire (*dum*) in a terracotta pot and eliminating the *bhoonna* (frying) process of cooking. It is generally a must in big family gatherings.

NAYYER RUBAB

Achrach. A seasonal Sindhi dish, *achrach* is made with minced meat, onions, spices, yoghurt, and sliced unripe mango. Since mangoes are seasonal, unless one has access to frozen unripe mangoes, this dish can only be made in summer before the mango season is in full force.

Adus pulao. A Hyderabadi speciality, *adus pulao* is basically an Iranian dish which is cooked with slight variations in Iran, Afghanistan, Pakistan, India, Egypt and Greece. *Adus pulao* (*adus* means black lentils) is a mix of black lentils, fried raisins, dates, meat, and plain rice. The dish comprises plain rice and black lentils cooked separately, with various spices. It is served generally with the lentils completely dry and mixed with fried raisins and dates. When it is dished out, the raisin-lentil mix is spread over the plain white rice and served with steamed/roasted chicken or lamb, green salad, pickles, and yoghurt.

Some people use saffron to give a golden yellow colour to the rice. A very common variation of *adus pulao* in Pakistan is plain white rice served with black lentil curry and pickles in summers.

NAYYER RUBAB

Afghan refugee. The cuisine of the refugees from Afghanistan, like that of the Pakhtuns, is neither too spicy nor too pungent, and yet, is not bland in taste. The peculiarity of this cuisine is its unusual predilection for using animal fat, so much so that even barbecued meat is accompanied with fat pieces. Afghans are as famous for their hospitality as the Pakhtuns of Khyber Pakhtunkhwa, and it is unthinkable that a visitor would be turned away hungry from their doorstep. They drink green tea practically throughout the day, accompanied by *gur*.

Akhni. Unlike most types of *pulao* (rice dish), this Memon community's rice dish is made in red masala instead of green, and the mutton and rice are cooked with red chillies, potatoes, onions, tomatoes, yoghurt, and a lot of aromatic spices. Turmeric is also used, so the rice is yellow in colour.

Akoori. A Parsi version of spicy scrambled eggs, *akoori* is made with tomatoes, onions, coriander, spices and, of course, eggs. It is normally enjoyed with *karak pav/pao* (crusty bread) at Sunday brunches.

Another Parsi version of *akoori* is made with greens, generally spinach, topped with fried or full-boiled eggs. *Akoori* sandwiches are also popular for taking along to picnics. *Bharuchi akoori*, which along with scrambled eggs also includes potatoes and dry fruit, is another popular dish. In winters, green fresh garlic is added to the scrambled eggs.

ZARNAK SIDHWA

Alcohol. Although alcohol consumption is prohibited in Islam, Muslims did generally imbibe liquor from ancient times. As early as *c.*2000 BC, the Indus Valley Civilisation seems to have practised not only alcoholic fermentation, but even distillation. A distillation assembly had been put together using clay objects commonly found at Harappan sites. Numerous liquors are mentioned in Vedic literature with the sources for fermentation, including sugarcane juice, pulp, molasses, honey, and coconut water. The fruits used included grapes, mangoes, date palm, bananas, apricots, and pomegranate. Extensive drinking was also noted around AD 600 in Kashmir. Even during the Mughal rule, the first Mughal emperor, Babar had periodic bouts of abstinence, when he would break his flagons and goblets of gold and silver, and give away the pieces, only to resume drinking later. While Akbar rarely drank wine, Jahangir on the other hand, by the end of his reign,

would imbibe twenty cups of double-distilled liquor in a day. Shahjahan drank in moderation, and Aurangzeb was a strict teetotaller who issued severe prohibitory orders on all his subjects—Hindus and Muslims alike. Today, although alcohol is sold in licenced shops in Pakistan, it is officially illegal for Muslims to purchase it. Hence, after the once ubiquitous wine shops and open consumption of liquor was banned in Pakistan in 1977—ironically as a political stunt by the then prime minister, Zulfikar Ali Bhutto, who used to drink regularly himself—the serving of alcohol in public places in the country has become covert affairs.

SHANAZ RAMZI AND NAYYER RUBAB

Almond (badam). Derived from the old Persian term *vadam*, *badam* or the almond (*Prunus amygdalus*) is of Central European/West Asian origin, along with other related *prunus* species like the cherry, plum, peach, and apricot. In Mughal times, though fairly plentiful by the time of Akbar, they were always expensive.

Almonds are extensively used in Pakistani epicurean cuisine, both in enriching savoury dishes such as *biryani* and *qorma*, as well as a garnish for desserts such as *shahi tukray*, *kheer*, and *halway*. They are used either ground or slivered, roasted, blanched, or in their original state. They are also used to make sherbet or as a flavouring for pink tea.

Alsi ki pinni. *Alsi*, flaxseeds or linseeds as they are also called, are seeds of a plant which grows up to a metre high and bears blue coloured flowers in the early months of the year. In the northern parts of Pakistan, they are known as *alsi kay beej*. *Alsi ki pinni* or flaxseed *laddu* is a delicious winter snack prepared with ingredients known for protecting one's body from cold, cough, and other winter ailments. Traditionally, in Pakistan, *alsi ki pinni* are given to pregnant women and breastfeeding mothers. It is a traditional Punjabi sweet, and is a combination of wheat flour, clarified butter, jaggery, cashew nuts, almonds, pistachios, and raisins.

The seeds themselves and the oil extracted from them both have numerous therapeutic uses. They are a rich source of micronutrients, dietary fibre, manganese, vitamin B1, and the essential fatty acid, alpha-linolenic acid also known as ALA or Omega3. The seeds come from flax, one of the oldest fibre crops in the world known to have been cultivated in ancient Egypt and China. Ground *alsi* can be added in various dishes like chutneys, curries, and a variety of sweet dishes.

In Pakistan, *alsi* is grown on marginal and sub-marginal lands under irrigated as well as rain-fed conditions of the Punjab and Sindh provinces.

KAUSAR AHMED

Amchoor. Also known as mango powder, this flavouring (*Mangifera indica*) is made from unripe mangoes, which have been sliced and sun-dried, then ground to a powder. *Amchoor* is mainly used to impart a tart, fruity sourness to fish and vegetable dishes, although it is also used as a meat tenderiser.

Amirti. The word *amrita* itself means 'manna' or the food of the gods, and this dessert does not disappoint. Resembling the *jalebi*, the *amirti* or *imarti*, is a Bengali dessert. The batter of ground *urad* (white lentils) is coloured with saffron and piped into hot oil in symmetrical loops and layers that give it the appearance of a rose. It is then immediately soaked in pre-prepared sugar syrup that not only allows it to absorb the sweetness but also increases its size. The end product is soft and oozy and of a deep orange colour.

NAYYER RUBAB

Anar dana. Some wild forms of pomegranate grown in some areas of Kashmir and Murree Hills, boast a sour taste and are usually utilised to make *anaar dana* (dried pomegranate seeds resembling tiny raisins). These are used in making a number of savoury dishes, including some pulse and vegetable entrées, for their sweet and sour flavour. Ground dried pomegranate seeds are also often used to make chutneys. The seeds and pulp are separated from the rind of the fruit and dried in the sun for 10 to 15 days, during which time they turn a reddish-brown. The spice is marketed in this form and often ground before use.

Anar gosht fry. *Anar* (pomegranate) is abundantly found in Balochistan region but is an expensive fruit which is extremely popular as much for its nutritious value as its tantalising flavour. As its name suggests, *anar gosht fry*, is a meat-based dish that has pomegranate seeds as one of its ingredients. The word *fry*, when used for a curry, entails a lot of cooking of the meat till it is completely tender. A popular way of cooking is to soak the meat (ideally mutton) in freshly squeezed pomegranate juice for four to six hours before preparing the curry base with onions and desired spices and adding the meat and the juice along with yoghurt.

However, water must not be added while cooking, as the curry paste has to remain thick. The paste comprises regular curry spices as well as tamarind paste, *kewra* (screw pine), nutmeg, and, of course, pomegranate seeds. Once the oil separates from the spices, meat is added and cooked on low heat while stirring continuously. A wonderful winter dish, it is eaten with *chapati*.

ZUBAIDA TARIQ

Anday ka qeema. This dish is a delicious take on a scrambled version of a spicy vegetable omelette. Onions are sautéed, chopped tomatoes are added to it, and then beaten eggs are stirred in. The trick is to keep stirring the ingredients continuously till the egg appears like mince. Optionally, capsicum and/or any other vegetable could be added to suit individual tastes. A twist of lemon on top gives an appealing tangy flavour.

Garnished with diced green chillies and coriander, this is not just a delicious holiday breakfast served with *paratha* or toasted bread. It is often eaten at dinner, too, and is a cost-effective, go-to meal in households operating on a tight budget or in times of emergency when one may not have an entrée ready and unexpected guests drop by. Also known as *ghotala* or *khagina*, the *ghotala* version has boiled *urad ki daal* stirred in along with beaten eggs.

SHAHA TARIQ

Anday wala khana. A Khoja speciality, this rice-based dish incorporates *chana* (gram lentils) or *arhar daal* (pigeon peas) cooked in masala, as well as potatoes and boiled eggs that have been lightly fried. It is made with the gravy mixture placed in a layer over the boiled rice, before being put on *dum*.

Anglo-Indian. The term Anglo-Indian was used for the first time in the Indian census of 1911 to denote persons of mixed ethnicity. In 1935, the Government of India Act formally identified them as 'A person whose father or any other male progenitors in the male line is or was of European descent but who is a native of India.' The Indian Constitution in 1950 retained the key points of that definition when Anglo-Indians were listed as an official minority group. The Anglo-Indian community traces its origin to the earliest contact between Europe and India. The discovery of sea route to India by the navigator, Vasco da Gama, in 1498 and his landing at Kozhikode led to the establishment of the Portuguese rule in Kozhikode and surrounding areas. As early as 1510 the Portuguese governor, Afonso de Albuquerque, conquered Goa and encouraged his countrymen to marry Indian women to help establish Portuguese authority. The offspring of these marriages were known as Luso-Indians.

When the British East India Company gained dominance over India, a large number of their officials and soldiers settled down in this country. At that time, the Board of Directors of the Company did not allow their families or wives to travel along with them. The English women were also not willing to undertake the long and strenuous sea voyage for a country that was culturally altogether different. In the 18th century, the British East India Company following the previous Dutch and Portuguese settlers, encouraged its employees to marry local Indian women. The Company even paid a sum to every mother of an offspring of cross-cultural union on the day the child was christened. The children of such unions were known as Eurasians. In the 19th century, when Suez Canal was constructed, the distance between Britain and India was considerably reduced and so was the travel time; hence, British women started travelling to India. The mixed marriages dwindled and their offspring came to be rejected and were treated with disdain and called *kutcha butcha* (half-baked bread). Gradually, the Luso-Indians who had retained their culture, got merged with the community of mixed British and Indian descent. Over the years their segregation from European community and marriage among themselves gave rise to a culture that was a mixture of European and Indian. In the early 20th century, they were placed in a broader ethnic category under the rubric Anglo-Indian. The cuisine, dress, speech, and religion of the Anglo-Indians were totally different from the native population. They were more Anglo than Indians; only dark complexion betrayed their origins.

The Anglo-Indians developed a distinctive cuisine which is a fusion of English and local cookery. The bland British food was made tastier by adding indigenous spices. Jhal frezi/jalfrezi is their staple; other typical dishes include mutton vindaloo and pepper water.

ANJALI MALIK

Anise. A sun-loving plant with feathery, serrated leaves and delicate umbels of creamy white flowers, the seeds of anise are light brown, oval and have a strong liquorice taste. Anise (or aniseed), though very similar to fennel seed, is not the same. The botanical name of anise is *Pimpinella anisum* while the botanical name of fennel is *Foeniculum vulgare*. Both anise and fennel belong to the Apiaceae family.

Anise is a little sweeter than fennel seed. It is a spice native to the Mediterranean and Southwest Asia. It is being cultivated in northern and eastern parts of the subcontinent since the time of Muslim invasions. The slender, aromatic seeds are often served after a meal as a mouth-freshener and digestive. They are slightly roasted for this purpose.

French traveller Francois Bernier (AD c.1665) mentions carrying sweet biscuits flavoured with anise during his travels in India.

BISMA TIRMIZI

Apple. The second largest crop—after dates—of Pakistan's largest province (area-wise), Balochistan, also known as the fruit basket of Pakistan, is apple. Two kinds of apples are grown here: red delicious and golden delicious. One can find multiple shades of red, green and golden among them. A symbol of health, beauty and love, apples in Pakistan are popular both for eating raw and cooking. Pakistani apples are renowned for their flavour, if not for their size and looks.

Apples can be preserved and cooked in many forms like jams, jellies, pickles and chutneys. They have substantial amounts of pectin, which makes jam-making easy. In Pakistan, apples are also used in fresh juices, fruit *chaats* and fresh fruit salads. Boiled with little sugar, they are often added in custards, trifles, tarts, and pies.

In this region, apples have been grown from time immemorial; grown in high altitude areas (about 1,300 metres above sea level), original wild apple trees were found in Khyber Pakhtunkhwa and Balochistan, besides other areas. The old Silk Route played an important role in the cultivation of this fruit. Amir Khusrau mentioned apples in the subcontinent in about AD 1300. They were given attention by the Mughals in their efforts to grow temperate fruits of high quality at suitable locations.

NAYYER RUBAB

Apricot. A walnut-size, sweet and aromatic fruit, apricots (called *khobani* in Urdu) grown in China for the last 4,000 years, is now grown in many countries, including Pakistan. In Pakistan, it is grown in Balochistan and Khyber Pakhtunkhwa provinces. Wild apricots can be found in Kashmir as well. The smooth, velvety, yellow skin apricot with a tint of orange is the first fruit of snowy mountain areas in spring. Their white flowers fill the valleys and give message of good fortune to growers.

Full of fragrance and sweetness, golden orange apricots are a summer delicacy in Pakistan. In the northern areas of the country, deciduous fruits, including apricots, are primarily produced as cash crops. They are eaten fresh in season, and a great deal more are dried in the sun for eating throughout the long, cold winter. The dried apricots are pureed and mixed with snow to make ice cream. As with apricot jam, the ice cream requires no sugar because the apricots are naturally sweet. The Hunzakuts, who live in the Himalayan Mountains of northern Pakistan, have cultivated and valued this fruit for over 1,500 years, and their apricots, both fresh and dried, are famous. In fact, the longevity of their lives and clear skin have been attributed to their heavy consumption of apricot and its powdered seeds.

Popular in the rest of the country as well, apricots are not only consumed fresh, but also used for cooking purposes. A dessert made with slight variations by many communities in Pakistan, is apricot delight or *khubani ka meetha*—a very popular sweet dish in Hyderabadi cuisine, and a common feature at weddings. Dried apricots are also commonly used in *biryani* (layered meat and rice dish) to add a sweet and tangy touch to the existing aromatic and spicy flavours.

Apricot chutney is prepared with vinegar, salt, red chilli pepper, strips of ginger, garlic cloves, raisins, and blanched almonds and stored in jars to last the whole year. Apricot oil is extracted from the kernels through a laborious and time-consuming process; it is of two types: bitter and sweet. The sweet oil is used for cooking, while the bitter one serves as a beauty product for skin and hair.

An excellent source of vitamin A, and a good source of vitamin C, copper, dietary fibre, riboflavin, calcium, phosphorus, niacin iron and potassium, two types of dried apricots are available in the market: one with kernel which is dark brown and is used in preparing some rice dishes and curry, and also served with cream, while the other, which is golden orange, is without the stone, treated with sulphur dioxide, and used as dry fruit. Dry apricots are also valued in the northern areas for their ability to provide extra oxygen to the consumer, thus helping them cope with breathlessness and blood pressure problems.

KAUSAR AHMED AND NAYYER RUBAB

Arab rule and culinary influences. During the mid-7th century, the maritime routes were dominated by the Arabs under the leadership of the Umayyad General, Muhammad Bin Qasim. They entered Sindh and Multan regions via the Arabian Sea and the western port of Bhambore which lies to the east of Karachi. Many Hindus living in Sindh quickly converted to Islam, but the Arab empire did not spread much farther into India at that time.

The impact of Islam on the cuisine of the country after the arrival of the Arabs began with numerous raids mainly for booty and plunder between AD 998 and 1030 by the Arab, Mahmud Ghaznavi, followed by the conquest of Sindh and the Punjab by Mohammad Ghori in the decade after AD 1182.

The Arabs shaped the culinary, social, and cultural landscape of this region. To the somewhat austere Hindu dining ambience, the Muslims brought a refined and courtly etiquette of both group and individual dining, and of sharing food in fellowship. Food items native to the region were enriched with nuts, raisins and clarified butter. A largely nomadic people, the Arabs often used the barbecue and spit roast to cook lamb, mutton and poultry; cook meat with bones; or make kebabs by mincing meat, with only a little pepper, sumac, cardamom, saffron, fresh herbs, and salads. This bland cuisine was not acceptable to the subcontinental palate which was used to far greater spice in their food.

As habits changed, the predominant Hindu diet of grains, legumes, and vegetables was influenced by the Arab love for meat. As more locals began to expand their diet, the traditional Arab barbecued meats were infused with local spices resulting in the present-day spicy kebabs. The strongest of these influences can be found in the cuisines of the coastal Sindh and Balochistan regions.

The Arabs are said to have brought 'lighter' spices such as cinnamon, saffron, cardamom and asafoetida (*hing*) along with pistachios, almonds, sultanas, and coffee to India. Other Arab culinary influences on Pakistani cuisine can be seen in the food cooked with a combination of sweet and savoury flavours, the use of nuts in rice, dry fruit, and fresh salads.

Some of the Pakistani recipes that have strong Arabic background include desserts stuffed with nuts/dry fruit and rice, and dishes such as *tireet* (meat soup). There is also a more modern influence, especially in the big cities, of chicken and mutton *shawarmas* with pitta bread, *qehwa* (green/mint tea), and the culture of smoking a *sheesha* (pipe) with food.

SUMMAYA USMANI

Arhar (*Cajanus cajan*). A legume now grown throughout the tropical regions of the world, *arhar* is commonly known as pigeon pea in English. Owing to it being resistant to drought and its generally hardy nature it is suitable to be grown on poor land by small farmers. Two main varieties are distinguished—var. *flavus* and var. *bicolor*. The former is known as *toor*, and the latter as *arhar* in Urdu. Old Sanskrit names for the pigeon pea are *tuvari* and *adhaki*; hence, it is likely that the distinction is of long standing. In fact, the origin of *arhar* goes back to prehistoric times. Archaeological evidence shows that this legume was domesticated in the eastern part of the subcontinent along with rice some 3,500 years ago. It is also mentioned in the *Rigveda*.

The *arhar* plant is grown in the tropical and sub-tropical regions of the subcontinent, South-East Asia, Africa, and Latin America. It grows well on semi-arid land and can survive drought conditions. The plant is quite adaptable because the coarse bush is deep-rooted. The *arhar* plant grows up to a height of three to ten feet. It has pointed, slender, trifoliate leaves and yellow flowers. The flowers turn into pods that are similar to English peas. They are green and pointed with a bit of a reddish tinge. Several pods are produced in clusters on a straight stem.

Each pod of *arhar* has seven to ten peas which are greenish brown in colour when whole, but they are usually eaten skinned and split which reveals their yellow interiors. It has great symmetry and more flattish shape. The peas are eaten in or out of their pods when green, and also dried or ground into flour. They have a mild nutty flavour.

Arhar is a rich source of proteins, minerals, and vitamins. It has a variety of other uses as well, such as a cover crop and as livestock feed. It is the first seed legume plant to have its complete genome sequenced. It contains a high level of protein and important amino acids, methionine, lysine and tryptophan. *Arhar* plants enrich the soil with vital nutrients such as nitrogen.

Arhar is a common lentil used in Gujarati households. It is used in making *daal gosht* which is a combination of four kinds of lentils and mutton, and in making *khichra*, a combination of four types of lentils, ground wheat and mutton, and *khichri*, a mix of *arhar daal* and rice. Some people add onions, garlic, ginger, and tomatoes to this *daal* to make it tastier.

ANJALI MALIK

Aromatic. Aromatics include vegetables, herbs, and spices, as well as whole grains and oil-rich nuts and seeds mostly used in cooking for their flavouring properties, rather than consumed as food. Examples of aromatics are: green chillies (*Capsium frutescens*) or *hari mirch*;

garlic (*Allium sativum*) or *lehsan*; ginger (*Zingiber officinale*) or *adrak*; herbs such as curry leaves (*Murraya koenigii*) or *kari patta*; fenugreek (*Trigonella foenum-graecum*) or *methi*; mint (*Mentha*) or *podina*; bay leaves (*Laurus nobilis/cassia lignea*) or *tej patta*; and fresh coriander (*Coriandrum sativum*) or *hara dhania*. All now vaunted as 'superfoods', these aromatics are not just blessed with ample nutrients but also contain agents that actively combat diseases. These ingredients are at the heart of Pakistani cooking, making it both immensely flavourful and incredibly healthful.

Arrowroot (ararot). A starch which is usually made from the swollen roots of *Maranta arundinacea*, the true Pakistani arrowroot can be eaten whole, boiled, or roasted. However, it is fibrous, and better when reduced to starch by pulverising and washing the roots. There are two varieties, red and white, of which the first is considered superior.

Arrowroot starch is a delicate product, with remarkably fine grains, and is, therefore, a traditional invalid food. It makes a light-textured, translucent paste without any flavour of its own, and sets to an almost clear gel. In the past, it was frequently used as a thickener for soups and sauces and was preferred over cornflour which would make them undesirably opaque. It is also lighter than cornflour and less obviously starchy. In recent years though, for some unfathomable reason, its importance has diminished.

Aryan. Broadly speaking the Aryan civilisation followed the Harappan civilisation. Nomadic tribes living in the steppe grasslands near the Ural Mountains in Central Asia, who called themselves Aryas, were postulated to have fanned out following climatic changes to reach as far west as Ireland and as far east as the Indo-Pak subcontinent. Three tribes formed the chief migrant groups. One of these was the Ailas or Aryans, who eventually came to dominate the whole of northern Indo-Pak; the second was the Dhaityas, and the third consisted of the Manva or Dravidians, an even earlier ethnic stock. Another small group with affiliations to Central Europe and Iran entered the region and settled in the land of the seven rivers, Saptasindhu. The interaction between these two groups of migrants was one major detriment of the Vedic and later Hindu culture of the country.

Whereas the Harappan civilisation had been largely urban, that of the Aryans was predominantly agricultural and pastoral. Barley was the major grain eaten by the Aryans. It was fried in clarified butter and consumed in the form of cakes dipped in honey called *apupa*. The modern-day Bengali sweets *pua* and *malpua* (known as *malpura* in Pakistan) preserve both the name and the methodology of this preparation.

Rice, which later dominated the Aryan food system was cooked in water or milk and either eaten on its own or accompanied by curd, clarified butter, sesame seeds or *mung*. Some spices and aromatics such as turmeric, fenugreek, ginger, and garlic were cultivated in Aryan times. Others like pepper and cardamom came from South India, and asafoetida from Afghanistan.

Asafoetida. Asafoetida, or *hing*, derives its name from its distinctive and almost repulsive stench. The first part of the name, 'asa' comes from the Persian *a za*, meaning mastic, while the Latin *foetidus* means stinking. It is a dried gum resin derived from the sap of roots and stem of ferula species, a giant fennel that exudes a vile and unappetising odour.

Introduced into the cuisine from Afghanistan, this spice is less widely used in Pakistani cuisine though it is widely used in Indian food; asafoetida powder is a crucial ingredient in Indian vegetarian cooking. In fact, its usage in Pakistan is limited to the cuisine of Hindus.

It complements most commonly used vegetables, such as potatoes, onions, cauliflower, peas, and quick cooking greens. Since it has a very pungent taste and unpleasant smell, it is always used in very small quantity and fried before adding other ingredients into the oil. Usually, one of the first aromatics added to a dish, its initial pungent and camphorous funk mellows out and is replaced by musky aroma as it fries for a while in butter or oil. It is also used for tempering dishes just before serving. Asafoetida is normally used in preparing pickles, fish, vegetable, lentils, and nimco. The most popular road-side food item in Pakistan served with *hing* water is *gol gappa*, also known as *pani puri*.

Asafoetida is made by cutting the plant stalks close to the roots just before flowering and drying the milky liquid that oozes out. Initially, the liquid is whitish and then turns into light yellow, the colour of asafoetida when used in cooking. Reputed to help digestion, asafoetida is also prescribed for respiratory diseases, such as whooping cough and asthma. In the days of yore, it was also believed that it enhanced the musicality of voice, so the singers of Mughal court would have some asafoetida early in the morning before practising their singing.

NAYYER RUBAB AND KAUSAR AHMED

Ashak. Basically, an Afghani dish that has become very popular in Khyber Pakhtunkhwa as well, it is made of *gandana* greens that are boiled, drained, and re-boiled several times before being stuffed in flour wrappers, folded into triangles (like those used for *samosa* in other parts of the country), steamed or re-boiled, and served with yoghurt.

Ashura. *Haleem* and *khichra* (meat and whole wheat dishes), although popular dishes round the year, are particularly associated with Ashura, the tenth day of Muharram (the first month of the Islamic calendar), marking the martyrdom of Imam Hussain—grandson of the Prophet (PBUH)—his family and compatriots. In commemoration, many Muslims spend this day in fasting and worship. The fast is usually broken with either *haleem* or *khichra*, both of which are high-energy foods. For the same reason, they are also popular items at *iftars* in Ramazan, as they provide instant energy.

Believed to have been introduced to the subcontinent by Persians, *haleem* has several variations, and in Anatolia, Iran, Northern Iraq and the Caucasus region is known as *keshkek* and *harisa*. However, *haleem* comprises meat and wholewheat, and may or may not include pulses, while *khichra* incorporates four kinds of pulses, wholewheat and meat.

B

Bactrian. A very modern society, Bactrian existed between 600 BC and AD 600, and occupied Bactria, also called Bactriana, an ancient country lying between the mountains of the Hindu Kush and Amu Darya (ancient Oxus River) in what is now part of Afghanistan, Uzbekistan, and Tajikistan. The Bactrian land was especially important as it served as a meeting place not only for overland trade between East and West but also for the crosscurrents of religious and artistic ideas.

At the height of their power the Bactrians ruled almost all of what is now Afghanistan, parts of Central Asia, and a large area that is now part of Pakistan. The Graeco-Bactrian kingdom was founded when the Graeco-Bactrian king Demetrius invaded the subcontinent early in the second century BC. After the Greek conquest of Bactria and the Persian Empire, the Hellenistic influence on the culture of ancient Central Asia and ancient north-western India was considerable. Hellenistic traditions were especially evident in art, architecture, coinage, and script.

In the first century AD, the new Bactrian leaders extended their rule into north-western India. In fact, the Greeks in the subcontinent were eventually divided from the Graeco-Bactrians centred in Bactria (now the border between Afghanistan and Uzbekistan), and the Indo-Greeks in the present-day north-western subcontinent. The most famous Indo-Greek ruler was Menander. He had his capital at Sakala in the Punjab (present-day Sialkot). The Indo-Greeks ultimately disappeared as a political entity around AD 10 following the invasions of the Indo-Scythians, although pockets of Greek populations probably remained for several centuries longer during the subsequent rule of the Indo-Parthians and Kushans under whom the country became a centre of Buddhism, leaving its mark on the culture and cuisine of the country, wherever its influence was felt.

BISMA TIRMIZI

Baghar or tarka (tempering). Derived from the Sanskrit *bagharna*, this technique is commonly used in the preparation of *daal* and *dahi ki karhi* (yoghurt-based curry) and generally marks the end of a cooking process. It involves shallow-frying of different whole spices and/or flavour enhancers, one after the other, in very hot oil or fat and then pouring the oil along with the contents over the prepared dish. The temperature of the oil is crucial, because if the oil gets too hot, the spices will burn, while if it is not hot enough, the flavour of the spices will not be released. The whole spices used are those that generally pop in oil to release their flavours and aroma (cumin, fenugreek seeds, mustard seeds, whole red chillies, etc.), while flavour enhancers used are those with a very low water content (mostly sliced onion, curry leaves, and chopped garlic). The ingredients of *baghar* release their flavour as they hit the oil, and the dish is then covered for a few moments while the ingredients are allowed to brown gently so as to allow the full flavour to be infused. *Baghar* is sometimes performed at the beginning of the cooking process in which case, the rest of the ingredients are added to the oil later.

SHAHA TARIQ

Bagharay baingan. Originating from Tashkent, *bagharay baingan* were introduced into the subcontinent by the Mughals and eventually became a prominent and regular part of Hyderabadi cuisine. In fact, the dish became so popular over time that it has come to be regarded as integral to Hyderabadi cuisine along with *mirchon ka salan*. It is especially popular in summers and often a must at festivities.

Bagharay implies that the dish is garnished with smoking hot, spiced oil, while *baingan* is eggplants. Small and tender eggplants are partially quartered and stuffed with a spicy, sour, sweet, and salty mixture (a ground combination including coconut, peanuts, tamarind, jaggery, and mustard seeds) and cooked on low heat in a rich and creamy gravy. A final *baghar* or pouring of hot oil flavoured with spices gives the finishing touch to the dish.

It is a great side dish with Hyderabadi *biryani* and/or *puri*. It could also be refrigerated and served cold. The availability today of packaged spice mix for this dish, which is otherwise laborious to prepare as it requires the grinding of a variety of ingredients, has made it infinitely easier and quicker to prepare it.

ZUBAIDA TARIQ

Bajindak. A speciality of Hazaras, a community settled in Balochistan, *bajindak* is a dish of green vegetable similar to spinach. *Bajindak* ripens in spring when it is cooked with garlic and eaten as a health sustaining food.

Bajra (pearl millet). *Bajra* is the Urdu word for *Pennisetum americanum*, which, despite its name, originated in western Africa, where many wild forms still exist. The *bajra* crop is believed to have come to the subcontinent quite early, just before 2000 BC. Especially popular among the Gujaratis, *bajra* is their staple dietary item used to make flatbread.

Rich in fibre, proteins, vitamins, and essential minerals, *bajra* is a healthful, gluten-free alternative to wheat. In Pakistan, *bajra* is consumed in the province of Punjab as well as by the Gujarati communities settled in Sindh, especially in Karachi. Its health benefits are many and it is preferred in many rural households because of its availability, low price, and being a main source of energy, protein, vitamins/amino acids (except lysine and threonine), and minerals.

Millet is a very rich source of phytochemicals and micronutrients as compared to other major cereals, such as wheat and rice. Pearl millet is reported to be rich in resistant starch, soluble and insoluble dietary fibres, minerals, and antioxidants. It contains about 92.5 per cent dry matter, 2.1 per cent ash, 2.8 per cent crude fibre, 7.8 per cent crude fat, 13.6 per cent crude protein, and 63.2 per cent starch.

BISMA TIRMIZI

Bajray ki roti. A Gujarati favourite staple, *bajray* (or millet) *ki roti* is a dry-weather yield and, hence, very much part of the diet in Rajasthan and other arid areas. Since the *roti* tends to be thick and dry, when served at breakfast it is always accompanied with butter or clarified butter, and yoghurt drink. At lunch, it is frequently accompanied by fish curry.

In the Gujarati community, *bajray ki roti* is a winter favourite, as it is considered a heat-producing staple. It is often used as an essential ingredient in winter delicacies such as *lassan* (made with green garlic and *bajray ki roti*) and *muthia* (made with an assortment of winter veggies, mutton, and *bajray ki roti*).

Bajra is gluten-free and full of nutrition such as protein, calcium, iron, and phosphorus.

NAYYER RUBAB

Bakarkhani. Kashmiri *bakarkhani* has a special place in Kashmiri cuisine. It is believed that it most likely originated in the Middle East and eventually spread to Kashmir. It is similar to a round *tandoori naan* (flat bread baked in a clay oven) in appearance, but crisp and layered, and sprinkled with sesame seeds. Traditionally, *kandurs* or *bakarkhaniwalas* (bread-makers) ignited their *tandoors* (open, lined, large, spherical clay ovens) around midnight to have the bread available by morning. In order to make the bread, *bakarkhani* dough of white flour, and *mewa* (dry fruits) is kneaded well and stretched thin by hand over the entire span of a wooden board. It is divided into small portions, and after spreading *ghee* (clarified butter) over it, flour is strewn on, the dough is folded, and the process is repeated several times. Each dough portion is then rolled out into a *roti* and sesame seeds are spread on it. The *roti* is baked in the *tandoor* and during the process of baking, milk may be sprinkled on the dough. Nowadays, however, in place of *ghee* and milk, molasses solution is often added so that the colour of the bread turns reddish. The Kashmiri *bakarkhani* is typically consumed hot for breakfast.

However, *bakarkhani* is also believed to have originated in Dhaka, Bangladesh, and the story of its origin is a far more romantic one. As stated in *Kingbadantir Dhaka* by Nazir Hossain, back in AD 1700 when Dewan Murshid Quli Khan came to this part of Bengal, a small boy named Aga Bakar Khan accompanied him. Growing up, Aga Bakar fell in love with Khani Begum, a dancer of Arambag. But their love was doomed and Khani was killed by another man who desired her, leaving a bereaved Bakar to mourn her for the rest of his life. Legend has it that he named this especially prepared bread, *bakar-khani*, after his and Khani Begum's names.

Unlike the Kashmiri *bakarkhani*, this one is made of flour kneaded with milk, *ghee*, and sugar, and cooked in a *tandoor*. *Ghee* is then applied on the *roti* and holes are pierced on it. It is normally eaten with *aaloo gosht*.

Baking. A method of cooking food that uses prolonged dry heat, baking is normally done in an oven, but also in hot ashes, or on hot stones. The history of baking in the subcontinent goes back to the Indus Valley Civilisation as breads would be baked in traditional clay ovens called *tandoors*. Although this medium is still commonly used all over the country for baking flat, leavened breads, Pakistan gradually transitioned into using basic gas ovens, and professional, high-quality ovens in urban areas.

While the most common baked item in Pakistan is bread, many other types of foods, including desserts, have now begun to be baked as well. The history of dessert baking in Pakistan goes back to the birth of the country with the launch of the first bakery that baked a cake for a reception in Karachi for the founder of Pakistan, Quaid-i-Azam Mohammad Ali Jinnah, in 1947.

Modern day bakers in Pakistan have kept up with the West in innovating techniques and perfecting the art of baking designer cakes and pastries. Over the past several years, Pakistan has become popular for its variety of baked items, some of which are rarely found elsewhere in the world, like the quintessential Pakistani lemon tart. There is also now an array of gourmet bakeries and innumerable home bakers creating items which are not only flavourful, but a visual treat as well.

The evolution of baked items served in trendy and modern settings of cafes and coffee houses is perhaps responsible for one of the most competitive industries in Pakistan, which only seems to be progressing each day.

KAUSAR AHMED

Balochistan. On the west of the Indus plains lies Balochistan, the largest province of the country in terms of area—about 343,000 sq. km. It is also the most scarcely populated of Pakistan's provinces—the cause of under-population being its extremely tough terrain. Compared by geologists to the rugged landscape of the planet Mars, Balochistan's terrain has, for centuries, imposed strict limitations on economic activities. In recent years though, with the development of the province's rich mineral resources, the situation has been changing.

Balochistan derives its name from one of its three principal ethnic groups, the Baloch; the other two being the Pakhtuns and the Brahuis. Some historians believe that the word 'Baloch' is derived from the name of Belus, king of Babylon, while others are of the opinion that Balochs are of Turkman lineage. The nationalist Balochs, on the other hand, ascribe their origin to the earliest Muslim invaders of Persia.

The Baloch, like the Pakhtuns, are a tribal population whose original territory extends beyond the national borders. Over 70 per cent of the Baloch in the world live in Pakistan, with the remainder residing in Iran and Afghanistan.

The Brahuis—said to be of Dravidian stock—by contrast, believe that they are indigenous to Balochistan, although according to one school of thought they are of Turko-Iranian origin. Both the Baloch and the Brahui make their homes in the vast upland deserts stretching southwards and westwards from Balochistan's capital Quetta, to the Arabian Sea. They are predominantly pastoral nomads, breeding sheep, goats and cattle.

The Pashtu-speaking peoples of Balochistan, which include Afghan refugees, are concentrated exclusively in the relatively fertile hills and valleys to the north and north-east of Quetta. From there they continue northwards in an unbroken chain through the tribal belt of the frontier to Peshawar and beyond.

Yet another distinct ethnic group in Balochistan is the Makranis; according to one theory, they have been given this name because they live on the Makran coast that stretches from Karachi to the Iranian border. The Makranis are a fishing community and according to a folk-tale about their origin, their ancestors were fishermen from Ethiopia who were blown far off-course by a storm and ended up in Balochistan. However, according to some historians, they could be the genetic legacy of the African slaves who were brought to the Indo-Pakistan subcontinent by the Arab and European invaders. Historians feel that there is also the possibility that Makranis are the descendants of the earliest humans who arrived in Pakistan along the coastal route out of Africa.

Another ethnic group in Balochistan is the Hazaras, a Persian-speaking community about whose origin very little is known. It is believed that they migrated in the 1880s from central Afghanistan into British India and settled to the east of Quetta. According to some researchers Hazaras are Mongolian in origin and are descendants of Changez Khan, a theory supported by the similarities in the language and words that the Mongols and Hazaras use even today. Another plausible theory is that Hazaras were Buddhists who actually lived in Afghanistan at least since the time of the Kushan Dynasty some 2,000 years ago.

By and large, the food in Balochistan tends to be non-spicy and simple, concentrating more on nutrients than on spices. Since they were originally a nomadic people, they didn't have too many utensils on them, and the cooking process did not entail too much frying. Eating on *dastarkhwan*s rather than at tables remains the norm.

Balti cuisine. The Balti of Baltistan—sometimes referred to as 'Little Tibet'—use spices and ingredients in their cuisine that are similar to those used in other Pakistani dishes, such as Mughlai. There is often a base of garlic, ginger, and onion, while the spices used include coriander and cumin, as well as fragrant spices such as star anise, cardamom, clove, and saffron which originate in neighbouring China and Iran. However, while Balti cuisine employs flavours that are similar to other Pakistani and Central Asian cuisines, because of the unique fusion of influences from the surrounding cultures of Iran, China, Tibet, and Afghanistan, it is distinct in its method. The techniques resemble Chinese wok-cooking, involving fast stir-frying of pre-cut ingredients which is similar to the cooking of Szechwan's spicy cuisine. There are also slow-cooked dishes, where it resembles its next-door neighbour, Tibet, which also fuses subcontinental and Chinese influences in its cuisine. While most Balti dishes are dry, some do have gravy similar to other Pakistani food, thanks to the wide-ranging origins of Balti cooking that can also be traced to the ancestry of the Mirpuris, the tastes of the Mughal emperors, the aromatic spices of Kashmir, and the 'winter foods' of lands high in the mountains.

In Balti cuisine, traditionally, pieces of *naan* or other flatbread are used to scoop up food directly from the pot in which it is cooked, while it is still sizzling, rather than serving the food in plates. The pot is a wok-like vessel known as a *karhai* in other parts of Pakistan but is called *balti* (bucket) in Baltistan and in many other cultures in the Himalayan regions. In fact, it may be possible that the term *balti* for the pot came from the Balti people's use of this particular pot in their cooking. Its concave shape concentrates the heat, just like a wok does, allowing fast cooking without using a lot of wood.

In the summer months when it is possible to grow vegetables, Balti eat whole-wheat *roti* cooked slowly on the *tawa* (iron griddle) and re-cooked over fire, with whatever vegetable that is easily available. In the winter months, however, when vegetables cannot be grown, the diet comprises fruits, spaghetti, *daal* and wheat-based items eaten with *shorba* (soup). Soups are also popular and eighteen variations of *bhalay*, a traditional Balti soup, exists, including the popular *traspi bhalay*.

Kashmiri tea is a popular beverage that is consumed at least twice a day.

Balti gosht. This meat dish is based on Kashmiri/Baltistani style of one-pot dry stews cooked in a two-handled, cast-iron pot known as a *karhai* or *balti*, resembling a bucket. *Baltis* generally incorporate a main ingredient combined with mild spices such as cardamom, cloves, cassia bark, and cumin together with flavour enhancers such as garlic, ginger, tomatoes, and onions.

Though there are many theories to its actual descent, the term *balti* is said to have originated in Birmingham, England where this dish now has cult status. One theory that prevails is that the current *balti gosht* is inspired by the dry curries of Baltistan, Northern Pakistan, and its present form was created by the Pakistani/Kashmiri immigrants who settled in Birmingham in the 1960s. Others say that it is simply a dish loosely based on the cooking styles of North Pakistan and the name given to the dish came about because of the shape of the pot in which it is cooked, the bucket or *balti* pot. This dish is relatively unknown to Pakistanis by its British name *balti*; however, similar dishes can be found in Pakistan that are commonly known as *karhai* or *handi*.

The flavours of *balti* are based on Mughal and Kashmiri style spices and cooking styles and could be made with a variety of meats such as lamb, mutton, and chicken.

SUMMAYA USMANI

Banana. Arguably the world's most healthful fruit, banana has become a major fruit crop of Pakistan, since after the fall of the eastern wing of the country. Prior to 1971, bananas were mainly grown in East Pakistan (now Bangladesh) and were considered a rare and expensive fruit in West Pakistan. Today, they are mainly grown in Sindh where the soil and climatic conditions are favourable for their successful cultivation.

Other than eating them fresh off the bunch, bananas are consumed in the country in the form of shakes, mashed to be given to infants as their first semi-solid food, and cooked with coconut in some communities to be eaten with *chapati* as the main course. They are also used in a number of desserts including custards, trifles, and banana fritters. Banana leaves are also used to wrap and serve fish in, especially by the Parsi community, as it is believed that it enhances the flavour. Bananas are a very good source of vitamin B6, manganese, vitamin C, potassium, dietary fibre, biotin, and copper.

KAUSAR AHMED

Banjan burani. *Banjan* is an Afghan word for eggplant, and *burani* is a style of presentation. *Banjan burani*, a luscious, flavoured Afghan eggplant side-dish, is made using the freshest ingredients. Adopted by Balochistan, but incorporating yoghurt instead of the traditional *khurood* (dried milk), in the Pakistani version, the eggplant is generally fried before baking or cooking with pureed tomatoes and pureed fried onions. Like most Afghan and Balochi dishes, *banjan burani* is mild in taste and even with the Pakistani twist, has minimum spices, retaining its authentic flavour.

As the eggplant and tomatoes cook, all the flavours and textures blend together. When ready, the eggplant preparation is placed in the centre of whipped yoghurt spiked with garlic and salt. It is served with flat bread, although it tastes just as well when eaten on its own.

Eggplant in yoghurt is eaten in many parts of the world, from the Mediterranean region to the subcontinent, with slight variations in the recipe. But, no matter what the method of cooking the eggplant, there is no denying that yoghurt and eggplant beautifully complement each other.

KAUSAR AHMED

Bannu kebab. Originating in the Mughal Empire, it is said that *bannu kebab* was named after Banno, one of the maharanis (a ruler's wife) of the Mughal era. The Mughal kitchen, which saw a fusion of cooking styles ranging from Persian, Central Asian, and subcontinental, gave birth to new and unique Mughlai flavours. These flavours were passed down through generations and became very popular roadside dishes in Pakistan, especially in the heavily crowded food street of Karachi, Burns Road. *Bannu kebab* is a prime example of one such dish.

Bannu kebabs are marinated boneless chicken cubes wrapped in egg, threaded on skewers and cooked in a clay pot or *tandoor*. This kebab is infused with a combination of flavour enhancers, which include cardamom, saffron, cashew nuts and dried fenugreek leaves. The secret to its succulence is that just when it is almost cooked, it is removed from the *tandoor*, smeared with a beaten egg and placed back in the clay oven. The kebab can be tastily ensconced in a *paratha*, accompanied by a few slices of onion with a gentle squeeze of lemon, or can be served separately with *naan* and chutney.

KAUSAR AHMED

Barfi. A Pakistani sweetmeat, *barfi* is inspired by the *pera*. *Barfi* is made principally of dried milk (*khoya*), the name coming from the Persian word for snow, presumably because plain *barfi* is white and might be thought to resemble snow. In its plain form, *barfi* is among the simplest of all local sweets. It is, however, common to improve its already pleasant taste by adding ingredients such as coconut, carrots, pistachios, or white pumpkin, and by flavouring with cardamoms. The prepared mixture is simmered until thick, left to cool, flattened and cut into small cubes or diamond shape.

Barley agriculture. Barley is one of the most ancient crops in the world. It is as ancient as agriculture itself. The earliest evidence of barley agriculture in the subcontinent has been found from around 6000 BC at Mehrgarh in Balochistan. At Mehrgarh the evidence of crop cultivation in period 1 (7000–6000 BCE) comes from the charred remains as well as from the impression of wheat and barley on mud bricks. *Rigveda* and *Atharvaveda* also refer to *yava* which is barley. From the *Yajurveda* it is learnt that barley was sown in winter and reaped in summer. The scientific name of barley is *Hordeum vulgare* and it belongs to the grass family. It is a short-growing seasonal crop and is drought tolerant. In the subcontinent, it is cultivated as a *rabi* season crop which means sowing takes place from October to December and harvesting from March to May. Barley crop can be grown on a wide range of soils but it is best grown in sandy and moderately heavy loam soils that have neutral to saline reaction and medium fertility. Only two or three irrigations are enough for optimum yield.

Crop rotation is beneficial in barley cultivation. Barley can be grown in combination with maize, millet, rice, sorghum, pigeon pea, sugarcane, cotton, and sesame. But this rotation varies from area to area depending on the quality of the soil.

Barley provides useful amounts of minerals such as copper, zinc, and phosphorus. It is rich in fibre, particularly the soluble fibre beta glucan and pectin—the types that can help lower high blood cholesterol. Barley improves immunity and is beneficial for anaemia patients. It prevents bone disorders, aids in digestion, weight loss, controls type-2 diabetes, treats kidney stones, prevents urinary tract infection and asthma, and protects against cancer.

ANJALI MALIK

Baryan. Basically, these are dried dumplings of a combination of soaked *mung* (green gram) and *chana daal*. The soaked pulses are seasoned with salt, chilli powder, ground cumin powder, and ginger. Spooned on an absorbent paper in little dumplings, *baryan* are ideally dried under a warm winter sun or alternatively placed in an oven. Once dried they can be stored for a long shelf life. They could be fried and added to a regular curry and left to cook on a low flame till soft and ready. Garnished with diced green chillies and freshly chopped coriander leaves, they make a delicious main course for a light lunch. They could be served with *chapati* or plain boiled rice.

SHAHA TARIQ

Basmati rice. This long-grain rice, grown in the Himalayan foothills, is aged for about a year, and has a wonderful, rich, aromatic flavour and fine texture. It cooks fast, and with lengthy rinsing and/or soaking prior to cooking, the texture is improved further. As it tends to elongate during cooking (rather than swell) and contains less starch than other long-grain varieties, it also produces distinct separate grains.

Bateesa/pateesa. A favourite traditional sweet in Pakistan, *bateesa* is very much a part of festivities. It incorporates the Middle Eastern and Afghani influence of using nuts to balance the sweetness but can also be made by simply mixing roasted refined flour and gram flour in equal portions with *ghee* into a moist mixture. However, the trick lies in the roasting and stirring which have to be just right to ensure a perfect result.

Sugar syrup is cooked separately on moderate flame till it gains thread-like consistency. The mixture is folded in into the roasted flour and stirred continuously to attain a flaky texture. It is then cooled, sprinkled with nuts and crushed cardamoms, cut into squares and refrigerated till ready to serve.

It could alternatively, also be made only with refined flour. This variety is lighter and flakier in texture.

SHAHA TARIQ

Bay leaf/tej patta (*Laurus nobilis***).** One of the most ancient of herbs, bay leaves (the leaves of the bay or laurel tree) or *tej patta* in Urdu, are often used in Pakistani cooking for their distinctive flavour and fragrance. The leaves are used in their fresh as well as dry form, and only develop their full flavour after weeks of picking and drying.

The bay leaf is thought to have originated in Asia Minor region, from where it travelled around the Mediterranean and parts of Asia until it came to Pakistan. Its history stretches back to the times of Greeks and Romans, who sincerely believed that the herb symbolised wisdom, peace, and protection.

Bay leaves typically work as a flavour enhancer and, used along with turmeric, is a standard component of Pakistani cuisine. They are used in food, especially rice dishes such as *biryani*, as a condiment, as well as in pickles, although they are not widely used in curries.

In the coastal areas, though, bay leaves are also used as a seasoning on fish gravies, lentils, and vegetable greens. It is sometimes also an ingredient in *garam masala*, which is used in many traditional dishes.

Bay leaves are only added in food for their distinctive flavour, and are not eaten raw, or with uncooked salads. The flavour of the bay leaf in all its aromatic sweetness is released when sizzled and cooked in oil. Bay leaves can also be roasted and ground into a powder form to provide a sharp flavour, but as with many spices and flavourings, the fragrance of the bay leaf is more noticeable than its taste. This spice is also used as a digestive aid and is supposed to be of assistance in cardiac disorders.

KAUSAR AHMED

Bean. Beans are one of the longest cultivated plants. It is a common name for large plant seeds of several genera of the family Fabaceae that are used for food consumption. In fact, it is a term loosely applied to any legume whose seeds or pods are eaten, and which is not classed separately as a pea or lentil. High in fibre and antioxidants, beans are not just good for the waistline, they may also aid in disease prevention. Although there are many kinds of beans, the ones most commonly used in Pakistan are red and white kidney beans (known as *lobia*), green *mung* beans, and fresh beans. Broad beans, also called fava beans, the size of a small fingernail in their wild state, are also found in the Himalayan foothills.

Beans are used in a variety of traditional Pakistani dishes, salads, and *chaats* (a variety of tangy snacks). *Lobia* curry is a popular bean curry in Pakistan, which is rich in proteins, and consisting of aromatic flavours and spices. Cluster beans or *gawar ki sabzi*, eaten plain or with potatoes also constitute a very popular dish, as do French beans.

KAUSAR AHMED

Beef. Beef is the culinary name for meat from bovines, mainly cattle, and the third most widely consumed meat in the world. Beef, harvested from cows, bulls, or steers, is an extremely popular protein used in Pakistani kitchens, and an essential ingredient in certain dishes. It is consumed shredded, whole, cut, and, most popularly, ground. Kebabs made of ground beef are a common item in Pakistani cuisine; one can find countless varieties of kebabs such as *seekh*, *behari*, *shami*, and *chapli* all across the country.

Once considered a poor man's meat, beef, and barbecued meat, play a more important part in Pakistani cuisine than in other South Asian cuisines. Aside from kebabs, there are a number of popular dishes in Pakistan that are ideally made with beef such as *nihari* (a slow cooked beef stew) and *koftay* (meatballs), and hunter beef.

KAUSAR AHMED

Beh (*Nelumbo nucifera*; Indian lotus). The lotus flower is an aquatic plant, the seeds, young leaves, and stem of which are edible. The stem of the lotus flower is widely used in Pakistani, Chinese, Vietnamese, and Japanese cuisines. In the subcontinent, it goes by numerous names—*kamal kakri*, *beh*, or *bheen*. The lotus stem's creamy white flesh has the crisp texture of raw potato, and a flavour, which is nutty and mildly sweet.

Both Kashmiris and Sindhis are well known for their love of the lotus and are avid eaters of this crunchy stem. Sindhis cook it in many unique ways such as *bhee patata*—lotus stem and potato curry; *bhee basar*—lotus stem in onion-based masala; *swanjhro ain bhee*—drumstick flowers with lotus stem.

The most traditional way of cooking lotus stem is in a clay pot; when they become soft and stringy, they are served with a dash of mint and coriander chutney. This *chaat* is known as *kuneh ja bhee*. One of the most famous *chaats* of the pre-Partition era, this pride of Sindhi cuisine is now almost a lost culinary heritage. The loss would be all the greater because not only is lotus delicious, it is also nutritious. The lotus plant is rich in iron, calcium, and vitamin C, whereas the chlorophyll present in the stalk acts as an active antioxidant to fight cancer-producing free radicals.

SUNITA ACHRIA

Bengali cuisine. Bangladesh came into being only in 1971, when the two parts of Pakistan, East and West, split after a bitter war. Before the formation of Bangladesh, East Pakistan popularised a large number of fruits and desserts, not to mention *paan* (betel leaf), for which the eastern wing was famous, in its western counterpart as well. The result was that after 1971, when trade between the two wings stopped abruptly, Pakistan (as West Pakistan came to be known) found itself without many of the food items its people had grown to love. Gradually, however, it began to grow the fruits that used to come from the erstwhile East Pakistan, such as bananas, coconuts, lychees, and pineapples, as well as its own betel leaf.

But it is Bengal's desserts that really won the hearts of Pakistanis and which remain to date the greatest influence on the country's cuisine. In fact, most Pakistani desserts find their origin in Bengali desserts. Adopted by the local gastronomy, they have become extremely popular, particularly in Karachi, where Dhaka-based sweetmeat shops had established branches.

After 1971, many Bengalis who were running sweetmeat shops or were working as cooks in homes or restaurants in Karachi, opted to stay behind as they were earning better than they would have in their motherland. They too, became instrumental in introducing many quintessential Bengali dishes to the country, and especially to Karachi.

Hence, with rice being staple in Bengali cuisine, boiled rice is a must in households that had their roots in East Pakistan. A number of other quintessentially Bengali dishes, or even ingredients, are common in these households, although seldom found in the other communities. A case in point is a special mix of masalas comprising onion seeds, fenugreek seeds, fennel seeds, cumin seeds, and nigella seeds collectively known as *panch phoron*—*panch* is five in Urdu and *phoron* means spices—often used for the preparation of a number of vegetable dishes, including potatoes.

Mustard seeds are also an integral ingredient in Bengali dishes used in a variety of ways—fried in oil, crushed to yield a pungent paste, or as a source of oil for cooking.

Certain savoury food items that are quintessentially Bengali have become popular with other communities that have been exposed to the cuisine. Fried Bengali stuffed snacks such as *kachoriyan* (inspired by the Bengali *daal puri*) and *singaray* (also known as *samosay*) for instance, have now become universal favourites.

Bengali dessert. Bengal is known as the land of sweet lovers, and Bengalis are famous for their love of *mishti* or sweets. It is commonly believed that this region, which once was known as Gour Banga, got its name from the production of *gur* (molasses). Most Bengali sweets are made from milk products and sugar, sometimes flavoured with spices, fruit, nuts, coconut, and other ingredients.

It is believed that Portuguese influence in Bengal in the 17th century resulted in the creation of innovative sweetmeats employing cottage cheese. The most quintessential Bengali dish is *sandesh*, which are small sweetmeats made by fermenting boiling milk with lemon juice, and flavouring it with sugar, rose water, and vanilla extract.

However, that said, most indigenous *mithai* (sweetmeats) of Pakistan is believed to originate from Bengali recipes, which are regarded as the basis of all Pakistani desserts, so much so that the ever-popular *halway* and *jalebi*, normally regarded as having Arab roots, are also of Bengali origin. *Rasgulla*, *chumchum*, and *ras malai*, quintessentially Bengali sweets, are also among the favourite desserts of Pakistan. In recent years, Karachiites have become acquainted with the Bengali pancake, *malpuay*—known as *malpuray* in Karachi— and it is now a sought-after dessert at elite weddings.

The Bengali tradition of making different kinds of pan-fried, steamed or boiled sweets, known as *piṭhe* or *pitha*, flourishes in Pakistan as well. These sweets indicate the coming of winter, and the arrival of a season in which rich food can be partaken of. The richness lies in the creamy silkiness of the milk which is mixed often with molasses or jaggery made from either date palm or sugarcane, and sometimes sugar.

KAUSAR AHMED

Besan. Gram flour or *besan*, made by peeling and grinding split grams, principally, brown chickpeas, is also known in the region as Bengal gram flour. It is made by milling, very finely, what is called *chana* or *chana daal*, husked and split.

Besan is rich in carbohydrates and protein and free from gluten. Its texture is fine, and it is deep yellow in colour. It is used to make a wide variety of snacks such as *pakoray*, *laddu*, *dhokray* (*dhoklay*) and *besani roti*. It is also used as a binding agent and to make batter for coating fried food. A vast variety of foods may be dipped in the batter and deep fried, such as potatoes (mashed or sliced), onion rings, green chillies, cauliflowers, and eggplants. The batter by itself is also deep-fried to yield a variety of crisp snacks, such as strings of *sev*, pellets of *boondi*, and Gujarati snacks like *gathiya*.

Besan ki bhaji. *Besan* is one of Pakistan's staple flours. Very popular for making dumplings and *dahi ki karhi*, it serves as a great alternative in the absence of any vegetable dish. *Besan ki bhaji* is made with *besan* as the key ingredient, serving as a simple side dish. Diced onions are fried golden and then covered evenly with a layer of *besan*. While continuously stirring the whole,

salt, chilli powder, and turmeric are added, followed by a little water, and the *besan* is then allowed to cook on low flame. Garnished with fresh coriander, it is a wholesome accompaniment to any main course.

SHAHA TARIQ

Betel nut. A popular stimulant in the subcontinent, betel nut is the fruit of the areca palm, *Areca catechu*, and, therefore, also known as areca nut. The nut contains a stimulating alkaloid (arecoline) and tannins which give it a pleasantly astringent taste. The usual way of consuming it is with the betel leaf in the form of *paan*, although many people like to chew it on its own or together with fennel seeds, as a digestive and/ or mouth freshener.

Bhaati. This is a meal served to mourners right after the funeral. Comprising lentils and pumpkin, this non-meat meal is imperative in some Muslim communities, as traditionally meat is not cooked in a household on the day a death has taken place, particularly in the meal served immediately after the burial. Interestingly, in the Bohra community also a simple meal comprising lentils is served, after a funeral, but it includes meat (*daal gosht*), boiled rice, and *firni* (rice pudding).

Bhakri. A flat, unleavened *chapati* made of wheat flour, *ghee*, and cumin or carom seeds, *bhakri* is a Gujarati speciality. It is cooked on a *tawa* and is very nutritious as it is made from whole grains and is gluten-free. Thicker than *chapati*, it has a biscuit-like texture.

Other food grains produced locally are also used for making *bhakri*. It could be made from *bajra*, *jowar* (sorghum), or rice flour. To make *bhakri*, salt, *ghee*, and cumin/carom seeds are added to the flour of choice. It is then kneaded with warm water to prepare the dough. This dough is flattened and then roasted on an iron griddle. Coarser than *chapati*, because it is made of coarse grains, its texture is crispy from outside but soft from inside. *Bhakri* is eaten with *achar* (pickles), chutney, yoghurt, vegetables, or just onions and chillies.

ANJALI MALIK

Bhature. A variant of *puri*, *bhature* is of Punjabi origin. The difference is that *bhature* is made with fermented/ leavened dough and incorporates additional ingredients, making it chewy in texture. Refined flour is mixed with semolina, yoghurt, oil/*ghee*, baking soda, sugar, and salt. Variations include ground *maash daal* or minced meat. Kneaded into a dough by adding water, it is left to rise and then rolled out into discs before being deep fried in crackling hot oil. They are traditionally served with *cholay* (chickpeas) and are a favourite at holiday breakfasts or with high tea menus.

SHAHA TARIQ

Bhel/bhel puri. Of Gujarati influence, *bhel* is a fond reference to the very popular snack of subcontinental, and now Pakistani, street cuisine, commonly known as *bhel puri*. Originally a Gujarati fast-food item, even among *chaat* experts, there is much disagreement today as to what goes into a genuine *bhel puri*. Nowadays, it is usually made according to consumer/producer preference, and the availability of ingredients. However, most recipes include puffed rice topped with *sev* (a thin, crispy, and slightly spicy fried snack made with *besan*), thin, crisp-fried discs of dough, fried lentils, chopped onions, diced tomatoes (optional), boiled cubed potatoes, and sweet and spicy chutneys. The sweet chutney is made with tamarind and dates, while the spicy one incorporates green chillies, coriander and mint leaves with lemon.

Optionally, raw sweet mango, *papri puri* (crispy fried *puri*) and roasted nuts can be added to give enhanced flavour. The trick is to mix in the chutneys just before eating as chutneys tend to soak in, making the dish a soggy mesh in no time.

SHAHA TARIQ

Bhindhi basar. A Sindhi vegetarian speciality, *bhindi basar* is a simple dish made with cleaned, washed, dried, and cut okra (*bhindi*) that is fried and then mixed into masala that has been fried with julienne onions and tomatoes. A variation is known as *bhindi basar patata* which also incorporates potatoes.

Bhoonna. The key to Pakistani cooking lies in the understanding and execution of five fundamental techniques, one of which is *bhoonna* or frying. *Bhoonna* involves the frying of ingredients (meat or vegetables) in oil or fat in an uncovered utensil, on high flame, whilst stirring constantly, till they change colour. An important feature of Pakistani cooking, *bhoonna* is crucial to the preparation of a large number of dishes and is usually done at the beginning of cooking a dish. Where this process is used, onions are added first to the oil/fat, and other flavour enhancers follow once the onions have browned to a desirable degree. During this stage, water is not added at all or added just sparingly to prevent the spices from burning; stirring is essential so as to prevent the ingredients from sticking to the pot. The process is considered to be complete when the oil starts to separate from the spices and the colour of the gravy changes.

This technique is adopted to kill the raw smell of ingredients and deepen the colour of the spices to richer hues. The process also allows the spices to blend together, and all flavours to intermingle and be imbibed by the rest of the ingredients. The constant stirring and frying during this stage of cooking helps to break down pieces of tender flavour enhancers, such as onions and tomatoes, till they are completely mashed, and the gravy is of a smooth consistency.

Bihari. The Biharis are an ethnic group originating from the state of Bihar in India with a history going back three millennia. Their ancestry can be traced to the Munda inhabitants of the region as well as to the Indo-Aryans.

At the time of Partition, many Muslim Biharis migrated to East Bengal (East Pakistan and subsequently Bangladesh), while a substantial number settled in Karachi (in then West Pakistan). After the formation of Bangladesh, a large number of Biharis moved to Karachi as refugees fleeing from the former eastern wing of Pakistan, thus increasing Karachiites' exposure to Bihari cuisine. Bihari cuisine is marked by their use of mustard oil for cooking as opposed to regular cooking oil.

Bihari kebab. A succulent and tender variety of charcoal grilled meat, *Bihari kebab* is perhaps the most popular Bihari dish in the country. This skewer of beef mixed with herbs, seasonings, raw papaya, and onions, is unique in the way that mustard oil is used in its preparation, while traditionally, garlic is not used.

One of the oldest establishments in Karachi that offers *Bihari kebab* is Al Kebab, located at Bahadurabad. Serving exclusively this kebab and *paratha* since the 1960s, it has only recently opened a franchise in the posh Defence area of Karachi.

Strangely enough, instead of eating it with *paratha* as is usually the case wherever *Bihari kebab* is prepared in the country, Biharis prefer to eat it with plain boiled rice and *daal*. Alternatively, it is also eaten with *bakarkhani*. Interestingly, it is also often eaten with *puri* or *paratha* made with the left-over marinade of the *Bihari kebab* and wheat flour.

Biryani. A term of Persian origin meaning 'fried', *biryani* refers to a spicy dish of layered meat and rice.

By the time of the second Mughal emperor Humayun's reign (1530–1540), the Mughal's court kitchens had begun to experience a fusion of cooking styles between Persian, Central Asian, and subcontinental cooking, marking the evolution of Mughlai cooking. Cooks in these kitchens were from Arabia, Turkey, Egypt, and the subcontinent, particularly from Sindh. It is during this period that *biryani* was invented—in fact, according to hearsay, Empress Nur Jahan invented it—although some attribute this invention to Mumtaz Mahal, wife of Shah Jahan. With the royal kitchens evolving the dish from a delicately aromatic Persian *pilau* into a highly aromatic, spicy rice dish with subcontinental flavours fused in, the *biryani* came into being. Truly reflecting the fusion of subcontinental and Mughal flavours and celebrating the Persian cooking techniques of *dum* and *bhoonna*, *biryani* is a dish in which meat is marinated in yoghurt, rich spices, onion, ginger, garlic, and almonds, and finished with steam-infused saffron. In fact, according to the book *Ain-i-Akbari* by Abu'l Fazl—which documents the culture of Akbar's reign—the Mughals used Central Asian and Persian spices, such as saffron, in lavish amounts when making this dish.

While the original Mughlai *biryani* was only meat-based, the Awadhi *biryani*, thanks to the nawab of Awadh, Wajid Ali Shah, incorporated potatoes in it, enhancing the flavour manifold.

A festive and celebratory dish prepared for weddings and religious festivals as well as solemn occasions, such as deaths and funerals, the traditional *biryani* was a layered dish of rice (it is essential to use Sella or Basmati rice) and mutton. In the modern-day *biryani*, however, the meat can be chicken, mutton, or lamb, while seafood and vegetables are also popular. Today, it is marinated in a yoghurt-based spice—onion/ginger and garlic paste—and then cooked in a pot. This curry is then topped with par-cooked rice that is further infused with flavour enhancers such as browned onions, almonds, and green chillies, and flavourings such as screw pine and saffron. The pot is covered with a tight lid or even sealed with dough, as is the traditional method. It is then cooked under steam (*dum*) over low heat on a stovetop or in the oven until all flavours are infused and the rice is cooked through. The exception to this method is the Hyderabadi *biryani* where uncooked rice and uncooked marinated meat are slow-cooked to perfection.

Present-day Pakistani *biryani* is a result of a fusion of flavours of the heritage cooking styles of the Muslims of the subcontinent. A plethora of different *biryani* styles, such as Bombay *biryani*, *danda biryani* made with mutton bong, and Hyderabadi *biryani* not to mention provincial recipes such as Sindhi *biryani* made with meat, potatoes, and dried plums make up the Pakistani *biryani* landscape. Every home in Pakistan has its own style and recipe of *biryani* that is usually a family recipe going back generations.

Additionally, *biryani* is a Pakistani 'fast food' popular with the masses, available in take-away places; it combines curry and rice to become a quick and easy meal for every day lunches or a one-dish meal at home.

SUMMAYA USMANI

Biscuit. Biscuits found in the subcontinent have a uniqueness in flavour indigenous to the essence and zest of the people of the subcontinent. When the colonists came to the subcontinent, they brought with them biscuits from their far-off lands, and the vibrant people of the Indus adapted this buttery European teatime snack with local spices and flavours to give it a *desi* flare.

The word biscuit is derived from two Latin words *bis* and *cotus*, which literally means twice cooked. In ancient times, the flour dough was first dried in an oven and then cooked for the second time. When first introduced to this baked delight, the British called it *bisquite*, while the Dutch called it *koekje*, meaning little cake, hence the American term cookies, for biscuits. The journey of biscuits is as delightful as its taste. It was initially created to be a travellers' food, nutritious, and easy to store and carry.

In 1660, the famous French traveller, François Bernier, describing his visit to Bengal, mentioned that in Bengal the supply of inexpensive sweet biscuits, flavoured with anise, to the crews of European ships was very common. This indicates that the very small-scale production of biscuits had already started in Bengal during the 17th century. The industrial production of biscuits was a later phenomenon and initially the Europeans imported these from outside the colony.

Gradually, from the second half of the 19th century, Europeans, Muslims, and lower-caste Hindus also started to establish bakeries and manufacturing workshops in the colony. Hence, when the British came to the subcontinent in the garb of the East India Company, they brought with them biscuits to charm the locals. Rich and upper-class natives were introduced to this baked delight, in its current flaky, buttery form. In the early 18th century the art of baking biscuits, on commercial basis in the region, took root while in the 19th century a *tandoor* was set up in Central Calcutta for making *desi* biscuits. Slowly biscuit-making and eating spread to the entire subcontinent.

Biscuit-making encouraged experimentation with flavours and with indigenous ingredients, such as almonds, cardamoms, saffron, anise, carom seeds and cumin, and within no time, the *desi* biscuit was born. The traditional *nankhatai* became perhaps the most typical local version of biscuit popular in the subcontinent.

The popularity of the biscuit caught on in such a way that it started getting transported to other markets within the subcontinent, including Karachi, and, expectedly enough, the subcontinental biscuit became a favourite to be consumed at tea time.

BISMA TIRMIZI

Bitter gourd. Thought to be a native of the subcontinent, the bitter gourd plant is first mentioned as *karivrnta* and later as *karavella* (Urdu *karela*) in early Jain literature (*c.*400 BC). Bitter gourd (*Momordica charantia*) is a tropical vine fruit belonging to the gourd family (Cucurbitaceae) and related to zucchini, cucumber, and squash. Green in colour, it is elongated and has a rough, bumpy skin. It is a tricky vegetable to cook because of its inherent bitterness. Kannada literature of the 16th century refers to the practice of debittering the bitter gourd by soaking it in salt water and washing it—a practice popular even today. Cooked dexterously, it can be a delicious vegetable that is especially popular because of its health benefits. In fact, bitter gourd is also known as nature's silent healer and is a valuable source of vitamin A and C, fibre, and folate.

In Sindh, apart from the more conventional style of cooking it as a vegetable curry, or mixing it with mutton and serving *karela gosht*, it is frequently cleaned out, stuffed with minced meat, tied with string, and fried (*qeema bharay karelay*) or stuffed with gram lentils and onion (*chanay ki daal ka karela*) and fried. Some even bake or steam it after cutting it into slices.

NAYYER RUBAB

Black cumin. Black cumin can either indicate a rare, dark variety of true cumin, or more commonly, a spice consisting of the seeds of *Nigella sativa*, native to the Levant. Despite being called black cumin, it does not resemble cumin in taste, nor is it botanically related. It is cultivated on a small scale in the subcontinent but is mainly collected from wild plants in forests. The seeds are small, dull black, roughly wedge-shaped, and pungent. They are used to flavour fried rice dishes,

as well as in the spice mixture, *panch phoron*, used to prepare certain Bengali-origin dishes. Black cumin is also sprinkled on bread and biscuits and used for flavouring vinegar and pickles.

Bohra cuisine. Bohras are a Shia Muslim community that originates from Gujarat, India. They trace their conversion to Islam from Hinduism in approximately AD 1100 when Arab Ismaili missionaries arrived from Yemen to Gujarat. The word Bohra (also spelled 'Vohra') is derived from the Gujarati word *vohorvu* or *vyavahar*, which means 'to trade'. As the name indicates, the community primarily comprised traders, as is the case even today.

Today, commonly known as Bohris, there are only 1.5 million of them in the world constituting a small, yet tightly-knit community. Regarded to be peace lovers and food lovers, the Bohris in Karachi are renowned for their cuisine which is influenced by several other foods such as Middle Eastern, Mughlai and Gujarati. Not only are they known for the unique taste of their manna but also for their unusual eating practices, which may be summed up by the saying 'Eat together, stay together.'

Their unusual eating style actually goes back to ancient times as Bohris believe this eating style was practised by Prophet Muhammad (PBUH). Traditionally, Bohris eat communally from large *thaals*, which are steel platters holding several *katoris* or small bowls, each one filled with a different item. The dining etiquette for eating from a *thaal* requires a minimum of seven people to be seated around it, while it is normally placed on the floor on a steel ring called *kundli*. The floor is covered with a large printed cloth called *jazam* over which a square cotton cloth called *safro* is arranged, and the ring is placed in the centre of the *safro*. Diners sit around the *thaal* on the *safro*, their legs tucked under the raised *thaal* and eat directly off the serving dishes placed in it. However, the *thaal*'s popularity among non-Bohris has resulted in a modernised version of it, with the *thaal* often placed on top of a dining table and diners serving themselves from it in plates.

Typically, the meal is initiated with a pinch of salt, believed to cleanse the mouth and cure 72 diseases, followed by a sweet dish. According to some Bohris, consuming sugar activates the metabolism and readies it to digest the *khaaras* (the savoury dishes) that come up next. On special occasions, they start their meal with *sonderu* which is rice cooked in clarified butter and sugar. The savoury dishes, eaten after the dessert, are unique and distinctive, and vary from the regular *karhai* or *salan* cooked in most households in Karachi to the more unusual fare. Each dish is placed in the centre of the *thaal*, and those sitting round the *thaal* take turns to avail of portions of the dish, until it is wiped clean, and another course takes its place. This is done to avoid wastage of food since wastage is highly frowned upon by this community. Accompaniments, such as *achar* and/or soup, are also placed on the *thaal*.

Last of the savoury items is the rice. Like all Pakistanis, this community too loves its *biryani*. However, other rice dishes invented by Bohris themselves are also very popular among the diners. Bohris believe rice to be a plant from Heaven and that it should be consumed by everyone even if it's only a spoonful as it protects one from 70 diseases. After the savoury dishes are consumed, dessert is served once again. Quaint as this custom is, today, eating out of *thaals*, even among many Bohris, is reserved for special or family occasions.

Another aspect of Bohri cuisine is that unlike most Pakistani foods, which are made with mixed spices or *garam masala*, Bohri cuisine has a base of green masala—made with ginger, garlic, and green chillies ground together—and hence, is lighter on the palate. *Dhungar* is often given to dishes to give them an irresistible, smoky flavour. Yet another interesting culinary-related fact about Bohris is that they do not eat fish unless it has been caught by one of their own, as they feel that fish too, should be *halal*. And they only eat fish with scales.

Boiling/tenderising. At the end of the *bhoonna* stage in the cooking process of most Pakistani dishes substantial amount of water is added to the pot which immediately brings the temperature down. What follows is the boiling or simmering of ingredients that need to be tenderised—such as meat, vegetables, rice, or lentils. Tenderising cannot be done in oil alone and requires a lot of water since the ingredients need to absorb it in order to soften. In cases where the ingredients release water when cooked, like spinach or chicken, extra water may not be needed. Characteristically, this stage of cooking is carried out on a very low heat with the pot covered. As the water content in the pot drops, the oil, which has blended with the water, separates, and resurfaces.

Boli. Also known as *bhalli*, *boli* is a much loved, simple dessert of the northern regions, particularly of Baltistan, where it is a Hindkowan favourite. It is unique in terms of its ingredients and is considered almost a delicacy. Its special ingredient is the first burst of milk that the cow/buffalo gives after delivering her calf. If taken on the very first day, it is quite watery and a dash of normal milk is added before boiling it. However, if taken on the second or third day, no addition of normal milk is required. Not only is this milk extra nutritious but delicious too. Boiled with a pinch of crushed cardamoms and sugar, it is cooled to set, and sprinkled with almonds (optional) to serve. It has a glassy, firm consistency and can be eaten like a pudding.

ZUBAIDA TARIQ

Bombay biryani. *Biryani* is by far the most popular cuisine in Pakistan. It is equally loved by all and is prepared for special occasions as well as on a regular basis—especially on weekends when the entire family is able to partake of the meal together—as a complete meal on its own. Its varieties are endless and their versions vary from city to city and community to community.

Bombay *biryani* is a slightly nutty, and sweet and spicy version of the regular *biryani*. In addition to the usual ingredients that go into making curries and other types of *biryani* it also incorporates dried plums, potatoes, and tomatoes. The meat (generally mutton, though increasingly chicken is also being used) is marinated with yoghurt, dried plums, and spices, and cooked with oil. Once it becomes tender, steamed, and fried potatoes are added to it. A layer of boiled rice (boiled with black cumin, cardamom, and cloves) is placed at the bottom of the pot and covered with chopped green chillies, browned onions, tomatoes, mint and coriander, and finally a layer of the prepared meat. The layers are then repeated and the top rice layer is sprinkled with either infused saffron or yellow food colour mixed with warm milk; the *biryani* is then put on *dum*. Bombay *biryani* is especially loved for its soft crunchy potatoes and plum-flavoured curry.

ZUBAIDA TARIQ

Bombay duck. Bomelon are small fish that the residents of Bombay used to treat with asafoetida and then hang up to dry in the sun. Fried until they were golden brown and crumbled over, they imparted a strong salty taste that the British in the subcontinent adored. They christened this seasoning Bombay duck as these fish (*Harpadon nehereus*) were known to swim close to the surface of the water. As early as the 17th century, the British living in Bombay were known as 'Ducks'.

A fish from Synodontidae family, bomelon is found in large numbers along the coast of Karachi as well and is available in fresh and dried form.

The dried Bombay duck is a popular condiment in the Hyderabadi style of cuisine in Pakistan. Although the fish is tiny in size, it requires thorough cleaning— it must be scraped clean and its head and tail cut off before frying so that it's sharp pelvic and pectoral fins, and small but many bones don't detract from the taste of the fish. The dried fish, when fried, leaves a strong odour and it takes a staunch foodie to be able to bear its pungent smell. But for those who don't mind it, the deep fried, crispy fish is a chewy and delicious accompaniment to *khatti daal* (tangy lentils) and rice. It is also a popular dish in Parsi cuisine where it is called *sookha boomla nu tarapori patio*.

SHAHA TARIQ

Bone marrow (nalli). Bone marrow is the soft, nutritious substance found in the internal cavities of animal bones, especially the shin bones of cows and calves, and goats. It is normally a part of meat dishes such as *gosht ka salan*, where the marrow is sucked out of the bone and eaten or used as an ingredient to dress beef dishes such as *nihari*, but also constitutes a dish on its own, such as *paya*, comprising goat trotters.

Boondi. Sweetened *besan* (gram flour) mixed with water plays an important part in making the tiny confections *boondi*. Dribbled through a perforated ladle into hot oil, the mixture forms pea-sized balls which are then coated in syrup.

Bosrak. A sweet dish of Afghani origin, popular with the Hazara community, this is a fist-shaped fritter made with flour and sugar, and deep fried in oil.

Bossari/busri. A rich *roti* prepared with *gur* and *ghee*, this Sindhi bread is normally a breakfast item, especially popular in winter. Similar to the *gogi ki roti* prepared in Khyber Pakhtunkhwa when a girl visits her parent's home for the first time after her marriage, this special bread is prepared by the bride's family on the day after the wedding.

Bottle gourd. A climbing plant that originated in Africa, bottle gourd has been in the region for so long that it has even been described in the *Rigveda*. Now called *lauki* or *kaddu*, *Lagenaria siceraria* is widely used since 2000 BCE as a soft vegetable. Long and light green in colour, its hard, dried shells find use as water bottles, blowing horns, and musical instruments such as those used by snake-charmers.

It is such a tasty vegetable to boot, that it is used both in savoury, and sweet dishes, and also eaten raw, mixed in salad or with yoghurt. *Lauki ki sabzi* is served on its own as a vegetable dish as well as cooked along with mutton in a curry, whereas it is also the main ingredient in delectable desserts like *lauki ka halwa*. Gourd is a valuable source of vitamin B and C and is full of good pectin.

NAYYER RUBAB

Brahui. Closely linked to the Baloch, with whom they have substantially intermingled and whose cultural traits they have absorbed, Brahuis are a Dravidian ethnic group believed to be a remnant of the inhabitants of the Indus Valley Civilisation. A variation of 'Barohis' meaning 'mountain dwellers' or 'highlanders', Brahuis live mostly in the rugged hills around the town of Kalat in Chaghi district in Balochistan, while a few reside in Sindh as well.

For many centuries, Brahuis ruled Kalat and enjoyed their independent status even during the British Raj, but in 1948 Kalat was finally incorporated into Pakistan. Known for their hospitality, the community has preserved its language, culture, customs, folk instruments, music, and food.

They cultivate wheat and millet, which are ground into flour and baked into unleavened bread. *Braisni roti*, made in Kalat till today, is bread that is roasted in a *tandoor* which is set in a wall, instead of in the ubiquitous *tandoor* which is in a pit. Rice is also eaten, but usually only on special occasions. Mutton, on the other hand, is an important part of the diet of the Brahuis. Food is often eaten from a communal platter. Dates, wild fruits, and vegetables are also part of the Brahui diet. Tea is drunk at meals and is also taken as part of various social ceremonies.

The popular Balochi dish *sajji* is among Brahui specialties as are other traditional Balochi dishes such as *khaddi kebab* (a whole goat stuffed with rice and dry fruit and cooked in a pit), *khurood*, *kaak* or *kurnu* (wheat dough wrapped around stone and cooked on fire), *tireet* (gravy made with *khurood* and eaten with small pieces of *roti* soaked in it) and the winter special dish *khadeet* (dried, whole marinated goat, consumed with rice).

NAYYER RUBAB

Braise. Braise is actually a Gujarati distortion of 'breast' and comprises mutton ribs. An exclusive and special savoury dish of Bohra community, it is especially served at weddings to the in-laws. Boiled in *hara masala*— Bohris cook food in green masala comprising garlic and green chillies, as opposed to the ubiquitous mixed spices used by other communities—and herbs, and then given *baghar* (tempering), usually of just black pepper, it is considered one of the best cuts of meat, and is eaten on its own, served without any staple.

NAYYER RUBAB

British colonisation and culinary influences. The effect of British colonisation upon the subcontinent from the start of the 18th century was the direct consequence of mingling of the British with the aristocratic locals, who had been excited to try the food of the rulers. Initially though, there was only disappointment on their part since the bland flavour of British cuisine left them rather unmoved. However, some local aristocracy took to the British ways relatively easily, as they ardently desired to appear 'modern'.

Hence, together with the introduction of Anglo-Indian style dishes in their cuisine, the British also influenced their culinary habits, dining table etiquette, and use of certain utensils and cooking methods. The use of cutlery, seating at dining tables with napkins on laps, and general dining etiquette so common now in major cities of Pakistan are thus the legacy of British colonisation.

Besides these changes the British were responsible for introducing sophistication into the cuisine and the concept of three-course meals to a people used to serving all the dishes of a meal at the outset rather than course by course, not to mention afternoon tea and cakes, and a concept of starters such as soup.

But it must also be said that the effect of British colonisation upon the subcontinent cannot be seen in isolation from the influences of local cuisine on that of the British. Even though British adaptation of subcontinental food gave rise to a hybrid cuisine in its own right in the region and has since been an integral part of both India and Pakistan's culinary heritage, it has also become popular in the UK with the British.

Of course, that was not the case from day one. When the British first came to the region (early 18th century) the food of the subcontinent displeased them immensely, as local spices did not appeal to the British palate. Hence, the initial aristocratic menus of the British did not feature curries, now so popular with them. With time and mingling with the local aristocratic people and a sense of a need to not appear as overbearing rulers, the British embarked on an attempt to bring the then backward and impoverished citizens, the perceived benefits of the first world. As a result of this, the British food, too, started to get a local flavour by virtue of their employing local cooks who, not being well-versed in the British ways of cooking, began to merge the spice element into certain British dishes, keeping their basic visual structure vaguely intact, such as in soups and rice dishes.

And thus, the British or Anglo-Indian cuisine in the subcontinent began to evolve, with English meat casseroles being thickened with flour, and flavoured with local masalas, and though these were a far cry from curries, they were not casseroles, either. Local cooks now learnt the art of roasting and grilling, but with Indian flavours. Rather than stuffing chicken with breadcrumbs and herbs, they plastered coriander, cumin, and pepper on it and created a masala roast. Leftover meat minced was usually made into cutlets by the British; the same was recreated with masalas and mashed potatoes to make *cutlass*.

What's more, the British practice of curing the meat is probably what gave rise to recipes like hunter beef in Pakistan, which is similar to the recipes found in the UK-published book, *The Scots Kitchen: Its Traditions and Recipes* by F. Marian McNeill.

The influences of British eating habits and their basic recipes that have been changed to suit Pakistani palates still exist today, both as a result of legacy and adoption of Western habits because of greater exposure through travels and the media.

SUMMAYA USMANI

Buckwheat (*Salajeet; Fagopyrum esculentum*). An herbaceous plant of the same family as rhubarb, buckwheat is grown for its seeds. Being hardy, it grows quickly even in unfavourable conditions, and is capable of producing two or even three crops a year; hence, it is mostly used in the northern areas of Pakistan where the climate is cold or soil poor.

The plant bears small clusters of seeds of a curious shape, triangular in cross-section with pointed ends. Buckwheat is similar to any typical cereal in nutritional value. It contains rutin, a substance which is considered to be beneficial for people with high blood pressure. The uses of buckwheat both in the form of husked whole grains and as flour are manifold. However, the flour has an unusual flavour which is not universally liked.

The leaves of wild perennial buckwheat grown in the Himalayas and Gilgit Baltistan are cooked as a vegetable.

Budauni pera. This is a sweetmeat, believed to have originated in Allapur, a small town, known for the excellent quality of its milk and milk products, located in Budaun, a famous district of Uttar Pradesh (UP), India. However, as legend goes, its origin must be attributed to a sweetmeat merchant Mamman Khan who came to Budaun to sell this special *peray*. This dessert was liked by everyone so much that they named it *Mamman kay peray*, but beyond Budaun they became famous as *Budauni peray*. Today, no matter where they are prepared and sold, they are known by this name, which has come to denote a style of preparation more than the place of origin.

The major difference between the more common white *pera*, and the light brown *Budauni pera* is that while white *pera* is made with dried milk but with moisture content, *Budauni pera* is made with evaporated milk boiled to a thick consistency (*khoya*) and stirred on low heat with sugar and other aromatic ingredients till it turns golden brown. When the mixture cools down, small flat balls are made with a thumb depression on top to place a piece of almond.

In Pakistan, a shop was set up by Al Haj Muhammed Ali Khan who moved from Budaun to Mardan after Partition; he called his outlet *Budauni Paira House* (since 1950). In Karachi there is actually a shop at Liaquatabad No. 10, called *Mamman kay peray* which only makes the one *mithai—Budauni peray*—and is famous for its high quality and taste.

NAYYER RUBAB

Buddhism. One of the world's largest religions, Buddhism originated in 6th century BC in eastern India as a reaction against the complex, ritual-ridden and expensive religion and caste-based society of the later Vedic period. It soon became popular because it addressed the needs of the new agricultural economy based on the use of iron ploughshare.

The founder of Buddhism, Siddhartha, was born in 563 BC at Lumbini, located at the foothills of Nepal. His father, Shuddhodana, was the chief of the Shakya clan of Kapilavastu. His mother Mayadevi, died soon after childbirth and so Siddhartha was brought up by his aunt Gotami and was, therefore, called Gautama. Siddhartha, being the Kshatriya prince, grew up amid great comfort and luxury. He got married to Yashodhara and had a son, Rahul. But he was very distressed by the miseries

of old age, disease, and death. He renounced the world at the age of 29 in search of the ultimate truth. After seven years he attained enlightenment at Bodh Gaya in Bihar. Henceforth, he began to be called Buddha or the Enlightened One.

Gautama Buddha established the monastic order (*samgha*) where the followers were admitted as monks (*bhikkus*) and nuns (*bhikkunis*). He devoted the rest of his life to the preaching of his doctrines. He died (*Mahaparinirvana*) at the age of 80 in 483 BC at Kushinara in eastern Uttar Pradesh.

Gautama Buddha preached *Ahimsa* or non-violence. He believed that cattle should not be slaughtered because oxen were required to pull the heavy iron ploughshare. But he did not categorically forbid his disciples from eating meat. The monks and nuns lived on alms, so whatever was put in their begging bowl they were to gracefully receive it and consume all food including meat and even rotten food. There was an exception though—if the monks got to know or suspected that the animal was slaughtered specifically to feed them, they were to refuse to take the meat. It is stated that those who take life are at fault but not the person who eats flesh. According to Buddha, those who do not wear silk, leather boots, furs or down…and do not consume milk, cream, or butter can truly transcend this world. Both physically and mentally, one must avoid the bodies and by-products of beings by neither wearing them nor eating them.

Buddha did not allow drinking of fermented liquors or strong drinks. He, however, allowed eight kinds of beverages to his followers: syrups prepared with ripe mango juice, rose apple, plantain fruit, grapes, honey, edible root of waterlily, coconut and parusaka fruit. Sometimes sugar and *gur* (jaggery) syrup was also prepared. All these beverages were taken in the evening as the followers of Buddha did not take their meals then.

The Buddhist monastic order realised the importance of food. Explicit rules were laid down as to what should be eaten and what should be avoided. There are different viewpoints regarding the dietary rules of various sects of Buddhism. Some sects of Buddhism do not allow the eating of five pungent spices, i.e. onions, garlic, leeks, chives, and scallions. They believe that if these five are eaten cooked, they increase sexual desire, and if eaten raw they increase anger. What's more, their foul smell deprived the eater the company of others. Asafoetida was also not consumed by Buddhists. However, Buddhist monks were allowed to use them in case of illness.

Buddha avoided two extremes: self-indulgence and self-mortification. He believed in the middle path and, therefore, advised the monks to be moderate in eating. They were asked to take as much food as was enough for maintaining the body and keeping it unharmed. No monk was allowed to take food more than what was necessary to sustain life. They were not allowed to store food in ordinary times. But some food-stuffs which were given to convalescent monks as tonics, such as *ghee*, butter, honey, oil, and sugar, could be preserved for a week. Buddha allowed the consumption of all food articles necessary to sustain life. However, the simplicity in food is emphasised in Buddhism.

The region that is today known as Pakistan once had a large Buddhist population, with the majority of people in Gandhara (present day north-western Pakistan) being Buddhist. The Swat Valley, known in antiquity as Uddiyana, was a kingdom tributary to Gandhara. There are many archaeological sites from the Buddhist era in Swat.

The Buddhist sage, Padmasambhava, is said to have been born in a village near the present-day town of Chakdara in Lower Dir District, which was then a part of Uddiyana. Buddhism was also practiced in the Punjab and Sindh regions. Most Buddhists in the Punjab converted to Hinduism from AD 600 onwards. However, Buddhism remained the faith practiced by the majority of the population of Sindh up to the Arab conquest by the Umayyads in AD 710. After the partition of Pakistan and India, the Buddhists fled to India. Gandhara remained a largely Buddhist land until around AD 800, when Pakhtuns invaded the region from Southern Afghanistan and introduced Islam.

ANJALI MALIK

Buffalo. While only considered a beast of burden in South-East Asia, in Pakistan the buffalo has also been a source of milk and meat since ancient times. The *Nilamata Purana* (6th century AD) mentions its use in Kashmir, and Ibn Battuta in the 14th century AD relished a porridge of de-husked *shama* grains mixed with buffalo milk. Another 14th century traveller noted that in certain dry tracts adjacent to the Sindh desert, fish and buffalo milk were abundantly available. In about AD 1600, Edward Terry commented that buffalo flesh 'was like beef but not so wholesome'. That said, buffalo milk is far richer in fat than cow milk.

Bumbaiya naan. With milk incorporated in the dough, *Bumbaiya naan*, also known as *sheermal* among the Gujaratis, is a soft, sweetish, spongy bread which looks more like a large round, flat bun. It is normally eaten with *qorma*, especially on Eid.

Bun kebab. Extremely popular and a great favourite with all ages, *bun kebab* is a very Pakistani version of a burger. Commonly available at roadside stalls, it is the mouth-watering local fast food that is partaken of by the rich and poor alike and is as popular as a snack as a main course.

Made with pink lentils and potato patty, the patty is coated with beaten egg and fried on a very hot skillet. The fried patty is then sandwiched between roasted buns; sliced onions, cucumber, and tomato are added for flavour, as are ketchup and green chutney. The vegetarian patty is substituted with a minced beef one for the benefit of meat lovers.

ZUBAIDA TARIQ

Bunda palla machli. *Hilsa ilisa*, the famous *palla* of Sindh, though a sea fish, ascends the Indus in order to spawn. The migration continues throughout February, March, and April. Fried, steamed, or baked in sand, this fish is delectable in spite of its numerous small bones, and is believed to boast the finest flavour in the East. After cleaning it and stuffing it with a paste prepared from a variety of spices and herbs, it is cooked on low heat. When baking it in sand, the *palla* is wrapped in cloth, and buried three feet deep in hot sand under the sun. It bakes, thus, for four to five hours, from late morning to early afternoon.

There are two folklores surrounding *palla* in Sindh. One attributes its popularity to King Jam Tamachi. According to the folklore the king was smitten by Noori, the daughter of a Sindhi fisherman. So enamoured was he by her that he was willing to give up his empire for her hand in marriage, while the entire fishing community was up in arms about the proposal. In order to try and woo the community, the king gifted the people lots of land, and whenever he visited them, he would be served *palla machli*, which became a special delicacy to serve to visitors.

According to another tale, when Muhammed Tughlaq invaded Sindh, he was offered *palla* fish. He liked it so much that he consumed huge quantities of it, which caused his death. That is why *palla* fish came to be known as 'Enemy Defeater'.

Burus shapik. Similar to *berikutz* but without the layer of herbs, *burus shapik* is *burus* (soft, home-made goat cheese) layered on a Hunzakutz traditional whole-wheat *chapati*, and then covered with another *chapati*. Its outside is covered with apricot-kernel oil; it is cut into slices and served cold and is very filling.

Burutz berikutz. *Burutz or burus* is a soft, home-made goat cheese, and *burus berikutz* is *burus* mixed with herbs such as coriander and mint, layered on a Hunzakutz traditional whole-wheat *chapati*, and then covered with another *chapati*. Its outside is covered with apricot-kernel oil; it is cut into slices and served cold and is very filling.

Butcher. This term is commonly associated with a person who slaughters cattle (cows, goat, sheep). In the subcontinent, particularly in Pakistan and India, and also in Arab countries including Iran, they are called '*qassab*'. In Pakistan they are also known as '*qasai*'. Till a couple of decades ago the community belonged to the lower income group, but with time the upper, educated class has begun to invest in hygienic, state-of-the-art butcheries. The commercial activities of butchers are mainly in the following sectors: purchase/sale of live stocks; slaughtering of animals; sale of meat; sale of hides/skins.

In Pakistan, in the Punjab province butchers are generally divided into eight major clans, such as Arbi, Bhatti, Khokhar, Goraha, and Suhal. The Qassab community found in Sindh migrated from Delhi and Haryana, and are mainly found in cities like Karachi, Sukkur, Hyderabad, and Larkana.

In Pakistan, all butchers selling mutton and beef follow the prescribed Islamic ritual procedure of *halal*, through which the animal is slaughtered by cutting its jugular vein, while proclaiming the name of Allah. Fresh meat used to be sold throughout the week but is now restricted to five days a week in the cities.

NAHEED ANSARI

Butter. Made from cream—an oil-in-water emulsion—butter is further concentrated so that the final product is more than 80 per cent fat. When cream is churned by a revolving paddle, this disturbs the emulsion, forcing the fat globules together until they join up into a continuous mass with water droplets trapped in it. After churning, the butter is further worked, also washed in plain water, to remove as much buttermilk as possible and improve the texture and flavour. This also improves keeping quality, as does the addition of salt, which discourages the growth of bacteria. In this form it stays for longer than fresh milk or cream.

In Pakistan, butter is made not only from cow's milk but also from water-buffalo's milk. Not a popular medium for cooking in Pakistan—unlike its clarified product, *ghee*—butter is generally used as a breakfast item, or for baking purposes. Salted butter is more common than unsalted butter.

Cabbage. *Brassica oleracea* or cabbage, the first cultivated vegetable in the diverse genus *Brassica*, is the ancestor of most of its numerous relations, such as cauliflower and Brussels sprouts. The variety most commonly found in Pakistan is hard and white or light green in colour. In its raw form it is used to prepare coleslaw. It is used to make vegetable curry, although the smell of cooking cabbage, which most people dislike, is quite pungent, coming from various sulphur compounds, and so is not a very popular dish on its own. It is also stir-fried and served as an accompaniment in continental dishes or as an ingredient in many Chinese dishes that are extremely popular in the country. Since for stir-frying, the cabbage is sliced into thin strips, it reduces the sulphurous smell; hence, it is most popular when served this way. The coating of hot oil seals the surface and reduces the emanation, thereby retaining more flavour, while the texture is appetisingly crisp.

Cake. A form of dessert that is typically baked, cake is commonly eaten as a tea-time snack, as well as served as a celebratory dish on ceremonial occasions, such as weddings, anniversaries, and birthdays. It has a porous texture as the mixture rises during cooking. Typical ingredients for cake are flour, sugar, eggs, butter, or oil, a liquid, and leavening agents, such as baking soda and/or baking powder. Common additional ingredients and flavourings these days include dried, candied or fresh fruit, nuts, cocoa, and extracts such as vanilla, with numerous substitutions for the primary ingredients.

The history of cakes can be traced back to the 13th century. Cakes originated in ancient Egypt as round, flat, unleavened breads that were cooked on a hot stone. In ancient Rome, basic bread dough was sometimes enriched with butter, eggs, and honey, which produced a sweet and cake-like baked item.

The history of cakes in Pakistan, however, goes back to the integration of the Persian culture and cuisine in the subcontinent, thanks to the series of invasions that took place here. They introduced the very popular fruit-cake, slices of which would be sold by men on bicycles who would keep them in trunks in the rear of their cycles.

The advent of the British era—when the plain pound cake gained popularity—resulted in 'plain cakes' becoming a significant part of the evening tea, with locals beginning to enjoy dunking cake in their tea.

Over the years the cake market in Pakistan has tremendously evolved with many bakeries, cafes, and home-based bakers now serving and taking orders for freshly-baked cakes and offering a large variety of options which range from plain cakes to flavoured cakes, and cheese cakes to cream cakes for special occasions. Floral wedding and designer cakes in various shapes and with intricate patterns have come to be in vogue in Pakistan, with an array of professional cake designers springing up in all major cities.

Today, cakes are a work of art and may be filled with fruits and preserves or dessert sauces like pastry cream, iced with buttercream or fresh cream, and decorated with fondant, piped borders, chocolate, or marzipan.

KAUSAR AHMED

Caramel custard/crème caramel/egg pudding. Similar to the French crème brûlée, crème caramel is essentially a boiled custard. Caramel syrup is poured into the container before the custard is put in, and the custard is subsequently turned out before serving. Introduced to the region by the Portuguese whose speciality was fragrant egg custard, a style of dessert entirely new to the subcontinent and a hot favourite with the British during colonial rule, this was one of the first desserts to be adopted by the local people who would call it 'putin' as they couldn't pronounce pudding. With the caramelised sugar topping, caramel custard has milk, eggs, and sugar as its main ingredients. It is usually cooked in a double-broiler to ensure indirect heat or baked in an oven.

Cardamom (*Elettaria cardamomum*; elaichi). The dried fruit of a perennial herb, cardamom is the third

27

most expensive spice after saffron and vanilla. It belongs to the ginger family (Zingiberaceae). Originally introduced to the cuisine by the southern part of the subcontinent and later featuring prominently in dishes of Mughal origin, cardamoms add fragrance and flavour to various dishes and teas. They have been an article of trade in the region for about a thousand years.

Cardamom pods can be used with or without their husks and have a slightly pungent but aromatic taste. They come in two types—green and black. The green ones are regarded as 'true' cardamoms, while the larger black or brown ones come from some other species and are regarded as 'false' cardamoms. The fruits of the true cardamoms are three-angled and ovoid or oblong and are picked before they are fully ripe (when they would be apt to split) and cured by drying, after which they should be hard and of a good, green colour. Each fruit contains three cells in which there are numerous small seeds. These seeds, which turn from white to brown to black as the fruit ripens, provide the pleasing aroma of cardamom, and its warm, slightly pungent flavour.

The green pods grown in the subcontinent are considered the best in the world and are the more expensive variety; they are small in size and can be used in both sweet and savoury dishes. In Pakistan, this fragrant spice is used in rich curries and milk-based desserts. Tea and coffee are also often spiked with green cardamoms. The black ones, which are not true cardamom but from plants of the related *Amomum* and *Afromomum* genus, are cheaper, larger, coarser, and less aromatic, and only used for savoury dishes made with meat or vegetables or in pickles. Both the types are essential ingredients in *garam masala* (mixed spices). Cardamom pods can also be chewed as breath fresheners and digestive aids, and it is believed that they sharpen the mind.

Carom seed (ajwain). The seeds of *Trachyspermum ammi*, an umbelliferous plant related to caraway, carom seeds are pale beige coloured and look like a smaller version of cumin fruits. The seeds are considered a spice, which is used as a flavouring agent, as they are highly fragrant and smell and taste like thyme, but with a stronger flavour. They are normally used in seed form and are rarely used as powder. In Pakistani cuisine, carom seeds are used mostly to flavour vegetable dishes, and in pickles because of their preservative qualities. Possessing useful antioxidant and preservative qualities, they are believed to aid digestion, relieve symptoms of cold, and ease rheumatic pain. The seeds also yield an

essential oil, thymol, which is mainly used in toothpaste and for the treatment of ringworm infections.

Carrot (*Daucus carota*). An important root vegetable that has existed since prehistoric times, carrots were originally purple in colour and were indigenous to Afghanistan for almost 5,000 years. They came in colours such as red, yellow, black, and white, but not orange, until the 17th century when, reportedly, horticulturalists in the Netherlands decided to honour William of Orange, from the House of Orange, by creating an orange carrot. Many, however, believe that it was a coincidence and the orange colour was a mutation of the red and yellow carrot, with no significant link to the Royal House of Orange, as this orange carrot had already begun to spread far and wide into Europe, Middle East, and, of course, South Asia, with the coming of the Dutch East India Company to the subcontinent in the 17th century. The Mughal Empire was spreading and international traders were bringing in intriguing new goods for exchanges, barter and purchase, and the long, orange carrot is said to be one such treasure.

This new orange carrot was sweeter, prettier and of a non-sticky variety, making it popular among the cooks. The cooks in the subcontinent liked the new imported carrot and the sweetness that came with it, and since it was an era when new cuisines were being developed by expert chefs and connoisseurs, this kind of carrot seemed to be of a perfect variety to be used as the main ingredient in many desserts, along with sugar, milk, and clarified butter. The province of Punjab apparently took an instant liking to it, and started developing innovative new recipes, both sweet and savoury—from *gajar ka halwa*, *murabbay*, and *gajrela* (carrot cooked in milk), to *achar*, *gajar gosht*, *gajar matar*, and much more—making the carrot an instant hit all over the subcontinent, with both pauper and prince.

Carrot has remarkable nutritional and health benefits. There are good reasons to include carrots in human diet, since they are enriched with carotenoids, phenolic compounds, polyacetylenes, and vitamins and for this reason they may help reduce the risk of some diseases.

BISMA TIRMIZI

Cashew. *Anacardium occidentale*, or *kaju* in Urdu, is thought to be the native of north-eastern Brazil. Till the 16th century cashew was taken from there by the Portuguese to the East Indies, after which cultivation spread to the subcontinent. A small tree bearing a strange fruit, it has two parts: at the stem end, a cashew 'apple', and projecting from the other end of the apple, a smaller cashew 'nut'. When the apple is ripe, both the apple and the nut fall to the ground together. The nut is in a hard, double shell, between the two parts of which there is a caustic substance, so the kernel is difficult to extract. The usual way of treating the nut is to roast it whole, driving off the irritants, and making the shell brittle enough to crack without crushing the contents.

The nuts, which have a delicate texture and a mild almond flavour, are highly esteemed in the country. They are widely eaten plain, roasted with salt, or with tangy masala, as a snack or an appetiser, especially in winters. They are also occasionally added whole or ground to savoury and sweet dishes.

Cattle. A collective term that covers animals in the genus *Bos* of the family Bovidae, cattle are domesticated for various purposes, such as a source of milk and meat. In this region, cattle were first domesticated in Balochistan in *c.*5000 BC as is evident from excavations which reveal the hump-backed animals, while Indus Valley seals depict both the humped form and the ones with forward-pointing horns. The buffalo also appears to have been domesticated while the domestication of sheep and goats preceded that of cattle in the same area. All these were well-known species in the Indus Valley.

The history of cattle in the region shows their immense socioeconomic significance and reflects their value as draught animals—they were valued for their milk and meat, plus their dung which was used as fuel.

While once beef was regarded as a poor man's meat in Pakistan, with chicken taking the lead as the meat of choice, today, beef has become more expensive than chicken, second only to mutton. However, among the urban elite, who prefer to avoid red meat, chicken or fish versions of meat dishes are still preferred over beef— although there are certain beef dishes that gourmands would not dream of replacing with any other meat, as the taste is drastically compromised—such as *Bihari kebab, nihari, chapli kebab* and many more—and one sees that even non-red meat eaters do make the occasional exception to partake of these beef delicacies.

Cauliflower (phool gobhi). *Brassica oleracea* (botrytis group), commonly called cauliflower, is a variety of the common cabbage in which flowers have begun to form but have stopped growing at the bud stage. Introduced in this region after AD *c.*1850 for use by colonials, cauliflower has become a favourite vegetable in Pakistani cuisine because of its fine texture and ability to absorb flavours. Cauliflower is usually cooked along with other vegetables, such as green peas, carrots, and potatoes. As in cooking cabbage, care must be taken not to overcook cauliflower, or it starts to break down, giving off a characteristic sulphurous odour.

Cauliflower is rich in antioxidants that help prevent cancer and has an anti-diabetic reputation. It is also richer in calcium and contains more folic acid than almost any other vegetable.

Central Asia. The central region of Asia, Central Asia extends from the Caspian Sea in the west to the border of western China in the east. It is bound on the north by Russia and on the south by Iran, Afghanistan, and China. The region consists of the former Soviet republics of Kazakhstan, Uzbekistan, Tajikistan, Kyrgyzstan, and Turkmenistan.

The region was gradually Islamised beginning from the 11th and 12th centuries, and the process was virtually complete by the 15th century. The Mongols took over almost all of Central Asia in the 13th century, and their rule in the form of various independent khanates lasted until the conquests of Taimur (Tamerlane) about the year 1400.

It is believed by some that the term Mughal comes from a mispronunciation of the word Mongol, but the Mughals of the subcontinent were mostly ethnic Turks not Mongols. However, Babur (1483–1530), the first Mughal emperor, could trace his bloodline to Changez Khan. Post Changez Khan, the Mongol Empire split into four parts: Golden Horde of Russia (1242–1359), Ilkhanate of Iran and Iraq (1256–1353), Chinese Yuan Dynasty (1271–1368) ruled by Kublai Khan, and, finally, Mughal Empire of the subcontinent (1527–1707).

The establishment of the Mughal Empire was key in the evolution of the Muslim cuisine of the subcontinent. Mughlai cuisine is strongly influenced by the Persian and Turkic cuisines of Central Asia—the region where the early Turko-Mongol Mughal emperors originally hailed from—and it has in turn strongly influenced the regional cuisine of Pakistan.

Mughlai cuisine varies from extremely mild to spicy. It is often associated with a distinctive aroma and the taste of ground and whole spices. A Mughlai meal is an elaborate buffet of main course dishes with a variety of accompaniments.

Although the ruling class and administrative elite of the Mughal Empire could variously identify themselves as Turani (Turkic), Irani (Persian), Shaikhzada (Indian

Muslim), and Hindu Rajput, the empire itself was Indo-Persian having a hybridised, pluralistic Persianate culture. Decorated Indo-Persian cookbooks and culinary manuscripts adorned the personal libraries of the Mughal elite, serving as culinary guides and for aesthetic value.

One example was the *Ni'matnama*, a 15th century work illustrated with Persian miniatures. This was commissioned by Sultan Ghiyas Shah—a sultan of Malwa in modern-day Madhya Pradesh—and features Central Asian dishes such as *samosay* (fried meat-filled pastry), *khichri* (rice and lentils*)*, *pilaf* (rice-dish), *seekh kebab* (skewered and grilled meat and fish), and *yakhni* (meat broth) all of which are popular items of present-day Pakistani cuisine.

BISMA TIRMIZI

Chaakna (ojri). Goat's intestines and tripe curry, *chaakna* is the Hyderabadi name for this spicy stew of offal, which is more commonly called *ojri*. Since the meat that goes into this dish basically comprises spare parts of the goat that are often discarded, it is a low-cost meat entrée. Nevertheless, many people find it delicious and especially make it in spite of the hassle that goes into its preparation.

The tripe and the intestines have to be cleaned thoroughly which is usually a family-acquired technique. Basically, the intestines have to be washed under running water three to four times and the tripe has to be boiled and scraped with a brush or metal spoon and cut into small pieces.

A curry base is made with browned onions and ginger-garlic paste. Tomatoes are added to thicken and sweeten the curry. Spices include the basic red chillies, turmeric, black pepper, and *garam masala*, and bay leaves.

The cleaned and chopped intestines and tripe, and often chunks of liver and kidney, are added to the ready curry base and fried till they are perfectly blended. Desired amount of water is added to make the curry and then left on a low flame to cook. Half a cup of diluted sorghum flour is added in the end to give a thicker consistency to the curry.

Chaakna is a great favourite with the oldies who have grown up eating it but is not so popular with the youngsters.

ZUBAIDA TARIQ

Chaas (buttermilk). Also called *chhaachh*, *chaas* is the liquid left after the cream has been churned and butter removed. Much of the water, with milk sugar and proteins in it, is forced out in the form of buttermilk. In composition, it resembles a light, skimmed milk but it is also mildly sour as a result of the 'ripening' of the cream to make butter. In recent times, after a long period when buttermilk was in low esteem, more people have come to regard it as a healthful alternative to ordinary milk, having much less fat. It is normally drunk to accompany a meal or as a refreshing drink in summer.

Chaat. An Indic word which literally means 'lick', *chaat* is used to describe a range of snacks and fast-food dishes comprising assorted savouries such as *chana papri* (chickpeas with crispy fried dough wafers), *gol gappay* (hollow, fried crisp *puris* eaten with boiled chickpeas, also known as *pani puri*), *masalay wallay aaloo* (spicy potatoes), and *fruit chaat* (mixed fruits with *chaat masala*)—all dished out with sweet and sour chutneys and tangy sprinklers. It is believed that during the reign of the Mughal Emperor Mohammad Shah (AD 1719–48), *chaat* became a rage when the court hakim recommended highly spiced dishes to keep stomach problems and germs at bay. Today, it is one of the most popular snacks one can partake of. It can be consumed both hot and cold, depending on one's preference.

Chaats are popularly eaten at tea time, though occasionally even for lunch, and are a must in some form or the other at *iftar* (evening meal to break the Ramazan fast).

Chaat masala. *Chaat masala* is a mix of ground spices. It is added to make food spicy, sour, and tangy. The word *chaat* is derived from *chaatna* meaning licking in Urdu and Hindi, implying that its usage makes the food so tasty that people want to lick it clean.

The main ingredients of *chaat masala* are dried mango powder, black salt, cumin powder, coriander powder, pomegranate seed powder, mint powder, black pepper, red chillies, and asafoetida. The blend of all these spices gives a unique taste and flavour to *chaat masala*. People add these ingredients in different ratios according to their taste when making *chaat masala*, although it can also be readily bought off the shelf.

Chaat masala is used to spice up many types of food items. It is sprinkled over snacks, such as *pakoray* (fried dumplings of gram flour), *aaloo ki tikkia* (potato cutlets) and *cholay* (chickpeas and potatoes in tamarind chutney), and *dahi varay* (dumplings in yoghurt). *Chaat masala* is added to fruit and vegetable salads with a squeeze of lemon to make them tasty. Fruit juices and buttermilk are made delicious with this mix of spices. It is also sprinkled over fried cashew nuts and almonds. *Chaats* like *chana papri, bhel puri, sev puri, dahi puri,* and *fruit chaat* would not be half as delicious as they are if *chaat masala* were not added. The addition of *chaat masala* to food also helps in their digestion.

ANJALI MALIK

Chai (tea). The term *chai* is derived from the word *cha* of Mandarin Chinese, known in English as tea. The history of tea dates to 2737 BC when according to a Chinese legend, King Shen Nung discovered tea and realised that it was not just an aromatic beverage but had medicinal properties too. It became a popular drink under the Tang rulers (AD 618–906).

Chai is prepared from the leaves and leaf buds of an evergreen shrub called chahua (*Camellia sinensis)* meaning tea flower in Mandarin. Two leaves and a bud are plucked by hand and then dehydrated. They are then cut, twisted, and curled with the help of machines, before the process of fermentation begins. Different processing methods result in the creation of various varieties of tea, even though leaves for all types of tea are harvested from the same species of plant.

There are three major types of tea classified by processing methods:

1. Fermented or black tea which produces amber coloured full-flavoured beverage and is not bitter.
2. Semi-fermented or oolong tea which yields a slightly bitter, light brownish-green liquid.
3. Unfermented tea or green tea that results in a mild, pale greenish yellow beverage which is also slightly bitter.

Chai is the most popular beverage in Pakistan and is partaken of not just in the evening at 'tea time' but through the day, even in the scorching heat of summer. More than 109,000 tonnes of tea is consumed in Pakistan each year, making it the seventh-largest tea-consuming and third-largest importer of tea in the world (2014). It is the first drink of choice to be offered to visitors in any part of the country and is a symbol of Pakistani hospitality. It is a tradition and the lifeblood of the people and serves to strengthen business and social agreements. Perhaps, more importantly, the ability to make a good cup of tea is considered an important skill for every future wife. Among the rituals while looking for a bride and undertaking marriage negotiations, is the modestly dressed young woman rolling the tea

trolley into the drawing room and pouring out the tea she has prepared to everyone present. Tea crop is even represented on the state emblem along with wheat, cotton and jute.

To prepare *chai*, the processed tea leaves are boiled in water, then milk and sugar are added to make a very aromatic and tasty beverage. Strong, sweetened milk tea, spiced in many variations with ginger, cardamom, pepper, cinnamon, cloves, and other ingredients, is called *masala chai*. Lemon tea has also become an immensely popular drink. Tea is normally drunk hot, although iced tea has also gained in popularity among city dwellers. A variant of hot tea is *doodh patti* which is basically tea cooked in milk instead of water. The secret of the flavour is in allowing the milk to boil until it reaches the consistency of heavy condensed milk. In Pakistan, this is the most popular form of tea consumed in cities as well as villages.

While the British may have certainly played a role in boosting the popularity of a certain type of tea, they were by no means the first to introduce this beverage to the subcontinent, as the northern parts of Pakistan have been exposed to tea from time immemorial, thanks to its proximity with China, and invasions from Central Asia. In fact, *chai* or *cha* have been customary terms in Urdu at least since the early 17th century. What the British did was to popularise, among the local elite, brewed tea served in a tea pot, with milk and sugar served separately—a dainty exercise that was adopted by aristocratic homes or clubs, or high-end hotels. This kind of tea-drinking did not become popular with the commoners, so to speak, as it was too elaborate a process entailing the use of fine china in the form of tea pot, cups, saucers, milk pot, and sugar pot.

Hence, when it comes to tea, Pakistan is a melting pot: Pakhtuns and Baloch in the north-western and western parts of the country drink mainly green tea imported from Sri Lanka which is called *sabz chai.* Pakhtuns always take a supply with them when they travel. In the countryside they sometimes mix leaves and stems of opium poppy in their tea.

In Peshawar, the provincial capital of Khyber Pakhtunkhwa, green tea with a few drops of lemon, and lemongrass tea have become popular with young people, while in Quetta, the provincial capital of Balochistan, green tea is sometimes flavoured with poppy seeds. In the southern and eastern parts of Pakistan, the densely populated lowland provinces of the Punjab and Sindh, the subcontinental tradition of milk tea marked by the customs of the British colonial rulers, predominates.

This custom may originally date back to merchants who became acquainted with this type of preparation when dealing with the Mongols and Chinese who poured some cold milk into porcelain cups before adding hot tea to ensure that the fragile cups did not break. Anyone wanting black tea without milk simply orders *kali chai*. However, Pakistanis only forego milk for health reasons. Black tea imported mainly from Kenya—although the government is trying to increase the production of tea in the country—is generally drunk with heavy buffalo milk diluted with water. In the high mountainous regions of Central Asia, in the Pamir, Hindu Kush, Karakoram and Himalayas, people enjoy green tea with cow's or goat's milk, preferably with salt and a bit of butter. Tea is seldom sweetened here. Green tea brings with it its own set of benefits, as it helps regulate body temperature, controls blood sugar, manages blood pressure and helps fight tooth decay, depression, and Alzheimer's.

The mountainous region of Azad Kashmir is the home of a special Kashmiri pink tea (*Kashmiri chai*) which is slightly salted and flavoured with cardamoms. Strangely enough though, the best *Kashmiri chai* is not to be had in Kashmir!

Alongside imported tea, local varieties from Darjeeling, Assam, and the Nilgiri Mountains are sold in local teashops. However, they are only grown organically and are well processed for export to the European market.

Detailed research has concluded that tea decreases the risk of heart disease and various types of cancer. It also helps increase metabolism resulting in good digestion and weight loss.

ANJALI MALIK

Chakki. The term *chakki* for grinding stones is derived from the Sanskrit *chakra* (wheel, to turn) by way of the dialectical *chakka*. The *chakki* has two circular stones held slightly apart, either vertically or horizontally, for de-husking or grinding wheat, rice, and pulses. Animal and water power, used for centuries, was later replaced by oil engines and electricity. Health-conscious people in cities even today prefer to buy *chakki ka atta* (coarsely ground wholewheat flour) directly from the flour mills rather than from grocery stores to ensure it is freshly ground.

Chana papri/chana chaat/chola. One of the popular *chaat* items, *cholay* or *chana chaat* is a concoction of boiled chickpeas, potatoes, finely sliced green chillies, onions, coriander, and tomatoes, topped with tamarind chutney, sweet chutney, spicy yoghurt and *chaat masala*.

A slight variation, *chana chaat papri* refers to crispy fried dough wafers made from refined white flour and oil. In *papri chaat*, the *papris* are served with boiled potatoes, boiled chickpeas, chillies, yoghurt, and tamarind chutney, and topped with *chaat masala*. The *papri* provides the *chaat* with a crunchiness that enhances the flavour.

SHANAZ RAMZI

Chanwaran jo atto. In Sindhi, *chanwaran* is used for rice while *jo atto* means flour made from it. *Chanwaran jo atto* is ideally made with medium-sized rice grains dried and pounded in a flour mill until it reaches a fine grainy texture. Today, ready-made packs are also available and can be used comfortably without compromising too much on the quality.

Chanwaran jo atto is used in many traditional Sindhi recipes as it gives a nice, crispy coating as compared to refined flour.

ZUBAIDA TARIQ

Chapati/phulka. A form of *roti*, *chapati* is made of a thin disc of rolled-out, wholewheat dough (*atta*) and roasted dry on a flat skillet. When this is placed immediately, thereafter, on hot embers, or an open-flame, it puffs up to become a *phulka* that is best eaten piping hot. It is the staple food in most parts of Pakistan, India, Sri Lanka, and also among South Asian expatriates all over the world where it is cooked every day for meals to scoop up food such as curries. It is believed to have been consumed in the region since at least the time of Indus Valley Civilisation as carbonised wheat grains were discovered during excavations at Mohenjo-Daro, while at Harappan sites, flat metal and clay plates resembling the *tawa* have been found in plenty.

To make *chapati*, finely-milled wholewheat flour is mixed with a little salt and water and then kneaded into a soft dough and kept aside for at least thirty minutes for the gluten in the dough to develop. The method of making *chapati* is similar to that of making tortillas. After the dough is rolled out, it is cooked from both sides on a pre-heated iron griddle. *Chapati* can also be topped with *ghee* or butter. *Chapati* is made in different sizes (small, medium, and even large) but *phulka* is normally made in small size.

Stuffed *chapati* is also popular such as *aaloo bhari roti*, radish-turmeric *bhari roti* and vegetable stuffed *chapati* (gravy of mashed carrots, potatoes, peas, or fenugreek, slightly sautéed into a masala gravy).

NAHEED ANSARI

Chapli kebab. A gift from the dry fruit traders from Afghanistan who used to cross the Khyber Pass for trade, the Pakhtun favourite *chapli kebab* can trace its origin to the eastern region of Afghanistan. *Chaprikh* is a Pashto word meaning flat, and *chapli* is a derivation of this particular word; hence a flat, round kebab. A spicy, flat, round meat beef patty, the *chapli kebab* is a purely beef, and, at times, lamb fare, though some other kebabs are made using sheep, lamb, chicken, or goat meat. The Pakhtun recipe uses a perfect combination of beef and *atta*, thus this kebab in particular, is lighter in taste.

Fried in *ghee*, oil or animal fat called *dhal* in local Pashto, generous use of onions and tomatoes, and, in many cases, eggs, is the norm in *chapli kebabs*, which are spiced with *anar dana* (pomegranate seeds), roasted coriander, cumin, and ground red chillies. The ingredients used in the preparation of *chapli kebabs* are indigenous to Afghanistan, therefore the use of pomegranate seeds and dry coriander seeds, which make the *chapli kebab* so unique in taste.

Arguably Peshawar's most favourite food, there are more than 2,000 *chapli kebab* shops in and around Peshawar city alone and people come from far and wide to partake of the delicacy.

Chapoti. A Khow staple, *chapoti* are thick, round bread cooked on an iron pan and then broiled in the fireplace.

Chapshuro. A traditional dish of Gilgit-Baltistan, *chapshuro* is a minced meat and dough-based dish which is as delicious as it is unique. With the mince cooked in a little oil with onion, tomato, and spices, and then placed in the centre of a rolled-out flour dough, and covered with another rolled-out dough, *chapshuro* looks like a cross between a stuffed pizza and a pie. The edges are pinched together in such a way that they form an inch-wide border round the stuffed portion, and the *chapshuro* is then lightly roasted from both sides on an iron griddle. Once it turns a lovely golden brown, the *chapshuro* is ready to be cut all along the one-inch pinched border so that it comes off like a lid over the mince. The top layer then functions as a *roti* to scoop out the mince, ready for eating.

Chargha A Lahori speciality, *chargah* is a delicious, deep-fried whole chicken that has been marinated first with lemon juice and then overnight with spices and yoghurt. It is best eaten without any accompanying staple and frills—by breaking off the pieces with the fingers and digging one's teeth directly into the meat.

Chawal ki roti. A *chapati* made from rice flour; it is a staple food mostly for people living in small towns and villages in Sindh, though in recent times it has also begun to be consumed in urban areas. Since Pakistan produces different varieties of rice in substantial quantities, the rice-producing agricultural areas have *chapati* made from rice flour as their staple, as opposed to wholewheat flour which is more common in the Punjab and in the bigger cities.

Chawal ki roti is generally served with spicy or mild spicy vegetables such as *bhindi ki sabzi*, meat curries, and with different kinds of lentils as well as with various types of chutneys. *Chapati* made from rice flour tends to be thin and soft and very light to eat. It is gluten-free and is very easily digested.

NAHEED ANSARI

Chewra. A Gujarati spiced snack made from parched rice, *chewra* goes back to ancient times when it was known as *dhanah* (mentioned in *Rigveda*) and was made of beaten or parched barley. A parched and flattened product is obtained through soaking the grain in water, roasting it in hot sand so that the grain swells but does not burst, and finally pounding it in a mortar.

Charaka lists not only parched barley but also parched pulses such as *mung*, *masoor*, and *matar* under the generic name *bhrstadhanya*. But it is *chipita*, the other Sanskrit word for parched grains, which survives in *chewra* today. *Chewra* was one of the many savoury snack items called *nasto* that used to be popular among Gujaratis in the days of yore.

Today, extremely popular in Asian and African cuisines, and a favourite snack among nearly all communities of Pakistan, *chewra* is a savoury snack mix ideally suited for serving with tea or on its own. A national brand called Nimco, established in the 1950s has helped to popularise this and other Gujarati snacks to such an extent that a large variety of similar mixes are now being prepared under its brand name, and few remember to call this particular mix by its original name, *chewra*. This mix consists of a variety of dried and deep-fried to crispness ingredients made with gram flour and beaten rice, and mixed with peanuts, raisins, almonds, groundnuts, and herbs. All ingredients are marinated in a traditional blend of spices including mustard seed, coriander, salt and cumin. There is a sweet variety too which uses the same ingredients with sugar or *gur*.

SHAHA TARIQ AND SHANAZ RAMZI

Chha bhalay. A soup popular in the mountainous north of Pakistan, *chha bhalay* is a hearty, organic vegetable soup cooked with *chha* seeds (pearl millet), turnips, onions, carrots, and fresh mountain herbs.

Chicken. Chicken is the most common type of poultry in the world. As a meat, it *has* been depicted in Babylonian carvings from around 600 BC. In Pakistan, poultry was kept as backyard enterprise to meet household needs and consisted of '*desi*' chickens that were bred organically. In the early 1960s, the need for commercial poultry was felt which resulted in the form of a national campaign to enhance the production of poultry in the country, and 'farm bred' chickens became the norm.

Initially, because of the high costs involved in breeding chickens commercially, it was regarded as a rich man's meat in cities and was only cooked on special occasions or for special guests. Today, chicken is cheaper than the other meats available in the market and has replaced them in dishes that used to be primarily made with beef or mutton, such as in *nihari*, which was once only prepared with beef while chicken *nihari* was unheard of, and *biryani* which was primarily prepared with mutton. Another reason for the growing popularity of chicken is increasing health awareness among city-dwellers and their subsequent avoidance of red meat, especially by elders in the family.

Hot favourites made exclusively with chicken are barbecued items like *tikka* and *malai boti*. Broast chicken and *tandoori* chicken are also popular chicken dishes not made with any other meat, though many chicken dishes are now also popular of which alternate meat versions exist, such as *qorma*.

But even today, though many people have reservations about its health benefits because of the way they are bred, no formal meal in Pakistan is complete without '*kukar*' (poultry) being present on the dining spread. It is hence, a must at every wedding, whether in the form of *qorma*, or *biryani* as well as on every other festive occasion.

Chicken corn soup. A popular Chinese soup introduced to Pakistan by the many Chinese restaurants that had opened up in major cities of Karachi, chicken corn soup has been adopted so widely by the population at large, that it is even sold at wayside *rehris* (push carts) on the streets of Karachi. This broth is made with sweet corn, shredded chicken, and cornflour.

Chicken fried rice. A Chinese speciality comprising boiled rice that is stir-fried with finely chopped vegetables such as carrots, peas and spring onions, boiled and shredded chicken, and egg, chicken fried rice is a complete meal on its own. Vegetarian options without the chicken are also popular.

Chicken karhai. Chicken/mutton *karhai* is one of Pakistan's most popular dishes, widely consumed throughout the country. Originally made from mutton (goat meat) or lamb, *karhai* made with chicken has now become more popular, especially in the urban centres where people generally are more health conscious and avoid red meat. Although, traditionally, *karhai* was made without onions and only incorporated tomatoes and green chillies, with a minimum of spices, cooked in animal fat—the fresh meat is thought to provide the fat base for the cooking—these days there are all kinds of *karhais*—*karhai green masala*, *Peshawari karhai*, *black pepper karhai*, etc.—some with onion, and some even without tomato, which was once regarded as an essential ingredient in *karhai*. The two things that they all have in common is the utensil in which it is cooked and served—*karhai* (wok) from where the dish gets its name—and the almost dry nature of the dish, with barely any gravy, and only meat pieces in abundance. It is meant to be savoured directly from the *karhai* and consumed with hot *naan*.

NAHEED ANSARI

Chicken makhni. Succulent chicken pieces prepared in a combination of cream, tomatoes and aromatic spices, this composite dish is a culinary star that tickles palates across the world. Known as *murgh makhani* in Urdu, the genesis of butter chicken is inextricably tied to the evolution of another gastronomical favourite, the *tandoori chicken*. The man allegedly behind the creation of *tandoori chicken*, Gujral, migrated to Delhi after Partition, where he came up with the idea of *makhni* chicken for his restaurant, made from leftover *tandoori tikkay*. He deduced that a tomato gravy, lush in butter and cream, would soften his leftover chicken, and served it as such. The combination proved to be a masterstroke and thus, by accident or an act of genius, the butter chicken was born, which is now a favourite on the subcontinental menu.

BISMA TIRMIZI

Chickpea (*Cicer arietinum*). A small legume, first grown in the Levant and ancient Egypt, chickpea is now an important food in many parts of the world, especially Pakistan, where it is the most important pulse, known as *chana*. It makes a popular form of *daal* which is a main meal item almost throughout the country. Whole chickpeas are known as Bengal gram.

Chickpeas are high in protein and, therefore, more nourishing than other peas. They are known to increase sperm and milk and help to treat kidney stones. The chickpea plant's height varies from 8 inches to 20 inches, having small feathery leaves with white flowers with blue, violet, or pink veins. One seedpod contains two to three peas. The following are the varieties of chickpeas:

1. *Kala chana*—originated in Turkey, and is grown mostly in Turkey, the subcontinent, Ethiopia, Iran and Mexico. It contains small, dark seeds and a rough coat. It is efficacious for people with blood sugar problems because of markedly high fibre content as compared to other varieties. *Chana daal* is this kind of chickpeas, split, with the skin removed. *Kala chana* is served both as curry with eggplant and potatoes in it, as well as a *chaat*.
2. Bumbai chickpeas—are also dark but little bigger than *kala chana*.
3. *Kabuli chana* or *sufaid chana*—is light coloured, large and with a smooth coat, and was introduced in the subcontinent in the 18th century. Believed to have been brought from Afghanistan, it was given the name of *Kabuli chana* or the more obvious, *sufaid chana*.
4. Green chickpeas—*chana daal*, also known as *hara-bhara daal*, is prepared from green chickpeas.

Fresh chickpeas should always be boiled for 10 minutes and then simmered for about 30 minutes. However, for dried chickpeas, the cooking time would be anywhere between 90 to 105 minutes, but if pre-soaked for 12/18 hours, cooking time could be shortened. Chickpeas may be pressure-cooked or cooked at 90° C (194° F).

Chickpeas are used to make a variety of dishes in Pakistan, and is especially popular in *chaats*, and as a breakfast dish. Mature chickpeas are often mixed in cold salads, cooked in stews, and ground to make *besan*, while unripe chickpeas are also picked out of the pod and eaten as a raw snack; the leaves are eaten as a leaf vegetable in salads. Roasted chickpeas are a popular wayside snack, while cooked chickpeas are also a popular breakfast item.

NAHEED ANSARI

Chikki. The origin of *chikki* can be traced to Gujarati cuisine, as a similar brittle-type candy made from sesame seed (*shaskuli*) finds mention among the earliest works from Gujarat, in Jain literature in Sanskrit from the 7th to the early 14th century. That said, the etymology of '*chikki*', according to an article 'In Search of Lonavala Chikki', written by Amruta Byatnal, may be traced to this small town in Maharashtra. According to the writer, back in the early 1900s when the railway line had just started operating between Mumbai and Lonavala, a modest *mithai* shop owner, Maganlal Agarwal used to sell a crude version of *chikki*, called *gur dani*, made with peanuts, jaggery, and clarified butter, at his shop. The railways decided to sell packaged *gur dani* in the train. Thrilled by the exposure, Maganlal renamed the candy *Maganlal Chikki*. Though the name *chikki* stuck, it was the name of the town rather than Maganlal that it came to be known as and *Lonavala Chikki* became famous.

Mostly a winter's favourite sweet snack, and popular with all age groups, students can be commonly found enjoying it in schools and colleges, making it one of the most highly sold products in the school canteens.

Many kinds of *chikkis* are available, with the one main basic ingredient varying, while the other two ingredients remain constant. The basic ingredient could be pistachios, roasted sesame seeds, puffed rice, cashews, dates, dried and roasted coconut, roasted chickpeas, or almonds but the peanut *chikki* is the most universally loved.

Chikkis are very easy to make. Jaggery is dissolved in little water to make thick syrup and then mixed with peanuts or whichever main ingredient is being used, roasted, and poured into a flat pan. Using a flat rolling pin, the ingredients are then rolled out, and rectangular cuts made immediately, while the spread is still hot. When cooled, it is cut into pieces and packed in cellophane or in airtight containers to retain their crispness till consumed.

LAL MAJID

Chilli (*Capsicum frutescens*; mirch). A general term—derived from the Nahuatl language—for a wide range of fruits of the genus *Capsicum* (but not including the vegetable capsicum), chillies vary in size, shape, and colour, and most of all in taste, which ranges from relatively mild to very pungent and extremely hot. Most are long, thin, and pointed but there are many other shapes too, and sizes vary over a wide range.

There is no mention of the chilli in the subcontinent's literature before the 16th century, though now it is hard to imagine what food tasted like without them, considering that it has become such an important ingredient in most local foods. In fact, the word for green chilli in Urdu, *hari mirch*, as in many other languages spoken in the subcontinent, is simply an extension of the word for pepper, *kali mirch*. It is believed that the chilli became part of various recipes soon after the first voyage of Columbus and Vasco da Gama after which the plant was introduced to Europe and subsequently to the subcontinent through the Spaniards and Portuguese. Prior to that, black peppercorn was used as the basic spice.

In Pakistan, the most important distinction is between green and red chillies. Certain dishes require the incorporation of green chillies, while others are dependent on red chillies both for the flavour and the colour of the dish. For example, an intensely red coloured but non-pungent variety of chilli grown in Azad Kashmir, known as *Kashmiri mirch*, is used throughout the country to add a rich red colour to a dish without making it spicy. Still other dishes may use both red and green varieties—for instance, red chillies in their powdered form as part of the *masala* going into the dish, and green chillies for garnishing. As for the varied sizes in which chillies are available, the general rule is 'the smaller, the hotter', the hottest chillies being the little green ones.

Chillies are used for flavour and not merely for hotness. Even people who encounter the taste of chillies for the first time in a mild form, will usually agree that its flavour is subtle and attractive, and its gentle warmth stimulates not only the taste buds but appetite and digestion as well.

Chillies, even the hottest, are often eaten fresh and whole with a Pakistani meal, as well as used ground in cooking as an ingredient, or chopped up as a garnish. They may also be dried or roasted before being used in cooking—the different processes affect the flavours differently. They not only impart their own richly aromatic flavour and spiciness, but also have the ability to bring out the flavours of ingredients around them.

Fresh chillies are packed with vitamins A, B, and C. They are also potent stimulants to the system, have antibacterial properties, and help normalise blood pressure. Astonishingly, eating hot chillies in a hot climate can help keep the body cool, as they encourage sweating.

Chinese cuisine. China is bordered by fourteen countries including Pakistan—the others being Korea, Vietnam, Laos, Burma, India, Bhutan, Nepal, Afghanistan, Tajikistan, Kyrgyzstan, Kazakhstan, Mongolia, and Russia.

A Chinese meal usually comprises a starchy food, accompanied by at least one, if not several animal or vegetable products-based dishes. This model, which holds true throughout all Chinese territories, is executed differently in different regions and in different social classes. A contrast is drawn, in general, between North China, an area where wheat is the staple, and South China, where rice predominates, with a line between the two drawn by the Blue River, but the situation is made more complex because there are other starches besides wheat and rice. Specific regional preferences are nowadays completely blurred in certain areas by the rising standard of living. These days, the culinary division of China most often recognised, distinguishes four great cooking styles.

The identification of tastes plays a particularly important role in the appreciation of Chinese cuisine, and it is quite often one, or several dominant flavours which give a regional cuisine its character. The inhabitants to the north are reputed to like strong smells, such as those of garlic, vinegar, and soy sauce. In Sichuan, spices are liked, particularly the hotter and more pungent ones, while in the lower plains of the Yangtze, dishes with a delicate and subtle flavour are prepared. While Cantonese cuisine cannot be reduced to a few dominant flavours, it marries all flavours beautifully.

Three aromatic ingredients are practically indispensable to the Chinese cuisine—fresh ginger, spring onions, and soy sauce—which give Chinese food its quintessential aroma. Stir-frying can be regarded as the most emblematic method of Chinese cooking. It includes frying the various ingredients of a dish very rapidly over an extremely intense heat, most often separately, one after the other, then reassembling them with their seasoning before serving them. Raw items do not belong to any Chinese category.

Both its proximity to Pakistan and the fact that the country is so densely populated, has historically been a source of encouragement to the Chinese to immigrate in search of better living standards and lucrative work options. During the 1940s many Chinese Muslims fled unrest in China and settled in Karachi.

However, although currently, the Chinese community in the country is primarily of non-Muslim origin—their ancestors were Buddhists, but subsequent generations followed other religions or none at all—about 30 per cent are estimated to have converted to Islam. Most Chinese in Karachi are second generation immigrants—most of the oldest generation having passed away—while the third generation has migrated to other countries. Not surprisingly, the Chinese were instrumental in popularising Chinese cuisine in the country, particularly Sichuan and Cantonese styles that have a penchant for spices.

Chinese specialities in Pakistan. From the four broad types of identifiable Chinese cuisines, the Sichuan and Cantonese styles have become the most popular in Pakistan, and not surprisingly. The Sichuan Chinese cuisine in Pakistan has been adapted to suit Pakistani tastes, incorporating Pakistani seasonings and techniques of cooking, and doing away with some authentic Chinese ingredients. These dishes have become so popular that even restaurants specialising in Pakistani cuisine have Chinese dishes on their menu! The ubiquitous fried rice and chicken corn soup are classic examples of this, even sold on wayside pushcarts in Karachi.

However, there are certain Chinese dishes that are patronised by the Chinese community which have not become too popular with locals, such as *jiaozi* (also known as *gau gee*). These are steamed dumplings made with thinly rolled dough boasting vegetable or minced meat filling. It is particularly popular at the Chinese New Year. Another speciality that few Pakistanis have acquired a taste for but remains a favourite with the Chinese is *dim sum*—small individual portions of food usually served in a steamer basket.

Chow mein. One of the two prominent Chinese dishes—the other being the somewhat similar *chop suey*—*chow mein* comprises boiled noodles mixed with meat and vegetables. A typical Chinese meal will invariably have either *chow mein* or *chop suey* served as one of the main dishes, with the former being more popular, especially among families that have elderly people as well as children, since they find the soft noodles a lot easier to eat than the crisp, deep-fried noodles that make up *chop suey*. Interestingly, *chop suey* even comes in an 'American' version, served with fried egg placed on top of the meat and vegetables mixture arranged on the noodles.

Christmas. A festive season for Christians celebrating the birth of their prophet, Jesus Christ, who is also one of the prophets revered by the Muslims, Christmas is celebrated in a somewhat subdued manner by the minority community in the Muslim-majority country of Pakistan. Christmas bazaars which begin from October, hosted by various women's associations like BWA (British Women's Association) or consulates, selling lots of edible goodies, particularly associated with Christmas—such as mince pies, carrot cake, ginger cookies, marzipans, home-made candies, and jams—along with decoration items, set the tone of celebrations in small pockets.

While Christmas cakes are still made by a number of bakeries and hotels—aside from the traditional carrot cake, orders are taken on any flavour of choice—one can spot artificial Christmas trees adorning the foyers of many restaurants and hotels. However, most of the celebrations in public spaces are dining-based, and merriment in the form of drinking and dancing is restricted to private parties.

Interestingly, the Punjabi Christians in the country celebrate the birth of Christ in much the same way as Muslims celebrate Eid. Dessert in the form of *sewain*, *kheer*, *neuri*, and *goja* (made from semolina and dry fruits), custard, or cake is prepared to be shared with friends and family.

Luckily for the Christian community in Pakistan, Christmas coincides with the birthdate of the founder of the nation, Mohammed Ali Jinnah, and, hence, it is a public holiday, allowing at least room for celebrations and holiday spirit on 25 December.

Churi/churma ladwa. The Punjabi *churi* is a traditional sweet/dessert whipped up by using leftover *roti/parathay*, and normally eaten at breakfast. It comes to fruition by coarsely crumbling and pounding the leftover or fresh bread, and stir-frying it with clarified butter, sugar, nuts, jaggery or honey. Clarified butter and bread, not to mention nuts, are said to keep the body warm; therefore, this fine rustic dessert is readily made, and frequently consumed in the Punjab in winters. Mostly children are coerced to eat *churi* because it provides warmth from inside, beefs up immunity, and is believed to prevent winter cough and cold. *Pinni churi*, shaped as balls, is served with clarified butter and castor sugar or coarsely ground jaggery.

Churma, a slight variation, is a popular delicacy in Haryana and Rajasthan. Rajasthani *churma* is mostly served with *daal*. Shaped into balls (*ladwa* or *laddus*), it is coarsely-ground wheat crushed and cooked with clarified butter and sugar and is high in calories. Traditionally, it is made by mashing millet (*bajra*), or wheat flour *roti* and jaggery in clarified butter. Most Punjabi households consume *churma/churi* prepared from *chapati*, *paratha*, and/or *puri*. It is made both sweet and savoury.

BISMA TIRMIZI

Chutney. The Anglicised version of the Urdu word *chatni*, chutney comes from *chaat na*, meaning 'to lick'. So, essentially chutney is an accompaniment that is regarded to be finger-licking good. It is a spicy relish that is meant to add attraction to less piquant food, such as rice or *daal*.

Chutney can be made either by grinding fresh herbs, such as ginger, chillies, mint and coriander leaves, and spices, or by cooking them. The ground herbs and spices are mixed to a paste with garlic or tamarind or lime or desiccated coconut. Chutneys are always vegetarian and have a sour, tangy taste, even when they include sweet fruits, such as mangoes, and apricots and plums. Variations include mango chutney, apricot chutney, herb chutney, coconut chutney, green chutney (made with grated coconut, green chillies, lemon juice, and mint and coriander leaves), tomato and green chilli chutney, and sweet date and tamarind chutney. In the colonial times it was used to denote a preserve, usually of mango slices, slightly spiced and placed in sugar syrup.

Cinnamon (*Cinnamomum verum*; dalchini/daar cheeni). The term is loosely applied for both, cinnamon which is a dried bark of a tree indigenous to Sri Lanka, and *Cassia lignea*, which though closely related, is thicker and coarser and its taste is less delicate. In Pakistan, *cassia* is used and marketed like cinnamon.

The delicately flavoured bark of *Cinnammomum zeylanicum*, the cinnamon tree also yields the *tejpat* leaves used as an aromatic flavouring. The Urdu word *dalchini* for the product means Chinese bark, probably because it was once imported from China.

In Pakistani cuisine, cinnamon or *cassia* is used both in its stick form (strips of bark rolled together), and ground to a powder, and is popular for its flavour and the aroma it imparts to the dishes. As a culinary ingredient, ground cinnamon is used as part of *garam masala* used to season meat, poultry, fish, and rice dishes. On its own, cinnamon sticks are used to add fragrance to such simple village fare as a dish of boiled rice and lentils, as well as to the elaborate dishes of aristocratic cuisine such as *biryani*. It is also used to flavour desserts, teas, and coffee. Since cinnamon is delicate in taste, with a very warm and sweet flavour, it is best to purchase it in small quantities, because it loses its aroma and taste very quickly.

Cinnamon infused in warm water is effective for common cold. It is also used in making toothpaste and perfumes. Cinnamon is held to be a natural system cleanser and an aid to digestion. It is also antibacterial and helps regulate sugar levels. It contains manganese and aldehyde which aids bone, muscle and tissue development. It is also prescribed to people suffering from arthritis.

SHANAZ RAMZI AND NAYYER RUBAB

Clove (*Eugenia caryophylus*; laung). Believed to be present in the subcontinent since a few centuries before the start of the Christian era, cloves are dried, unopened flower buds of an evergreen tree which belongs to the myrtle family. The tree is small and evergreen and may live for a century or more. It flowers twice in the year, and it is the fully-grown but still closed buds which are harvested to be dried and marketed. Handpicked when pink in colour and dried till they turn brown, cloves are an important culinary spice. This spice resembles small nails, and therefore its name, since clove is derived from the Latin word '*clavus*' meaning nails.

Cloves lend their warm pungency to many sweet and savoury dishes and are usually added whole in Pakistani cooking. Cloves are used to flavour curry and give taste and aroma to rice (plain white rice, *pulao*, *zarda*, and *biryani*). It has a long shelf-life if stored in a cool, dark place away from light. Ground cloves form part of most *garam masala* mixes.

The essential oil from cloves has long been used as a natural pain-killer, particularly against toothache. It also aids digestion and relieves flatulence and is used as an antiseptic. Cloves are also known for lowering cholesterol levels in the blood. They are also a good air freshener and if placed in a cupboard or between clothes, help to keep the clothes smelling fresh.

SHANAZ RAMZI AND NAYYER RUBAB

Coconut (naryal). The Sanskrit term *narikela* (Urdu *naryal*) for the coconut is believed to be an aboriginal word, derived from two words of Southeast-Asian origin, *niyor* for oil and *kolai* for nut. In Sanskrit, the *narikela* only surfaces after *c*.300 BC in the *Ramayana*, *Mahabharata*, and *Vishnu Purana*.

The coconut tree (*Cocos nucifera*) is a member of the Arecaceae family (palm family) and the only species of the genus *Cocos*. It is the most useful tree in the world. Coconut, in its entirety, may be considered a fruit that offers multiple benefits. Its flesh provides a high-calorie diet, while its water is nourishing; its hairy fibre can be spun into a rope, and the hard shell could be turned into fuel. The coconut is also used in medicines and chemicals.

In Pakistan, the coconut is famous for its sweet water and jelly-like meat that is both healthful and extremely tasty. Apart from its popularity as a fruit, it is also valued for its oil, commonly found in almost every Pakistani home. Coconut oil is widely used not only in cooking, but also for skin and hair nourishment, as a natural remedy for many ailments, and in homemade beauty products. Often, the flesh is used to make coconut milk or cream, by soaking it in hot water. The first soaking process produces the thicker cream and subsequent soakings give the thinner milk. Coconut milk is used to prepare a number of dishes popular in certain communities including *kuku paka* and *khow suey*.

Desiccated coconut, a popular ingredient in many Pakistani dishes, is made from the white part of the kernel only, after the brown skin has been removed. It is sterilised, frayed out with water into a wet pulp, dried and sieved into grades.

LAL MAJID

Coriander (*Coriandrum sativum*; dhania). A plant of the family Umbelliferae, coriander is also known as cilantro. The plant reaches a height of 60–90 cm and has a branched stem and finely divided leaves. The seeds are two semi-globular fruits joined on the inner sides, giving the appearance of a single, smooth globe. The Sanskrit word for the seed, *dhanyaka* (from where the Urdu *dhania* is derived), first occurs in Sanskrit in Panini's grammar (*c*.600 BC). They are yellowish brown and have a mild fragrant aroma and a sweet aromatic taste, and carry no flavour of the roots, stems, or leaves. The seeds are used as an aromatic spice—either whole, coarsely ground or in a powdered form—in a large number of Pakistani dishes and are an essential item in *garam masala* commonly used to cook savoury dishes. Ground coriander seeds are often mixed with ground cumin to form *dhania-zeera* powder used in most curry dishes in Pakistani cuisine for flavouring.

The leaves of this beautifully fragrant herb are used in Pakistani cooking much the same way as parsley is used in Western cooking, both as an ingredient and as a garnish. Blended fresh coriander is an essential ingredient in green chutney and in some curries as well.

The leaves serve as a topping for many savoury dishes. Its zesty flavour goes well with green chillies and, therefore, it is used in most dishes that incorporate the latter.

Coriander is known for its beneficial effect on the digestive system and for treating insomnia. The plant is particularly effective as a diuretic and as a cooling agent to break fevers.

Court cuisine (nawabi cuisine). During the Mughal rule, when rulers and nobles became rich, banquets became even more sophisticated than ever before. New dishes, which the Mughals brought from Central Asia, were introduced, and together with Iranian influences on their cuisine another flavour was added to the Mughlai dishes. Court cuisine, in a nutshell, is a Mughal style of cooking merged with Persian and subcontinental flavours, which reached its zenith at the court in Delhi. When the Mughal Empire began to weaken, craftspeople and artisans moved to the new culture capitals of Lucknow and Hyderabad, and from there into the employ of neighbouring rajas in the princely states of the subcontinent.

Chefs were encouraged to experiment and innovate. Historically, rulers and the nobility used cuisine as a tool to display their generosity as well as their unique styles of cooking in the royal kitchen. It was customary for rulers to host banquets for nobles and vice versa, and no expenses would be spared in getting lavish menus prepared. Hosts vied to win the hospitality stakes. Each *nawabi* kitchen employed hundreds of chefs, many of whom cooked only one type of dish each—thus one specialised in various kinds of kebabs, another in *biryani*, and so on. The nobility would invite their peers to a meal where savouries were disguised as sweets or an entire banquet was crafted out of sugar.

Ibn Battuta has a good deal to say about the dining customs of the sultans, which were perhaps unique to Muslim royalty. A certain formality was observed as a ritual. Before dinner, the chamberlain would stand at the head of the dinner carpet and bow in the direction of the sultan, a cue for others present to do the same. Then all would sit down to eat and would be brought gold, silver or glass cups filled with fine sugar-water perfumed with rose-water (sherbet). After the sherbet was consumed, the chamberlain would call out *Bismillah* (In the name of the Allah) and everyone would begin to eat. Everyone would have a set of all the various dishes comprising the meal before him, and at the end of the meal, jugs of barley drink would be served, following which *paan* and nuts would be passed around. Then the chamberlain would again call out *Bismillah*, upon which all would stand up, bow as before and retire.

According to Ziauddin Barani, the author of *Tarikh-i-Firoz Shahi*, the competition was so great among nobles of the Sultanate to host elaborate feasts that in order to outdo one another in their display of pomp they would often take loans from moneylenders and Multani merchants. Interestingly, a thousand dishes were sometimes served—and that did not include breads and desserts. Two types of meals would be offered at the court—one for the nobility and the other for the commoners.

Crop rotation. This is the repeated cultivation of specific crops, in a planned order and on the same field, to prevent the fertility of the soil from being adversely affected. Even during ancient times, agriculturists, through experience, knew that producing the same crop year after year on the same field leads to the degradation of soil. They were also aware that cultivating a sequence of specified crops over several seasons could prevent this situation. So, in the early days, deep-rooting legumes, such as *arhar*, were sowed in regular sequence to maintain productivity, prevent soil degradation and nutrient depletion.

Crops consume large quantities of nitrogen, phosphorus, and potassium from the soil, and if the same crop is cultivated on the field continuously then the yield decreases. In order to increase the productivity of the soil it becomes necessary to keep the land fallow, or allow an interval between crops of different seasons, or add manure and fertilisers as nutrient. Rotation of crops which includes deep-rooting legumes to provide nitrogen, a sod crop for the maintenance of humus, a crop for weed control and fertilisers saves the situation.

In crop rotation, crops of the same family and root system (shallow or deep) should not follow each other. Crops requiring heavy tillage operations and leguminous crops must be included in the rotation. At regular intervals green manuring and forage crops should be grown. The succeeding crop should belong to a different family than the previous one. The rotation may vary from two or three years or longer period. Well-planned rotations make the farm a more effective year-round enterprise. It leads to more efficient handling of labour power and equipment. Market risks are

reduced and the ability to meet livestock requirements is improved.

A typical scheme selects rotation of crops from three classifications: cultivated row crops (corn, potatoes), close-growing grains (oats, wheat), and sod farming (cloves). A simple rotation would be one crop from each group with a 1:1:1 ratio, i.e. corn followed by wheat and then cloves. The varying effects of crops on soil, and on each other, and in reaction to insect pests, diseases and weeds require carefully planned sequences. Crop rotations should occur every four years as short rotations are not likely to provide the best crop balances and long rotations may introduce complications.

ANJALI MALIK

Cucumber (*Cucumis sativus*; kheera). One of the oldest cultivated vegetables, grown for some 4,000 years, cucumber may have originated in the subcontinent. It grows on the banks of rivers and on their dry beds. Bitter wild forms are still found in the Himalayas, and occasionally a cultivated fruit will still taste bitter, which is why as a precaution, steps are generally taken in the kitchen to debitter cucumbers before peeling and cutting. The top and bottom ends are sliced off and the exposed ends are vigorously rubbed with the removed caps till they give off a white froth. Then the exposed frothy ends are also removed, and the cucumber is now debittered and ready for cutting as required.

Like other *cucurbits*, cucumbers have a very high water-content—96 per cent. The cucumber is often eaten raw with salt or a dip, or in a salad. It is also often grated or chopped and dressed with yoghurt to make *raita*.

Cumin (*Cuminum cyminum*; zeera). Cumin seed or cumin for short, is a spice consisting of the dried, seed-like fruits of *Cuminum cyminum*, a pretty little annual herb of the parsley family Umbelliferae. *Zeera* seeds or powder are an essential component of curry spice and *garam masala*. There are two main varieties of cumin fruits or 'seeds' as they are often referred to— light brown (*sufaid zeera*) and black (*kala zeera*). The smaller, thinner black cumin seeds, native to Pakistan, have a stronger and sweeter aromatic flavour and are more expensive than the light brown variety.

The flavour of cumin, like that of most seeds, is greatly improved by roasting or frying before use, and so generally the fruits of the light brown cumin are roasted and powdered to form the spices for almost all savoury dishes, and are often mixed with ground coriander seeds to form *dhania-zeera* powder, used in most curries. However, they are also used whole and coarsely ground in many dishes and are widely used for flavouring lentils, vegetable curries, pickles, and breads. They also have the reputation of being a good digestive when roasted. They reduce free radicals in the blood, while their daily consumption promotes liver function, which is essential for detoxification.

Curry leaf (kari patta). Similar in appearance to bay leaves but very different in flavour, curry leaves are dark green leaves of the curry tree which is indigenous to Pakistan, Sri Lanka, and India. Its botanical name is *Murraya koenigii*. This tree is about 4–6 metres tall with a trunk which has a diameter of about 40 cm. The leaves of the tree have pinnate of about 10–20 leaflets. Each leaflet is 2–4 cm long and 1–2 cm broad. They are also called 'sweet *neem* leaves' because they look like *neem* (eucalyptus/*Azadirachta indica*) leaves but are not bitter like them and, in fact, have a distinct curry-like aroma.

These leaves are highly aromatic and are widely used as spice and condiment to flavour curries, vegetarian as well as non-vegetarian. The function of curry leaves corresponds, to some extent, to that of the bay leaf in Western countries. It is most commonly used in *baghar/ tarka* (as tempering). Curry leaves, whole or broken up, are sautéed in hot oil till they become brown and crisp, along with mustard seeds and dry red chillies and then added to dishes like *dum aaloo*, *dahi vara*, and coconut chutney to impart a distinctive, multi-spice flavour. Whole leaves are usually removed from a cooked dish before it is served.

In Pakistan it is profusely used along with onions and other spices for making curries and savoury dishes, whether of vegetables, mutton, chicken, fish, or beef. Here, the leaves are added in the first stage of making the dish.

The leaves retain their aroma when dried, and can be bought in semi-dried, dried, or powdered form, although they are, surprisingly, not an ingredient in curry powder.

Besides having flavouring property these leaves have great food and medicinal value. It is one of the most ancient herbs used in alternate medicine. Ayurveda considers curry leaves as rich in various nutrients which help in keeping the body and soul in good health.

Scientific research has shown that curry leaves are anti-oxidant, anti-bacterial, anti-dysentery, hypoglycaemic and hepatoprotective. They have anti-tumour, anti-microbial, anti-inflammatory, anti-trypanocidal and mosquitocidal properties.

ANJALI MALIK

Cutlet. The word cutlet originated from the French word *côtelette* and is known to be first used in the year 1682. Since then, it has found its place in almost all cuisines of the world, be it French, British, American, Russian, or Pakistani. Historically, a cutlet represents a small piece of meat (diminutive of cut).

During the British Raj, a cutlet specifically referred to leftover cooked meat (mutton, beef, fish, or chicken) minced and shaped into round or oval patties. Mashed with potatoes, the patty would be dipped in egg and then coated with bread crumbs and shallow-fried for a golden finish.

Over the years, local versions of cutlets—*cutlass*—began to be made with minced meat cooked with spices—onion, cumin, black pepper, *garam masala*, cilantro, green chillies, and red chilli powder—and then mixed with mashed potatoes. To date, they remain popular in urban centres of the country.

BISMA TIRMIZI

D

Daal (lentil). Whether the word is used to denote an ingredient, or a dish prepared from it, *daal* is one of the principal foods of Pakistan, and consumed both as a main course or as a side dish depending on the affordability of the consumer. Splitting pulses with simultaneous de-husking in a stone grinder or *chakki* yields two clean halves, called the ingredient *daal*. At least half a dozen types are in common use—these include *masoor, mung, arhar, maash,* and *chana.* Lentils vary in flavour and texture, as well as in the time required for cooking. Many prefer to soak the *daal* before cooking it, which reduces cooking time. They can be cooked in myriad ways from thick, medium, or thin preparations, which are regular accompaniments to *roti* and rice. One of the most common types of *daal* is made from *chana*. The split, medium yellow, chickpeas are larger than the grains of other types. Mixed *daals* together with meat form the delicacy *daal gosht* or the Parsi speciality *dhansak*. *Daal* can also be combined with rice to form *khichri* or *masoor pulao*. Whole pulses with a binder like *besan* are fashioned into deep-fried *varay* and used to stuff *kachori*, while the flour of certain lentils is used to make many fried snacks.

Aside from being relatively affordable, *daals* are a nutrition powerhouse. *Chana daal* is high in iron and has a number of benefits, for example, it reduces the risk of breast cancer, and prevents osteoporosis and migraines. *Masoor* is loaded with antioxidants that ward off illnesses. It is an excellent source of calcium and vitamin A and has a high content of potassium. *Mung daal* contains phytonutrients that boost immunity and is rich in vitamin C. *Maash* or *urad* is also rich in iron and is anti-inflammatory, while *arhar* contains high quantities of folic acid.

Daal bharay parathay. In the subcontinent, wholesome, homemade *chapati* is a staple at practically every meal, but when the household wants to add oomph to the meal, especially breakfast, a wide variety of *parathay* are served; these are shallow fried on concave iron griddles.

It is unclear as to when the *paratha* came to be, but it is believed that it originated in the northern part of the subcontinent, allegedly as far north as Afghanistan. The stuffed or *bhara paratha* is a delicious variant of the plain *paratha*. While stuffing can be of anything, from minced meat, to mashed potatoes, to shredded chicken, *daal bharay parathay* have a stuffing of cooked lentils.

BISMA TIRMIZI

Daal chawal palidu. A Bohra speciality, *daal chawal palidu* (rice with soup of seven lentils) is one of those rice dishes that are rarely made in other communities. Normally served at dinner on festive or religious occasions, this dish is part of the *thaal* feast that Bohras partake of as a thanksgiving celebration, on *pehli raat*, the eve of the new Islamic calendar (eve of first Muharram). The *palidu* comprises gourd (*doodhi*) cooked with onions, *masala*, gram flour, and mangosteen until it becomes a thick paste. It is eaten with cooked *arhar daal* and boiled rice, layered alternately in the pot before cooking.

Daal dhokri. This is a traditional dish of Gujarati cuisine which is a complete meal on its own. The *dhokri* is prepared with wheat flour and gram flour rolled out into a hard dough and then cut into diamond shapes before being immersed in a thick white lentil gravy with *masala*, peanuts, jaggery, and tamarind as the base ingredients. Healthful, easy to prepare, and filling, the dish has a sweet and spicy taste of aromatic spices and crunchy peanuts.

Daal gosht with meethay chawal. Made with a combination of four lentils—*chana, mung, masoor,* and *arhar*—boiled together and mixed with meat curry, this Khoja dish of *daal gosht* is uniquely often eaten with sweetened rice (*zarda*) by the community.

Daal ka hasma. A Bohra community's version of shepherd's pie, *hasma* means mixture, so any mixture of food constitutes *hasma*. It is usually made of leftovers; at the end of a meal all leftover food in the *thaal*—the platter from which a Bohri family eats its meal together, directly out of the serving dishes—is mixed together to make *hasma* in order to ensure that everything is eaten, to prevent wastage. *Daal hasma* is made of leftover *chapati* and rice mixed with *daal* of liquid consistency (made from mixing three lentils—*chana*, *mung*, and *masoor*). The mixture is then smoked to give added flavour. Other food items, such as leftover meat and gravy, freshly cut onions, and tomatoes or *achar* can also be added to the *daal hasma*.

Daal makhni. Made with lots of butter and cream, traditionally this *daal* was cooked over charcoals on low flame for hours, giving it a creamy texture. When cooked at home these days, more moderate amounts of cream or butter are used. Lentils and beans have to be soaked overnight for at least eight hours and gently simmered on low heat along with ginger, garlic, and *garam masala*. These are then combined with a tangy *masala* base which includes onions, tomatoes, dried mango powder, or even pomegranate seeds.

Dahi bara/vara/bhalla. The origin of present day *dahi varay* can be traced back to *c.*500 BC where mention of the deep-fried pulse preparation, *vataka*, first occurs in Sutra literature. In a book titled *Manasolla* from the early 12th century, there is a recipe of *vatakas*. A sweet and sour snack, this item comprises spongy, deep-fried lentil dumplings immersed in smoothly beaten yoghurt, and sprinkled with *chaat masala* and tamarind chutney. It is believed to be a Gujarati variation of an ancient dish from Dravidian times in South India, called *vartaka* which was made of beans, soaked overnight, and then skinned before being pounded and deep-fried. The Gujarati *varay* are numerous and are among the many *farsan* (salty snack) items eaten with a major meal or as a snack.

Dahi ki karhi. Gram flour curry with dumplings of fried pulse, this Gujarati, ideal summer afternoon dish uses diluted yoghurt as its base, while the usual flavour enhancers and aromatics are also incorporated in it. It has to be continuously stirred to achieve the right blended perfection. Once the curry comes to a boil, fried dumplings of gram flour are added. To finish the dish a tempering (see *baghar* or *tarka*) of hot oil with curry leaves and cumin seeds is poured on top. It is

served ideally with *bhuni khichri* (a rice and lentil dish) and papadams.

SHAHA TARIQ

Dalcha. While *daal*, a lentil dish made in many different ways, is the poor man's main course, with the addition of meat (chicken or mutton) or vegetables it is elevated to a special occasion dish known as *dalcha*. Pink lentils and gram lentils are most commonly used to make *dalcha* as other varieties tend to become sticky when cooked and cannot maintain a smooth curry-like texture. Mutton *dalcha*, and *lauki khatta dalcha* (bottle-gourd sour *dalcha*) are the two most popular types of *dalchas*. For the mutton *dalcha*, meat is cooked with curry spices and instead of adding water as in the case of regular curries, boiled lentils are added and simmered till spices are fully absorbed. Garnished with flavoured oil, usually with curry leaves and whole red chillies, it is a great Hyderabadi dish to serve with steamed rice or *roti*. For the vegetable version, the lentils are cooked with curry spice mix, and once it is of smooth consistency, chopped vegetables are added along with curry leaves and tamarind juice. It is brought to a boil and then left to simmer and garnished with hot oil to be served with steamed rice.

SHAHA TARIQ

Damido/anday ka mesu. A winter popular dessert made with eggs, sugar, chickpea flour, and clarified butter, *damido* or *anday ka mesu* is similar to another popular dessert, *Mysore pak*, made in South India. Especially popular with the migrant community now settled in Karachi, *anday ka mesu* is often made at home, though it is also available in most *mithai* shops.

NAHEED ANSARI

Daniwal qorma. *Daniwal qorma* is usually made with mutton and freshly ground cilantro, a generous amount of fried onions and creamy yoghurt. It is one of the dishes forming the backbone of *Wazwan*. The word 'daniwal' refers to coriander in the local Kashmiri language. However, unlike other *qorma* dishes that have a spicy, nutty, and creamy yoghurt-based gravy, *daniwal qorma* is an exception. It is a light and mellow yoghurt-based curry infused with aromatic flavours of clove and cardamom, instead of the spicy *masalas* used in *Mughlai qorma*.

BISMA TIRMIZI

Darbesh. A Pakhtun speciality, *darbesh* is a dessert made with semolina, jaggery and crushed dry fruit. These are cooked and set in a tray and cut into squares before serving.

Dastarkhwan. A Turkish/Persian word meaning tablecloth or spread, *dastarkhwan* is a term used all over Central Asia for the traditional/specific space devoted to serving and eating food. Traditionally, *dastarkhwan* is spread on the ground or on a low table, and the term signifies a neat and clean surface for serving food. When spread on the ground, as per tradition and customs, it is prohibited to step on it, particularly with one's shoes on.

The term is also used for small, square pieces of cloth used to cover bread and placed on the larger spread with other dishes. For the sanctity of the *dastarkhwan*, this cloth is not used for any other purpose.

NAYYER RUBAB

Date. The fruit of the palm tree (*Phoenix dactylifera*) is called date. The plant is regarded as a universal provider which is said to have 800 distinct uses. Three main types of dates are grown—soft, hard, and semi-dry. Pakistan is the only country in South Asia which grows dates on a commercial scale. There are more than 160 varieties of date palm in the country. Date production in Pakistan ranks third in fruits, while the same is the case for exports. Fresh Pakistani dates are exported in large quantities to a number of countries including India and China.

Not surprisingly, dates are grown in all the four provinces of Pakistan, with Sindh being the largest date-producing province followed by Balochistan, the Punjab, and finally Khyber Pakhtunkhwa. *Aseel* dates are premium dates of Pakistan, grown in Sindh. Visitors to Sindh, like Al-Idrisi in AD 1080 has mentioned the abundance of dates, denoting that its usage was once localised. The harvesting season for dates starts in July and runs until September.

The chief food value of the date lies in its very high sugar content, which can be 70 per cent by weight in a dried date. The fruit contains a fair amount of protein, plus vitamin A and some of the vitamin B group.

Most Muslims break their fasts in Ramazan with dates, as per the recommendations of the Prophet (PBUH), as dates are known to provide instant energy.

Degchi. The *degchi* is one of the most common utensils used in Pakistani cooking. It is a round, deep, broad-rimmed pot used for cooking curries, *daal* as well as rice.

The *degchi* was traditionally made of brass or copper, but now stainless steel and aluminium *degchi*s are quite common. It is a smaller version of the *degh* (cauldron), hence called *degchi*. The *degchi*'s round, thick base, makes it a versatile pot for cooking sauces, gravies, as well as milk-based dishes.

BISMA TIRMIZI

Delda. A Hazara speciality, a community in Balochistan, *delda* is made with split wheat and assorted beans.

Delhi Sultanate. A series of five different dynasties—the Mamluk dynasty, the Khilji dynasty, the Tughlaq dynasty, the Sayyid dynasty, and the Lodhi dynasty—the Delhi Sultanate ruled northern parts of the subcontinent between 1206 and 1526. Former Egyptian Muslim slave soldiers, Mamluks from the Turkic, and Pakhtun ethnic groups established each of these dynasties in turn. Although they had important cultural impacts, the five dynasties were not strong enough and did not last particularly long. The Sultanate ushered in a period of Indian cultural renaissance. The resulting Indo-Muslim fusion left lasting monuments in architecture, music, literature, and religion, though the same cannot be said of the cuisine of the period. Delhi was a backwater when it came to refined dining, the food lacking subtlety and balance between flavours, and regarded as being heavy and over-spiced. The Moorish traveller Ibn Battuta describes a royal meal at the table of Sultan Ghiyasuddin at Tughlaqabad, as a lavish spread comprising thin round bread cakes, large slabs of meat (sheep), round dough cakes made with *ghee* and stuffed with almond paste and honey, meat cooked with onions and ginger, and rice with chicken topping. In addition, there was *sambusak*, triangular pastries of thin bread fried in *ghee*, and stuffed with minced meat, almonds, walnuts, pistachios, onions, and spices, like the popular Pakistani snack, the *samosa* of today. Dessert comprised sweet cakes and sweetmeats, while the meal ended with *paan*. The Sultanate suffered from Timur's (founder of the Timurid dynasty) invasion of Delhi in 1398, and soon other independent sultanates were established in Awadh, Bengal, Jaunpur, Gujarat, and Malwa. The Sultanate provided the foundation for the Mughal Empire, which continued to expand its territory, and greatly influenced the cuisine of the region.

BISMA TIRMIZI

Desi chicken. This is a native domesticated fowl bred by local farmers on a small-scale in natural environments—

without much interference from large-scale mainstream farmers.

The chickens spend majority of their time in the great outdoors, running around and scratching the ground for worms or insects, supplementing their diet with household scraps. Living in natural habitat means competing and fighting for food, and trying to escape from predators, which manifests into the taste and texture of these birds, (muscle content). The meat is tender and quick to cook, has a low-fat content and higher muscle mass.

Desi chickens possess fewer toxins from free foraging, which means little to no health risks.

Although this variety of chicken is readily available in the subcontinent, for household consumption, its usage is mostly limited to rural areas, while city-dwellers prefer to use the more easily available and cheaper farm chicken.

BISMA TIRMIZI

Dessert. These, by and large, tend to be traditional milk-based puddings such as *sheer khurma* (made with vermicelli), *kheer* (made with rice), *halway* (a variety of sweets made with different ingredients), or even Western-style custard, trifle, and pudding. Seasonal fruit, dry fruit, or vegetable-based desserts are also common, and tend to be ubiquitously served when their main ingredients are in season.

Most households continue to cook Pakistani desserts such as *halway* and *sewain* (vermicelli) in *ghee*, despite the common belief that it has a higher cholesterol content as they feel that only *ghee* can provide the right flavour to these special traditional dishes.

Although during weekdays desserts are usually not included in the lunch menu, they are a part of the meal on weekends and special occasions, adding a festive touch to the menu. However, *mithai*, the *desi* option to pastries in Pakistan, are popular at any time of the day, more so after meals or as part of tea-time snacks. In fact, with *mithai* being an important part of the Pakistani lifestyle—there is rarely an occasion when it is not served—it is not surprising that sweetmeat shops catering mind-boggling varieties have sprung up practically throughout the country. (See *mithai*)

Over the years the cake and Western dessert market in Pakistan's urban centres has tremendously evolved as well, with many bakeries, cafes, and home-based bakers now serving and taking orders for freshly-baked cakes and offering a large variety of continental desserts, such as pavlovas, tarts, cheese cakes, mousse, tiramisu, and

much more. Hence, it is common to find households, particularly in the upper strata of society, indulging in these sweet treats and even preparing them at home for special occasions or when entertaining guests.

Dhaba. Wayside eateries have been part of this region's landscape even before Pakistan came into being. They came into existence to meet the needs of the truck drivers who plied their trade along the Grand Trunk Road in the pre-Partition days. Driving from Peshawar to Calcutta (now Kolkata) would be a long and strenuous exercise and they would need quick, hot food en route to sustain them through the journey, without wasting too much time. Since the drivers were mostly Sikhs the food was generally Punjabi fare, such as *aaloo parathay*, *daal makhni*, and *lassi*.

The etymology of *dhaba* is unclear, though some believe that the word is derived from 'dabba' (tiffin-box). By definition it is a simple establishment that caters to the working classes. By the 20th century these highway pit stops or *dhabas* were a firm fixture, the most famous one being 'Kesar da Dhaba' built in 1916 in Sheikhupura, which moved to the walled city of Amritsar after Partition. After 1947, truckers in Pakistan continued to frequent the *dhabay* on the highway but instead of *daal makhni* and other vegetarian dishes they started serving food preferred by their now main clientele, Pakhtuns, who dominated the intercity transport industry and are largely meat-eaters.

The proliferation of *dhabay* within the cities began with the movement of Pakhtuns to other parts of the country, especially to Karachi, after General Ayub Khan's coup in 1958. These enterprising people set up tea places in the city which primarily served plain *parathay*, eggs, and *doodh patti* to meet the breakfast needs of their fellowmen living on their own, and gradually started providing a limited, economical fare at other meal times as well.

However, over the years the *dhaba* culture has undergone a transformation of sorts, and now instead of the modest establishments frequented only by blue-collared workers, a number of glorified *dhabay* have also sprung up, which are essentially restaurants catering to families from upper classes but which have adopted the signature features of the original *dhabay* such as their location on main highways and *takhts* and charpoys laid out for informal seating. When the first of these, Cafe Habib, opened on the Super Highway in the 1990s, or perhaps even earlier, people travelled for at least a couple of hours from the far corners of Karachi just to eat the *dhaba* food on the roadside.

Then, a few years ago, one bright enterprising man, founder of *Chai Wala* started yet another trend in Karachi—that of upmarket *chai dhabay*—serving overpriced *doodh patti*—tea cooked in milk—along with *parathay* stuffed with a variety of interesting and unique fillings, such as Nutella, cheese, chicken *tikka*, and much more, in Karachi's posh Defence area. Before long, it was being thronged by youngsters from the upper classes. These *dhabay* only operate from the evening onwards and remain open till the wee hours of the morning, frequented by young and old, male and female, all clamouring for plastic chairs and rickety tables laid out on the gravel, or on make-shift parking spaces, waiting for their orders for what once used to constitute basic food at affordable prices by truckers.

SIBTAIN NAQVI

Dhaga kebab. A Dilliwalla speciality, this tenderised minced meat kebab dish derives its name from the thread used to wrap up the kebabs on skewers before they are barbecued.

Dhandaar patio. A lentil dish eaten with either fish or prawns, and rice, *dhandaar* is made by simply cooking well-blended pink lentils (*masoor daal*) with salt and turmeric. The consistency is kept thin so that it could be eaten with steamed rice or yellow *khichri* (rice and lentils dish). Traditionally, *patio* is made with fish—pomfret is preferred but otherwise any cut of fillet fish can also be used—however, prawns are a popular alternate. The fish or prawns are marinated with salt, turmeric, and red chilli powder. Onions are fried golden and ground *masala* comprising red chillies, cumin, ginger-garlic paste, tomatoes, vinegar and coriander is added to it and fried. The marinated seafood is then added, while jaggery and sugar are mixed in right at the end.

Those who avoid seafood cook the dish in the same way but add boiled eggs just before serving. This variation is popularly known as *lagan sera patia* (*lagan* means wedding in Gujarati) as it is mostly served on celebratory occasions, such as weddings and birthdays. Many Parsis also like giving the lentils a *baghar* or a *tarka* by shallow-frying some cumin seeds, chopped onion and finely chopped garlic in clarified butter. Once the tempering is ready, it is poured onto the lentils immediately and served.

ZARNAK SIDHWA

Dhansak. A Parsi speciality that is a variation of its Iranian counterpart, *dhansak* is a robust browned rice dish cooked with pulses. It has a unique spicy, sweet, and tangy flavour. At least three types of pureed pulses—and a maximum of nine—are cooked together along with pieces of fatty meat (mutton), tripe, vegetables, and spices.

In Parsi homes, *dhansak* is traditionally made on Sundays—as it takes long to prepare and sits heavy on the stomach—so that ideally it should be followed by an afternoon siesta.

Other than on Ghambar, a thanksgiving feast, *dhansak* is never prepared on auspicious occasions like festivals and weddings. In fact, it is associated with mourning, and is always prepared on the fourth day following the death of a near one, to mark the end of the traditional three-day abstinence from meat after the funeral.

Normally, a combination of four lentils (pigeon peas, chickpeas, pink lentils, and whole pink lentils), *dhansak* also incorporates potatoes, tomatoes, eggplant, pumpkin, fenugreek leaves, ginger, garlic, coriander leaves, green chillies and mint leaves. *Dhansak masala* includes coriander seeds, cumin seeds, red chillies, black cumin, mustard seeds, fenugreek seeds, black pepper, poppy seeds, cinnamon, cloves, bay leaf, star anise, mace, and nutmeg. Some Parsis only use pigeon peas, which are difficult to cook, hence soaking overnight is essential. A pressure-cooker is used to cook the lentils till tender. They are then mixed with spices, vegetables, and meat and cooked again. The meat is then removed and set aside, and the lentils blended well. The meat is added back in and the *dhansak* is allowed to simmer before it is ready to serve.

Although there is no vegetarian version of the recipe available, meat may be omitted, and a dish called *pulao daar*, which is actually the *dhansak daal* minus the meat, made. A combination of *dhansak masala* and *sambhar masala* is used in preparing this recipe. This dish is served on weddings and auspicious occasions.

Dhansak is always accompanied with caramelised brown rice (rice cooked in caramel water) and often, *kachumar*, a tangy local salad made with finely diced onion, tomato, and cucumber. *Gor imli kachumar* made with thickly sliced onions dipped in tamarind and jaggery sometimes replaces the regular *kachumar*.

ZARNAK SIDHWA

Dho do. A Sindhi speciality, *dho do* is a thick *roti* prepared with *masala* and garlic paste; it is served with mint chutney.

Dhokla/dhokra. First mentioned in AD 1066 in Gujarati Jain literature in Sanskrit as *dukkia*, the well-known steamed *dhokla* or *dhokra* is as popular a Gujarati snack today as it was in the days of yore, both with Muslim as well as with Hindus. *Dhokla* is a lemony, spongy, savoury, steamed cake made from rice and split chickpeas which are soaked overnight, mixed with curd, ground into a paste, and left to ferment. To make it flavourful, chilli flakes, coriander and ginger are added to the fermented paste, while baking soda is added to make the *dhokla* spongy, soft, and fluffy. The paste is spread evenly on a tray, steamed, cooled, sliced, and garnished with fresh cilantro, sesame, and black mustard seeds, and eaten with spicy red chutney. *Dhokla* was one of the many *farsan* items of Gujarat, which is eaten as part of a meal, or as a snack.

However, the same name is also ascribed to dishes in the Bohra and Memon communities, which are completely different from these steamed cakes. The Bohra *dhokra* for instance, is made of assorted vegetables and millet dumplings, similar to the Hindu *dhokri* and the Khoja *muthia*. The only difference between the Bohra *dhokray* and the other two dishes is that the Bohra *dhokra* also includes mince and drumsticks as opposed to no meat at all in *dhokri*, and mutton in *muthia*.

The *dhokra* of the Memon community, on the other hand, while also incorporating a variety of vegetables and fist-shaped rolls made of *bajra*, normally uses fish instead of mutton.

Dhokri wali kari. Another traditional dish of Gujarati cuisine, and a Memon speciality, *dhokri wali kari* is prepared with gram flour, onion, and yoghurt as the base ingredients of the curry. Soft *dhokri*, basically made with gram flour, boiling water and *masala*, are cut into pieces after being set in a pan, and then submerged in the prepared curry and cooked in it for a while. It is eaten with *khichri*.

Dhuan/dhungar (smoking). This technique imparts a smoky flavour to the dish and is particularly useful when there is no access to a barbecue or *tandoor* (clay oven). A piece of coal is heated until it is red hot and then put on top of a *chapati*, a piece of aluminium foil, or a small vessel and placed in the middle of the food to be smoked. Oil is immediately poured over the coal, which releases smoke, at which point the dish is covered tightly and set aside to allow the smoke to permeate the food. This technique is normally adopted at the end of the cooking process, giving the food a unique flavour, though sometimes it is done during the cooking process.

Dilliwallay. The Mughal era is unrivalled in its display of hospitality and its attention to style and luxury. Its cuisine is one of the many legacies bequeathed to the subcontinent by its rulers, perhaps more evident in Delhi than in any other city. Many of the specialities of Dilliwallay, brought with them to Pakistan, not surprisingly, are of Mughal origin. These include *bakarkhani, taftan, daal bharay parathay, nihari, shola, baryan, khandvian, kalmi baray, aaloo salan, shab degh,* and a lot more.

Diltar. Similar to *chaas*, consumed practically throughout Pakistan, *diltar* is a Hunzakutz yoghurt drink traditionally prepared in goat or sheep skin, which is vigorously shaken or rolled on the ground for a long time till butter is formed. This method of preparation is called taring. The buttermilk or watery milk left at the end is pure *diltar*. Salt, sugar, or fruits, like bananas, could be added for extra taste.

Diram phitti. A form of sweet bread—more like a moist cake than a crusty bread—made from germinated wheat flour or barley, *diram phitti* is a festive dessert indigenous to Hunza. It is popular at local weddings as well as in winter, and is savoured especially at Thummusheling, the festival related to the Vernal Equinox. What makes this dessert so special is that it is sweet without containing any sugar, as sugar is a relatively new import and is, therefore, not a part of any of the traditional dishes. To obtain this natural sweetness, the Hunzakutz use a special technique. Instead of drying and then grinding the freshly harvested wheat, the grains are kept moist. When the grains start to germinate and ferment slightly, they are ground into flour. This special fermented flour is then mixed with regular flour and used to bake *diram phitti*.

The legend goes that one of the Mirs of Hunza was warned of a conspiracy against his life from within his own ranks. He was told that the Diramiting tribe would take over his realm and that his only protection would be to slay every single male member of that tribe. So, the Mir ordered this by decree. But as soon as this decree was carried out, all crops became infected, threatening famine. Mir's only hope for salvation was to find a male Diramiting survivor, seeds sown from whose hands would secure the Mir's redemption and rid the crops of disease. This he did and kept his promise to protect the seed of the Diramiting, thereby, ensuring that life returned to Hunza soil.

A variation made with freshly cooked *diram phitti* is *diram shuro*. The *diram phitti* is mashed or crushed while still warm and fried in apricot oil, and then mixed in butter.

Do pyaza. A Mughlai dish which literally means 'twice onions'—as onions are added at two stages of the cooking process, *do pyaza* is made with meat, chicken, or prawns, but could also be purely vegetarian. According to one legend, this dish is a specimen of a particular gourmand's ingenuity. The gourmand was a *mullah* (preacher) and one of the famed 'nine jewels' in the court of Akbar the Great (the renowned Mughal emperor of India in the latter half of the 16th century). He maintained an open house, so that a steady stream of guests would arrive all evening, often many more than were expected. When he would realise that the food would be insufficient for all those who had dropped by, he would clap loudly to indicate to the cook that more onions should be added to the meat to make it go further. He discovered that doubling the quantity of onions made the dish, a rich aromatic, dry curry, even tastier. According to another legend, this dish was named after Emperor Akbar's minister, Mullah Do-Pyaza. The dish evolved further in Hyderabad and became a Hyderabadi speciality.

Dogh. An Afghani curd drink similar to *chaas* and *diltar*, the origin of *dogh* is traced to Iran. The word *dogh* is derived from *dooshidan*, which means milking. In olden days, Iranians made butter from full-cream yoghurt by placing the yoghurt in a leather bag or a big round pot and vigorously shaking it. After removing the butter, the remaining water from the yoghurt (*dogh*) would be consumed with food, especially in the summer months. A little salt and crushed mint leaves would be added to it for flavour. Nowadays, people make *dogh* at home by diluting yoghurt with cold water and adding little salt and dried crushed mint leaves, and even cucumber.

NAYYER RUBAB

Doodh ka sherbet. Once available freely in bottles at wayside restaurants, and as popular as the ubiquitous *lassi*, *doodh ka sherbet* is now more or less restricted to being served on special occasions at home in certain communities. A warm, saffron-infused sweetened milk with slivers of blanched almonds and pistachios, *doodh ka sherbet* is generally made to welcome the newly married Gujarati couple. In many communities, it is served to guests at engagement ceremonies or after the *nikkah* (marriage ceremony) has been performed.

Doodh khoya/mawa. Whole milk is evaporated to a solid consistency by boiling and thickening it in an open iron pan for several hours, over a medium flame to make *khoya/mawa*. It is often prepared at home from either cow or water buffalo milk or can be bought from the store. The ideal temperature to avoid scorching is about 80 °C (180 °F). The resulting milk solid is white or pale yellow in colour. It is used to make savoury dishes and desserts, has a slightly oily and granular texture and a rich nutty flavour. It is similar to ricotta cheese but lower in moisture.

If prepared in winter, it may be saved for use in summer, and may acquire a green tinge and grainier texture from a harmless surface mould. This is called *hariyali* (green *khoya*). With the advent of refrigeration, the production of *hariyali* is rare.

There are many varieties of *khoya* depending on the moisture content. Hard *khoya* or *batti khoya* (*batti* means rock) can be grated like cheese and is used mainly to make subcontinental *mithai* like *barfi* and *laddu*. *Batti khoya* is also most commonly used as an ingredient in making *qalaqand*. It has 20 per cent moisture by weight and can be aged for up to a year, during which it develops a unique aroma and a mouldy outer surface.

Granular or *daanedar khoya* is made by curdling the milk before evaporating it. The milk is coagulated with an acid like vinegar or lemon, during the simmering; it has a moderate moisture content. Its consistency is between *batti* and *chikna khoya* (oily *khoya*) which has 50 per cent moisture. Pindi, dry *khoya*, is used for preparing *barfi* and *pera*. *Dhap*, a less dried version, is used for preparing *gulab jamun*.

Like all dairy products, *khoya* is very good for strengthening bones and teeth, and is rich in calcium. Originating in the subcontinent, it is widely used in the cuisines of Pakistan, India, Nepal, and Bangladesh.

BISMA TIRMIZI

Doodh na puff. An extraordinary Parsi breakfast food, *doodh na puff* is made with fresh, whole milk that is covered with muslin and left to absorb dew overnight. It is whisked to a light froth in the morning, scooped up in a glass, and sprinkled with powdered nutmeg and cinnamon.

Doodh patti. Very popular throughout Pakistan, especially at roadside cafes, *doodh patti* is tea cooked in milk (*doodh* is milk while *patti* is tea leaves) together with sugar, instead of boiling it in water, and serving the milk and sugar separately—the way normal tea is served.

Originally a poor man's beverage, *doodh patti* was mainly served at roadside cafes across Pakistan, called *dhaba* where truck drivers on long hauls would break journey to refresh themselves with steaming hot *doodh patti* which would be both rich, and sweet enough to keep them awake. When consumed at breakfast, it is usually accompanied with different types of *parathay* and eggs, or with *aaloo-chanay ki tarkari* and *halwa puri*.

Gradually, *doodh patti's* popularity spread into the urban centres as well, and besides being offered at wayside kiosks, it became a regular feature at offices. With time it has come to be glorified, and now has become a sought-after feature at weddings and high-end parties, as well as at elitist *dhabas* serving the *doodh patti* at a premium price.

NAHEED ANSARI

Doodh ras. A Kashmiri dish made with lamb, *doodh ras* is a simple preparation in which pieces of lamb meat are boiled with whole spices wrapped in muslin, and then re-cooked immersed in a pot of boiling milk, lamb stock, and fried onion.

Doodhi falooda. This is a traditional Bohra speciality made with grated gourd, cream, and milk and served cold.

Doudo. A Hunzakutz speciality, *doudo* is soup cooked with home-made noodles and vegetables, such as potatoes and spinach, and thickened with whole wheat flour and eggs. It comes in many varieties such as *kurutze duodo* with *kurutz* (dried cheese), and the delicious *haneetze doudo* with nuts or crushed apricot kernels, garlic, and onion, and *chapsae doudo* with meat chunks. Since apricots grow in abundance in Hunza, apricot soup made with dried apricots, flour, and water is also popular.

Dried red chilli (sabut sookhi laal mirch). Constituting an important ingredient in Pakistani cuisine, dried red chillies can be used whole, or crushed, or in powder form. Whole dried chillies are usually fried in oil before use and are popular in *tarka* of dishes such as *karhi* and *daal*. They are extremely fiery and break easily once cooked, spewing their seeds into the broth; their effect can be toned down slightly by slitting them and shaking out the seeds before frying. The crushed and powdered chillies, however, do not tend to have the potency and flavour of the whole pods. Red chillies are healthy as they are low in sodium and very low in saturated fat and cholesterol. They are also said to be good for digestive ailments.

Dry fruit. Pakistan is extremely rich in the dry fruit industry. It grows fresh and dry dates, pine nuts (*chilgoza*) kernel, sweet and bitter apricot seeds, almonds, peanuts, figs, and raisins. Most of these are cultivated with variation in Sindh, Punjab, and Khyber Pakhtunkhwa. These are the quintessential winter snack—devoured plain, salted, or roasted—and a prime ingredient in making sweetmeats and many savoury items. In recent years, the active buying by exporters of dry fruits, such as peanuts, pistachios, cashew nuts, almonds, and figs, has increased primarily because of their increased domestic demand. Good quality shell almonds and walnuts are grown and consumed domestically as well as exported in large quantities.

Dry fruits are not only irresistible but also a powerhouse of macro and micro-nutrients, with high protein content, lots of fibre and healthy fats such as omega 3, 6, and 9. Pakistan exports sweet and bitter seeds of apricots to Turkey and India respectively, where the former is used in confectionary and sweet dishes, and the latter in herbal and homeopathic medicines. Fresh Pakistani dates are exported in large quantities to a number of countries, including India and China.

Modern new bakeries and *mithai* shops dot large urban cities and smaller markets, with both age-old trends and innovative new recipes heavily banking on dry fruit as a key ingredient. They are also popularly used to garnish a variety of desserts including *halwa*, *kheer*, ice creams, cakes, and puddings, as well as items like *Kashmiri chai*, and milk shakes. Pakistanis love their dry fruit in savoury items as well and use it as a key ingredient to oomph exotic entrees such as *qorma*, *biryani*, *bagharay baingan*, *mutanjan*, *pulao*, and roasted lamb, to name a few.

BISMA TIRMIZI

Dum (steaming). *Dum* involves cooking the dish in its own steam, and is a technique that originated in Persia, where the dish, prepared in a pot called *degchi* (also called *pateeli*) was sealed and buried in the hot sands of the desert to bring forth the best flavours. Another belief is that the technique became popular in the subcontinent in the 18th century, when the famine of 1784 made Nawab Asaf-ud-Daulah of Awadh provide jobs for his subjects by commissioning a monument that was to be built during the day and destroyed at night, thus ensuring a source of continuous employment.

During this process, large quantities of food—rice, meat and spices—were put in a gigantic cooking pot, sealed with dough, and cooked in large double-walled ovens. The resultant gentle steaming added a deliciously subtle flavour to the food, which would be fed to all the workers.

Regardless, this cooking technique has been in existence at least since the 1500s and has been documented in Abu Fazl's book, *Ain-i-Akbari*, in which various cooking styles in the royal kitchen and recipes have been mentioned. According to research, it is a cooking technique that was picked up by the formerly nomadic Mughals during their sojourn in areas such as modern Uzbekistan, Kazakhstan, Iran, and Afghanistan. It was a form of cooking popular in these areas, which allowed semi-prepared food to be cooked in its own steam by placing it in a heavy pot covered with a lid and sealed with a roll of dough wrapped all around its outer edges. The pot would be placed over very low heat—often just smouldering ashes—and live coals would be piled on top of the lid, with the result that the food would get 'baked' slowly with the gentle heat from above and below.

Today, this process is particularly used in the preparation of all rice dishes. Towards the end of cooking, when the rice is almost, but not fully, tender, the *degchi* is tightly closed (a weight may be added to the lid to ensure that the pot is sealed) and kept on a very low flame. An iron griddle may be placed under the pot to help distribute the heat evenly to its base. If a griddle is not available, the pot could also be placed in a warm oven. At this stage, the amount of water in the pot is minimal—just enough to moisten the rice and produce steam in the pot. Steam is produced at the bottom of the pot and as it rises, it fully tenderises the rice and separates the grains from one another, simultaneously imbibing a delicious, subtle flavour in the food. Probably the best example of a dish cooked using this technique is *biryani*. The process of steaming helps the aroma and flavour present in the spiced meat used in the *biryani* to be distributed evenly.

Dum aaloo. This was a popular dish at the grand Mughal courts, employing the *dum* technique of cooking. Mughals did not eat too many vegetables and among the few they did eat were potatoes, often cooked slowly and gently in a thick, dark sauce. This potato dish is made with favourite Kashmiri spices like fennel/anise and ginger powder. This dish is made by frying potatoes and then simmering them slowly in spices and yoghurt. It is eaten with rice.

Dum ke kebab. This dish is ideally made with *boti* (beef chunks) though *pasanday* (sirloin beef fillets) could also be used. A favourite practically all over Pakistan, it is basically a speciality of Hyderabadi cuisine. The beef is marinated with traditional spices, including roasted ground cumin and cardamom. Raw crushed papaya (with the peel) is added and the marinated beef is folded in yoghurt. Oil is added and it is then allowed to cook slowly over low flame with the lid on. Steam and heat do the magic. For a perfect finish, a burning piece of coal is placed on an aluminium foil inside the utensil and allowed to stay covered for five minutes to give it a smoky flavour. Served with freshly cut onion rings for garnish, *dum ke kebab* are ideally served with *naan* or *sheermal* (a rich, milk-based bread).

SHAHA TARIQ

Dum olav. A Kashmiri speciality and the region's version of *dum aaloo*, *dum olav* or Kashmiri *dum aaloo* is an extremely fragrant and light preparation with flavourful whole baby potatoes cooked in a delectable, thick yoghurt-based gravy, loaded with nuts (or nut paste), and dry fruit. Kashmiris make liberal use of dairy products and nuts in their daily meals.

NAHEED ANSARI

Dumpukht. The Persian word *dumpukht* literally means air-cooked (i.e. baked) and occurs in *Ain-i-Akbari* (AD 1590). Patronised by the nawabs of Awadh, *dumpukht* is a process of cooking using the *dum* technique (a cooking process over a slow fire, for a prolonged period); the effect was enhanced in later years by sealing the lid on the cooking vessel with wheat dough. Such long, slow, enclosed cooking results in the retention and permeation of the flavour of all the ingredients. This process is essential for making *pulao* even today, by slow cooking of rice and meats. A number of different kinds of dishes are made by Lucknawis involving this style of cooking, the most popular among them being the emptying out of the insides of a lamb and stuffing it with rice, almonds and raisins and then cooking it slowly in its own steam. Another dish employing this technique of cooking is made with a layer of cut-up potatoes topped with meat, yoghurt, turmeric, fat, and whole red chillies, and cooked overnight on low heat. Variations with pulses, called *namkeen* are also popular.

SUMMAYA USMANI

E

Easter Food. This cuisine is primarily for Easter Sunday, the day on which Christians believe Jesus rose from the dead. A day of rejoicing for Christians as it also marks the end of their long Lenten fast, and the beginning of spring, Easter is celebrated with Easter eggs, denoting rebirth and renewal. The Anglo-Indian and Goan Christians who used to reside in relatively large numbers in Karachi during the pre- and post-Partition times celebrated Easter with aplomb. A number of bakeries in the downtown Saddar area where most of the Christians used to live, would sell Easter eggs made out of chocolate shells just like in the West, marzipans, and hot-cross buns—the only time when they would be available. To date, although there are very few Anglo-Indian and Goan Christians left—most have immigrated—Easter eggs, both imported and locally made are sold at high-end bakeries and super markets, while one or two bakeries make the buns as well. Marzipans, though, are now made and sold the year round.

Eggplant/aubergine/brinjal (baingan). Eggplant, or *Solanum melongena* (known as *baingan* in Urdu), is botanically a fruit, although usually it is counted as a vegetable. Originating in the subcontinent, it comes in a variety of shapes and sizes (small and globular, large, and long), and colours (purple, green, yellowish, white, and striped, though purple is the most common here) and is found abundantly all over Pakistan. Eggplant is much favoured in Pakistani cooking because of its adaptability, fine meaty texture, and ability both to absorb and to blend strong added flavours. Cooked with its skin, as it is

digestible and highly nutritious, the eggplant is popular both as a vegetable curry, often combined with potatoes, and as a fried item, served in conjunction with yoghurt. The eggplant is rich in bioflavonoids which help arterial renewal and prevent blood clotting. It is also thought to be helpful in preventing some forms of cancer.

Eidul Azha. Eidul Azha, also known as Baqra Eid is a festive, religious occasion to commemorate Prophet Ibrahim's (as; Prophet Abraham in the Bible) readiness to obey God's commandment—to the extent of even willing to sacrifice his son. It is also one of the last rites of Haj (one of the five pillars of Islam, revolving around a pilgrimage). Goats, lambs, cows, and camels are symbolically sacrificed on Eidul Azha by Muslims in great numbers, and the meat is distributed among relatives, and the poor and the needy, while a portion is kept by the household to cook special dishes. Not surprisingly, barbecued mutton and beef are the order of the day and are served in conjunction with other delicious meat items such as *biryani* and *qorma*.

Eidul Fitr. Also known as Ramazan Eid, Eidul Fitr is a festive event that follows Ramazan—the month of fasting for all Muslims. To mark the occasion, special desserts of *sewain* and *sheer khurma* are prepared first thing in the morning in most homes and served to the menfolk as they return from offering Eid *namaz* at a mosque, as well as to all visitors through the day; it is the centre-piece of the Eid trolley, along with other delicious sweet dishes.

Falooda. *Falooda* (meaning shredded) is thought to be an adaptation of the Persian dessert *faloodeh* in ancient Persia, brought to the surrounding Middle Eastern countries and South Asia by Muslim travellers and merchants. The traditional Parsi-origin drink is made with *nishasto* prepared from *gehun doodh* (wheat milk powder) dissolved in water, while the version commonly consumed in Pakistan is made primarily with sago granules. In the Parsi version, *nishasto* is cooked till a thick gel-like consistency is formed, then it is poured through a colander over a large piece of ice, and stirred quickly, resulting in white droplets or tiny noodles. These are then left in the icy water and used as the main ingredient in the *falooda* drink. If wheat milk is not available, cornflour may be substituted. Just before serving the *falooda*, rose syrup or sherbet, milk, a few tablespoons of *nishasto*, very thin vermicelli, and basil seeds that have been soaked earlier, are layered in a tall glass, and topped with rose-flavoured ice cream. A popular summer drink, it is a favourite welcome beverage to serve the guests among the Parsis on Navroze, the festival celebrating the advent of spring (21 March). The more popular version found throughout Pakistan is made by mixing rose syrup with vermicelli and tapioca seeds along with either milk or water. In addition to these basic ingredients *sabja* or *takmaria* (basil seeds), tutti-frutti, sugar, and ice cream may be added. The rose syrup may be substituted with another flavoured base. Its variations are to be found throughout Pakistan.

ZARNAK SIDHWA

Falsa. Of indigenous origin, but with different beliefs about its discovery, *falsa (Grewia asiatica)* is a large, scraggy shrub believed to have been first discovered in Varanasi, India, and then taken by Buddhist scholars to the rest of the world. However, according to research, the fruit was named after Nehemiah Grew (1641–1712), an English botanist considered as the father of plant anatomy. The bushy tree is considered to be a native of South Asia, from Pakistan to Cambodia. It is cultivated commercially in the Punjab and around Bombay (now Mumbai), and on a small scale in the Philippines. The tree is small, covered with tiny hair, and grows to a height of five to six metres. It yields small, sour, purplish berries which are not only delightful to eat plain, or sprinkled with black salt, they are also popular as a refreshing acidic drink. Available only in summers, this is an expensive fruit—as the fruiting period is short and lasts only for three to four weeks—and is sold mostly by street vendors when it is in full-season in May and June; they make a killing selling it at exorbitant prices to those who want to beat the heat and quench their thirst in a refreshing manner. The fleshy, ripe *falsa* fruit provides water, ash, fat, sugar, vitamins A and C, minerals, carotene and dietary fibre, besides 724 calories per kilo. Medicinally, the fruit is an astringent and reduces stomachic inflammation and respiratory and cardiac problems. The ripe fruit is also good for the throat, and helps in blood disorders, fever, and diarrhoea, while the unripe fruit is used to treat biliousness. *Falsa* is digestive, prevents nausea, and reduces discomfort in the throat.

Fennel Seed (*Foeniculum vulgare*; saunf). Fennel has been widely grown in this region from early times. Similar in appearance to white cumin, these seeds have a sweet taste and are used for flavouring some curries, and vegetarian and fish dishes. Fennel seeds are also frequently chewed after a spicy meal as they are said to help the body digest fatty foods. They are believed to suppress the appetite as well. *Saunf* water is a home remedy for stomach upsets, while fennel tea is believed to improve cognitive function, alleviate depression, and delay the onset of dementia owing to high potassium content. Fennel contains trans-anethole, a compound that prevents retinopathy and glaucoma.

Fenugreek (*Trigonella foenum-graecum*; methi). A leguminous plant related to clover, fenugreek is widely cultivated as a condiment crop. Fresh fenugreek, available in bunches, has very small leaves, and is used to flavour both meat and vegetarian dishes. The dried leaves are also used for flavouring. Whole, dried, fenugreek seeds (*methi dana*), which are flat and yellowish brown, are frequently used as a flavouring in Pakistani curries. The flavour is almost unpalatably sharp but improves when the seeds are lightly fried. However, overheating makes them bitter. The seeds are also used in many ready-made curry powders and add relish and zest to all foods. They are particularly delicious with potatoes and are also used as a flavouring for pickles. Rich in vitamin A, fenugreek is considered to have the ability to cleanse the body of toxins. It is said to be anti-diabetic, effective in lowering blood pressure, and in improving the digestive, respiratory, and nervous systems.

Feyuk shaa moskut. This is a traditional Balti dish comprising mutton pieces cooked in a rich sauce of crushed almonds, walnuts and herbs. It is served with *chapati* or *palapu*.

Firni. Similar to *kheer,* except that *kheer* often has a liquid consistency, *firni* is made with milk, sugar, and ground rice, and flavoured with saffron, and always has a soft but firm consistency. Slivers of dry fruit such as pistachio, could be added for garnishing. Commercially, it is often set and sold in small, earthenware, shallow bowls, called *kulya,* containing just enough of the sweet stuff to whet the appetite.

Flavour enhancer. The use of flavour enhancers is widespread in Pakistani cooking, regardless of ethnic group, geographical region and socio-economic class of the household preparing the food. The five flavour enhancers most commonly used in Pakistani cooking are onion, garlic, ginger, tomato, and green chilli. One or more of these ingredients are found in almost every Pakistani dish, with onion topping the list.

Fresh-water fish. In Sindh, the most popular fresh-water fish despite its numerous bones is palla (*Tenualosa ilisha*). River fish is popular in the province of Khyber Pakhtunkhwa, especially with the fishermen residing in the Swat region where River Swat yields the best trout, along with River Kunhar. The banks of the Chenab are also home to delicious river fish. Reportedly, there are anywhere from 183 to 233 fresh-water fish species in Pakistan and Azad Kashmir, while just Chenab boasts 81 species. Most abundant river fish species of Khyber Pakhtunkhwa, Balochistan, as well as River Chenab include tilapia (*Oreochromis niloticus*), rohu or carp (*Labeo rohita*), mori (*Cirrhinus mrigala*), foji khaga (*Bagarius bagarius*), sangari (*Sperata sarwari*), dola (*Channa punctate*), mahseer (*Tor microlopsis*), trout, and khaga.

Fruit. Fruits that are either indigenous to southern Pakistan or have been here since recorded history include the jujube (*bair*), pomegranate, orange, lime, mango, sugarcane, falsa, guava, and grapes. Banana, jackfruit, lychees, and pineapples were essentially grown in the then eastern wing of the country (known as East Pakistan) and began to be cultivated in the present-day Pakistan much later, from late 1970s or early 1980s. The northern areas have an abundance of fruits such as cherries, peaches, apples, pears, plums, strawberries, and apricots. But it is the mango, regarded as the king of fruits in Pakistan, that is the pride and joy of the country. The average yield of mangoes is 11.20 tonnes/hectares and Pakistan's rank is fifth among the mango-producing countries of the world. There are many varieties which are grown in Pakistan, including: Sindhri, Langra, Chaunsa, Fajri, Samar Bahist, Anwar Ratole, Dasehri, Saroli, Tuta Pari, Neelam, Maldah, Collector, and Baigan Phalli. Each variety has its own unique taste and rating one kind superior over the other is purely a matter of personal choice and taste.

Fruit chaat. There are two varieties of *fruit chaat*—with fresh cream, and a basic variety. The latter is basically a cocktail of seasonal fruits along with generous doses of bananas, apples, and guavas. It is spiced with *chaat masala*, cinnamon powder, salt, black pepper with a dash of lemon for a zesty kick, and sugar. Extremely popular in summer months, and especially at *iftar* during Ramazan it is a refreshing tangy-sweet dish that is regarded a must at the *iftar* table in many households. The former variety has fresh cream poured on the fruits instead of being seasoned by spices and serves as a dessert as well as a snack.

Furfur bhalay. A flavourful organic vegetable soup of locally grown wheat and homemade pasta chunks cooked in a tasty chicken or mutton stock, *furfur bhalay* is a Baltistani speciality, only prepared in that region.

Gahambar. Gahambars are the six annual feasts celebrated by the Parsi community. These are large events aimed at bringing the entire community together to enjoy a meal. Long tables are placed parallel to each other with people sitting on one side only, so that people on the first table face those on the second, those on the third, face those on the fourth, and so on. The narrow channel in between the tables is meant to facilitate those serving the food. Instead of on a plate, the food is traditionally served on banana leaves. Various chutneys and pickles are served first, followed by *papeta ma gosht* (meat with potatoes) and hot *chapati*. This is often followed by *dhansak* and rounded off with Parsi custard.

Gajar batta. A winter speciality when carrots are in season, made by Dilliwallay and especially partaken of at breakfast, *gajar batta* may look and taste like *gajar ka halwa* made by other communities, but is prepared differently. It contains rice among the main ingredients, aside from sugar, grated carrots, and water, and can be simmered together till tender, or the carrots could be fried in oil first and then simmered. It is normally prepared at night and then eaten the following morning doused, as per taste, in either hot or cold milk, and cream.

Gajar ka halwa. Legend has it that the Sikhs from the Punjab introduced the *gajar* (carrot) *halwa* to the house of the Mughals. The orange carrot had already spread far and wide to Europe, the Middle East, and South Asia with the advent of the Dutch East India Company to the subcontinent in the 17th century. With international traders bringing new goods for trade with the Mughal Empire, the orange carrot is said to be one of the treasures introduced in Emperor Akbar's time to the Mughal Court. A Sikh cook in the royal kitchens of Emperor Akbar developed the *gajar ka halwa* recipe that became an instant hit with the Mughals who enjoyed its vibrant colour, flowery aroma, and slightly chewy texture. Made with carrots, *gajar ka halwa* is one of

the most popular desserts of Pakistan today, prepared especially in winter when carrots are in season, and more so in the Punjab. Made with shredded fresh carrots cooked in milk and cream, and mixed with sugar, the carrots are then fried in clarified butter. *Gajar ka halwa* can be eaten hot or cold depending on individual preferences and is garnished with slivers of blanched pistachios and almonds, and *khoya*.

Gajjak. A Gujarati winter candy popular in Pakistan, *gajjak* is a dry, crunchy sweet made from sesame seed and sugar or jaggery syrup. Since sesame is believed to have warming properties, it is rarely eaten in summer. The cooked mixture is allowed to set and then cut into rectangles. It is a favourite with all age groups, and along with dry fruit, is sold by street vendors.

Galavat kebab. According to one story pertaining to the origin of this aromatic and light *galavat kebab*, in the early 1900s, a small village near Lucknow called Kakori acquired fame for their melt-in-the-mouth, (hence its name, *galavat*) smoked mince kebabs served to the toothless pilgrims who would visit it, as the shrine of a Sufi saint was located there. The mince for the kebab was reputed to be made from the tendon of leg of lamb. The fat content was replaced by *khoya*, black pepper by white pepper, and a special mix of powdered spices was added to create the perfect blend. It is believed that the recipe was later taken to Lucknow, where this kebab became the speciality of a cook, Tunda—so called because he had only one arm after an accident—and hence came to be known as Tunda kebab. Later, immigrants to Pakistan brought the tantalising recipe with them.

Another legend is attached to this popular kebab. According to it, the recipe originated in the kitchen of one of Lucknow's famous nawabs, Asad-ud-Daula. Successor of Siraj-ud-Daula, Asad-ud Daula was known to be extremely fond of kebabs, with his special team of chefs dedicated specifically towards creating a new variety of kebab for him, every single day. As he grew old and lost his teeth, his chefs got together and produced a variety of kebabs that the nawab could consume. After a series of trial and errors with technique and ingredients, the chefs concocted what is now considered a culinary breakthrough—a kebab that would melt in the nawab's mouth without moving a single muscle—the famous *galavat* kebab.

Gandal ka achar. A traditional Punjabi pickle, *gandal ka achar* is prepared in winter when fresh mustard greens or *sarson ka saag* arrive in the market. Stems of mustard greens are called *gandal* in Punjabi. To make *gandal ka achar* (mustard greens pickle), thick stems of mustard greens are used, although the occasional thinner stems are also included. Some very young leaves attached to the very young stems could also be added. The process of making the pickle is simple. The thick stems have to be peeled and the leaves removed. After washing and cutting them they are boiled, strained, and set out to dry. The dried stems are then mixed with spices, vinegar, and mustard oil, and kept in air-tight jars in the sun for at least four days, till they are ready for consumption as accompaniment to any main course. The pickle is both unique-tasting and healthful.

Gannay ka ras (sugarcane juice). With sugarcane in abundance, pure sugarcane juice is a popular, refreshing street drink all over Sindh and the Punjab, especially in summer. In the Punjab, it is seasoned with ginger and lime, a trend that is now becoming popular in Sindh as well. Kiosks and wayside vendors exclusively selling sugarcane juice are not an uncommon sight in these provinces, while nearly all juice stalls in these regions offer *gannay ka ras* as well, throughout the year. Sugarcane is rich in antioxidants, so it helps fight infections and boosts immunity. It is rich in iron, magnesium, calcium, and other electrolytes, and, hence, it is great for dehydration. It helps cure common cold and other infections, and also fight fever as it boosts the body's protein levels.

Gannay ke ras ki kheer (rasawal). A Punjabi winter favourite, also known as *roh di kheer, rasawal* is made with sugarcane juice and rice, garnished with dry fruit and cardamoms. It is normally served in earthenware pots. This *kheer* is particularly favourite with Sikhs.

Garam masala (mixed spices). This is a combination of certain spices, and can be used either ground and dry roasted, or whole in Pakistani cooking. There is

no set formula but normally cumin, cloves, cinnamon sticks, black cardamom seeds, and black peppercorns are combined when making ground *garam masala*. Many people, particularly in the rural areas prefer to freshly grind their own mixed spices at home, although packaged *garam masala* is also popular these days with housewives who prefer convenience over quality. Bay leaves are often interspersed when using whole mixed spices. It is very potent in its powdered form and is used very sparingly and only at the end when the dish is almost ready, usually as a garnish. However, whole *garam masala* is generally used at the beginning of cooking a dish and lends a wonderful warmth and richness to the food. *Garam masala* is generally used with meat and rice but rarely with fish or vegetables, as the combination of powerful spices is considered too strong for delicate flavours.

Garlic (*Allium sativum*; lehsan). The most powerfully flavoured member of the onion family, and an indispensable ingredient in many dishes, the garlic plant's bulbs or heads have been used to flavour food since ancient times. A bulb contains six to more than two dozen cloves, each covered by a papery shell. The cloves have a pungent smell when whole but release a notoriously strong one when crushed. Generally, garlic is rich in minerals, containing, within the chemical complexity of its primary minerals, a relatively high amount of sulphur compounds. In addition, garlic contains trace minerals such as calcium, phosphorous, iron; and is rich in vitamins B1 and C. For as long as garlic has been known, it has been valued as much for its medicinal properties as for its flavour. Today, it is hailed as a 'superfood' with active health-giving properties. It is antiseptic and powerfully antibacterial when raw, and even when cooked, helps the body eliminate toxins and lowers cholesterol. It is reputed to cure many ailments including nose bleeds, skin problems, coughs, colds, bronchitis, and asthma. Probably native to Afghanistan, the garlic was despised as a food of the natives and foreigners by the high-born Aryans and it was forbidden on ceremonial occasions. In Pakistan, garlic is commonly used in curries, especially in conjunction with ginger in case of meat curries, while it is used on its own when cooking vegetables or fish items.

Garnish. In Pakistani cooking, the most common form of garnishing is chopped coriander, followed by sliced onions, green chillies and tomatoes. When garnishing desserts, ground cardamoms, almonds, and pistachios or slivered blanched almonds and pistachios, and currants are preferred. *Varq* (sterling silver leaf) used to be a highly popular garnish and was imbibed enthusiastically in the days of the nawabs, as it enjoyed the reputation of having aphrodisiac properties. However, over the years, inflation and health concerns have reduced its usage considerably.

Gatte ki sabzi/karhi. A popular yoghurt-based Gujarati dish, particularly eaten in the Thar area, *gatte ki sabzi/karhi* comprises gram flour dough hand-rolled into thick sticks or cylinders, cut into small pieces (*gatte*) and boiled or steamed. It is then immersed in beaten yoghurt or buttermilk that has been mixed with sautéed onion and masala paste and thinned with the water in which the *gatte* was boiled. The *gatte* is cut further into small, thick discs and cooked in the yoghurt curry till the curry thickens, and eaten with *chapati* or rice.

Gehar. This is a Hindu speciality mainly eaten at the Hindu Holi festival. *Gehar* is a dessert similar to a large *jalebi* (pretzel-shaped dessert), particularly eaten in Mirpurkhas and Hyderabad.

Ghalmandi. An indigenous dish of Chitral, a district in Khyber Pakhtunkhwa province, *ghalmandi* is made with milk and pure clarified butter. It has a filling of cottage cheese and local herbs sandwiched between two thick flat breads. The bread is covered with hot melted butter or walnut oil just before serving.

NAYYER RUBAB

Ghas ka halwa. A Khoja community dessert, *ghas ka halwa* is supposed to have a cooling effect, and, hence, is particularly popular in summer. Made with china grass that has been soaked and then boiled in water, the only other main ingredient used in it is sugar.

Ghatia. Gujarati savoury fried snacks that can be kept for days in air-tight containers, *ghatia* is essentially *besan*-derived (Bengal gram ground into gram flour) crisps in solid, cylindrical shape. Among the many ancient snacks prepared by Gujaratis and known as *nasto*, *ghatia* is now one of the many items eaten especially in Karachi and known by the new generic name of Nimco.

Ghatia salan. Made in the traditional style of *gosht ka salan* by frying onions and browning masalas before adding meat and water, the only difference in this Khoja

curry-based speciality is that *ghatia* (fried strips of *besan* dough) are added in it instead of meat.

Ghee (clarified butter). The original reason for making *ghee*, a name derived from the Sanskrit *ghrita, ghrta*, was to keep butter stay for long in the hot subcontinental climate. When butter, itself obtained by the churning of curd, is boiled down with constant stirring till all the water has evaporated and heating is continued till a strong, cooked flavour emanates, *ghee* or clarified butter is formed. It is allowed to stand for a while, then decanted or filtered through muslin to remove sediment. When left for long, *ghee* tends to separate into a mass of grains in a liquid medium which remains good for several weeks at room temperature. Regarded as the supreme cooking fat in Vedic culture *ghee* was prepared by melting and desiccating butter and was considered a commodity of enormous prestige. It was used for frying and as a dip to add relish to other foods. Both the Sultanate court and the later Mughal kitchens used *ghee* extensively; the *Ain-i-Akbari* (AD 1590) records that *ghee* for Akbar's kitchen came from Hissar. While it was the preferred, if not the only, medium of cooking in the days of yore, due to the debate on its health benefits or lack thereof—it was considered as being very high in cholesterol—it fell from favour as a shortening of choice for daily cooking, and was replaced by the ubiquitous oil, albeit reluctantly by the older generations, who were used to its superior taste. Over the years its use has been limited for cooking exotic, rich foods like local desserts, or frying of *parathay*, or preparing entrees like *biryani* and *qorma* when entertaining guests. Nonetheless, modern research has once again absolved *ghee* of its negative connotations and has concluded that saturated fats such as those found in *ghee* are good for one's health. *Ghee* not only reduces body fat in the long run, it also increases muscle strength and exercise endurance, and lubrication of connective tissues by breaking down LDL in the body, which triggers the metabolic rate, leading to faster food digestion and absorption. What is more, the presence of vitamin A in *ghee* prevents vision-related diseases.

Gilgit–Baltistan. Till recently, known as the Northern Areas, Gilgit–Baltistan is situated to the east of Chitral district, in the midst of the world's highest mountains and longest glaciers, covering an area of 72,971 sq. km. Sharing borders with China, India and Afghanistan, Gilgit–Baltistan was part of the Kushan Empire from the first to the 3rd century, and was occupied by Tibet, areas of China, and Afghanistan. Presently, the region consists of seven districts—the two Baltistan districts of Skardu and Ghanche, and the five Gilgit districts of Gilgit, Ghizer, Diamer, Astore, and Hunza-Nagar—has a population of nearly one million and is known for its scattered valley communities. Previously comprising Buddhist and animist population, this area converted almost entirely to Islam in the beginning of the 12th century. The staple food is wheat, while buckwheat and barley are also widely cultivated, and malt grasses are consumed. Those who can afford it, eat beef. Though they are mostly fruit farmers as apricots, apples, grapes, cherries, and plums grow in abundance, all the tribes have distinct identities and lifestyles. Among the ethnic groups living here are Baltis, Hunzakutz, Mughals, Kashmiris, Pakhtuns, Tajiks, and Mongols.

Ginger (adrak). Ginger is the perennial creeping plant of the Zingiber officinale family, with thick, tuberous rhizome, producing a stem of 60–120 cm high, with long, narrow, lily-like leaves. These are mainly consumed in the fresh ('green') state, but are also dried to provide an important spice, and ground into a paste to be used as a tenderiser in most meat-based dishes of Pakistan. In fact, fresh or dried ginger is one of the most popular and ancient flavourings used in Pakistan and is an essential ingredient in practically every curry of meat and chicken as it contributes a freshness and distinctive heat to meat dishes. Practically every recipe of meat dish of Akbar's court, mentioned in the *Ain-i-Akbari* (AD 1590), includes green ginger, and like Confucius, Akbar was known to have eaten fresh ginger with every meal as a digestive and carminative. Although it is usually known as root ginger, the part of the plant used in Pakistani dishes to flavour food is the rhizome or thickened underground stem. It is usually peeled and then blended into a paste or cut finely before use. Also used to spice beverages and curd dishes, ginger is a potent stimulant and aids the digestive process. Research shows that it alleviates travel sickness and vertigo. Infusions of ginger are also recommended against colds and sore throats. It is also reputed to help with anaemia and liver complaints.

Girgir aaloo. A Hunzakutz speciality, *girgir aaloo* is a combination of boiled whole *masoor daal* and potatoes, cooked with tomatoes, onions, and spices.

Goan food. Goa was a Portuguese possession—and the gateway to Portugal's empire in the East—for 450 years before yielding first to Dutch and then to British dominance. During this long period its culture was an interesting mixture of Latin influences and those of the Hindus and Muslims who represented the indigenous population. This was reflected in Goan food, which presented an interesting blend of Portuguese and subcontinental cookery. Thus, Goan dishes unite in their fiery sauces the culinary histories of three continents: Europe, Asia, and the Americas. Liberal use of vinegar (generally added to finish a cooked dish) is essentially European, but use of various local ingredients, and of the less-spicy Kashmiri chillies which impart an intense red colour, bespeak the local colour. The best-known example is probably *vindaloo*, originally a pork stew imported from Portugal but indigenised by the addition of local spices. Goan cuisine generally draws on fish, coconut and rice, with chillies forming central ingredients. When Sir Charles Napier occupied Sindh in 1843, many Goans who did not want to live under Portuguese rule moved to Karachi and were absorbed in the army as well as in civilian jobs. Some of them established bakeries which became extremely popular. Although most of them have now migrated to Australia, Canada, or the US, even now there are bakeries in the Saddar area—where Goans had initially made their homes—that make Goan specialities, especially at Christmas and Easter.

Goat. Goat meat is taken from the adults of the species *Capra hircus*, closely related to sheep. Adapted to mountain habitats, goats are sure-footed, able to climb steep cliffs to find food, and survive on tree bark and thorny scrub. There is evidence of goats and sheep being eaten during the Indus Valley Civilisation. Although goat meat and mutton are terms used interchangeably in Pakistan—in fact, to all intents and purposes, mutton in Pakistan means goat meat; it is goat meat that is popular almost throughout the country, and mutton (sheep meat) is popular only in Gilgit-Baltistan and Khyber Pakhtunkhwa.

Gola ganda. A popular summer favourite, *gola ganda* is a delightful concoction of shaved ice mixed with coloured syrups, fruit, and condensed milk (optional). It is served either as a popsicle or in a cup and is normally sold on push-carts on streets.

Gonglu (turnip). A Punjabi speciality, also known as *shaljam*, *gonglu* is a curry dish made with turnips and meat, normally served with white rice. Originally, *gur* was added to the dish at the tail-end of the cooking.

Gosh-i-feel/gosh-i-barra. Persian words meaning ears of elephant and ears of goat, respectively, *gosh-i-feel/gosh-i-barra* are Afghan delights, named such because of their distinct shapes, although the dessert is the same. Mostly prepared at home in Quetta—you will be hard put to find them being sold anywhere—they are made from flour, sugar, and oil, with crushed pistachios and almonds sprinkled on top. They are particularly popular on Eid and Navroze.

Gosh nu saag. The difference between *gosh nu saag*, a Bohri community's meat curry, and the ones normally made in the country—aside from the fact that it has a green curry base—is that most ingredients in this curry, including onions, are only partially cooked before the meat is added to it. In most meat curries, the ingredients are fried (through the *bhoonna* process) before the meat and water is added.

Gosht khara masala. Similar to brown stew, *gosht khara masala* is a Dilliwalla dish that incorporates whole spices rather than their powdered form. The only difference is that while brown stew is made with yoghurt, this dish uses tomatoes.

Gosht ki kari. A Khoja community speciality, *gosht ki kari* incorporates parboiled mutton cooked in lots of ground *masala* including *til* (sesame seeds), *khashkhash* (poppy seeds), *mung phalli* (peanuts), roasted gram and cashew nuts, roasted and ground onions, and tamarind. It is normally eaten with *baghara hua* (lightly fried) rice or *kark roti*.

Gram. A subcontinental term, gram refers to pulses which are whole rather than split—the latter are called *daal*. The word is of Portuguese origin, from grain (Latin *granum*), but does not apply to cereal grains, as one might expect. The term gram by itself, without an epithet, is taken to mean chickpea. Similarly, 'gram flour' means *besan*, which is made from chickpeas.

Grape. The fruit of the genus *Vitis*, the grape reached the subcontinent from Persia as far back as the 7th century BC, although, surprisingly, it receives only late mention in Sanskrit by Panini and Charaka in *c*.500 BC. Its use for making wine and spirits may have led to its suppression by puritanical rulers. Xuan Zang notes in the 7th century AD that grapes were brought from Kashmir. Babar encouraged grape cultivation, and by Akbar's time, grapes had become plentiful. In Pakistan, grapes are grown for consumption as well as for making juices, carbonated drinks, and raisins. A summer fruit, it is grown in all the provinces of Pakistan.

Greek influence. Pakistan lies within the region that was invaded by Alexander the Great in 327–323 BC, although archaeological evidence in northern Pakistan suggests that the Greek influence predates this invasion. It has been suggested that the symbols found on ancient Harappan seals, which in one interpretation are numerals, were later adopted in modified form as numerals by Greeks and others. Direct contact between Greece and the subcontinent was established with Alexander's invasion in 327 BC, followed by a stay of 18 months. At the time of the invasion, Ambhi (Omphis), the ruler of Taxila—now in the Punjab province of Pakistan—surrendered the city and placed his resources at Alexander's disposal. Greek historians, travelling with the invading army, described Taxila as wealthy, prosperous, and extremely well-governed. Many ethnically and linguistically distinct populations inhabit the region invaded by Alexander, at least three of which (Burusho, Kalash, and the Pakhtun) claim to be descendants of the Greek soldiers who invaded the subcontinent. However, a preliminary study using a limited number of genetic markers found no evidence for intermingling between the Greeks and Burusho or Pakhtun and provided ambiguous evidence of genetic blending between the Greek and Kalash populations. The earliest mention of a dish named *pilaf* can be found in the transcripts of history on Alexander the Great. It is believed that the young Greek conqueror enjoyed the reception he received at the hands of the locals of Bactria, an ancient country that lay between the mountains of the Hindu Kush and Amu Darya (ancient Oxus River) in what is now part of Afghanistan, Uzbekistan, and Tajikistan. The military forces accompanying Alexander savoured the Bactrian dish of rice and meat and took the recipe back with them not only to Greece, giving rise to the Mediterranean *pilaf*, but also to Pakistan, where the *pulao* has become a native dish.

Green chilli. Fresh green chillies and their riper red counterparts are used in Pakistani cooking both as an ingredient and as a garnish. Other than imparting their own richly aromatic flavour and spice, they also have the power to bring out the flavour of ingredients around them. They are an especially important ingredient in the cuisine of the Punjab and Sindh. Fresh chillies are packed with vitamins A, B, and C and are also potent stimulants to the system, which are highly antibacterial and help normalise blood pressure.

Green tea. Green tea has been consumed in China as a healthful, medicinal drink for the last 5000 years. Not surprisingly, it became popular with the communities settled in the northern parts of Pakistan as indeed in other neighbouring areas, including Tajikistan, to the extent that with the Pakhtuns of Balochistan it has become the most frequently consumed drink, taken almost on a daily basis with meals. Balochs now believe they are the only people who know how to make authentic green tea. Water is boiled with green cardamoms and sugar before adding the tea leaves, and allowed to brew. The beverage is traditionally served in small goblets without handles meant exclusively for serving green tea and was once considered a must at night time.

Greens (saag). Though largely a meat-eating nation, the average Pakistani does enjoy their cooked greens occasionally, though rarely consumes them raw. While all kinds of salad leaves are now available in urban centres, they are mostly consumed by the upper class or bought by high-end eateries. The most popular green vegetable in the country is *palak* (spinach), cooked generally with potatoes or at formal occasions, with *paneer* (cottage cheese), although *palak gosht* (spinach cooked with meat) is not, surprisingly, a combination that is very popular. In the Punjab, *sarson ka saag* (mustard greens) accompanied by *makai ki roti* (corn bread) is very popular in winter. Other greens include *bathua saag* and *cholai ka saag*. The green vegetables grown in Khyber Pakhtunkhwa are different from those found in other parts of the country, and hence some of the vegetarian dishes popular there are peculiar to that region only. *Kachaloo key patton ka saag* made with yam leaves in sesame seed oil; *panerak* (from the Malvaceae family), *tara meera saag* (wild water cress), *pishtaray* and *tawa* potato peels, are just some of the unusual greens that are popular in Khyber Pakhtunkhwa, cooked with garlic. Besides the unique taste of a well-cooked *saag* dish, these leafy green vegetables are very nutritious, packed with vitamin A, folic acid, carotenes, vitamin K, and flavonoid antioxidants that have immense disease preventing properties.

Guava. This is the fruit of the small, shrubby tree *Psidium guajava*, though there are several other species in the genus with good fruits, and the name 'guava' is applied loosely to most of them. Portuguese mariners introduced the fruit to the subcontinent and it became well-established in the region in the 17th century. Guava fruits vary in size, shape, and colour, even within the principal species, *P. guajava*. They range from the size of an apple to that of a plum, and may be round or pear-shaped, rough, or smooth-skinned, and greenish-white, yellow, or red in colour. The fruit has an outer and inner zone, the latter with many small, gritty seeds. The taste is acidic but sweet, with an unusual aromatic quality partly because of eugenol, an essential oil that is also found in cloves. Besides being eaten fresh, guavas are used to make fruit *chaats*, beverages, jams, and jellies. In Pakistan, they are grown abundantly practically all over the country—in fact, Pakistan is reportedly the second largest guava-producing country in the world, after India—and especially in Sindh, where Malir's guavas are famous for their taste.

Gujarati. With a very strong Jain influence in Gujarat even before the 6th century BC, it is not surprising that Gujaratis who settled in Pakistan (mostly in Karachi) are, by and large, very fond of vegetarian cuisine, even if they are meat-eaters. In fact, the dishes they are most known for, particularly their savoury fried snacks, are all vegetarian. Renowned for the simplicity of their lifestyle, this lack of fussiness is reflected in the Gujarati cuisine. Traditionally, Gujaratis eat from *thalis*, which are steel platters holding several *katoris* (little bowls) each one containing small quantities of different vegetarian dishes. Gujarati specialities include *khandvi*, a savoury, rolled crepe made with gram flour and yoghurt, and spongy *dhoklay* (savoury lentil, flour, or rice cakes). Gujaratis, who settled in Pakistan, hail from various parts of India and their cuisine, therefore, varies somewhat. Nonetheless, certain commonalities are to be found. A touch of sugar goes into most Gujarati spicing. In fact, Gujarati dishes tend to be a blend of sweet, spicy, and sour. Among the quintessential Gujarati savoury snacks that have become particularly popular in Karachi are *papar, ghugray, bhel puri,* and *pani puri,* while fried sweets like *khaja, laddu, kheer, pheni, sutar-pheni, gundh-paak* (which contains the aromatic resin *gu*) are popular Gujarati desserts.

Gulab jaman. Balls of milk powder (*khoya*) kneaded with flour, *ghee,* and warm milk, deep fried till they turn dark-brown and then gently boiled in medium-thick sugar syrup, *gulab jamans* are believed to have been introduced to the subcontinent in mediaeval times by Persian invaders. The sweetmeat derives its name from the Persian word *gol*, meaning flower and *ab* meaning water, referring to the rose water scented syrup (*gulab* also means rose in Urdu) in which they are boiled. The word *jamun* also reflects the deep colour of the subcontinental fruit by the same name. *Gulab jamans* are a highly popular dessert practically throughout the country and also very similar to certain desserts made in Bengal as well as in Arabia. They can be eaten hot, at room temperature, or cold.

Gundh phera. A Bohra community speciality made with edible gum, whole wheat flour, sugar and *ghee*, and enriched with pistachios, almonds, cardamom and saffron, *gundh phera* is a crumb-like dessert particularly popular in winter and regarded as a highly nourishing dish for young mothers.

Gundpaak. A Gujarati sweet which contains the aromatic resin *gund*, *gundpaak* is a very nutritious dessert generally made in winter; it is often served to nursing mothers. Made with whole wheat flour, jaggery, *gundh* (edible gum), almonds and milk, it is cooked into a mixture and allowed to set on a greased baking tray, then cut into squares.

Gur. Sweet in taste and honey-brown in colour, *gur* is the raw form of sugar made from sugarcane and at times referred to as natural sugar. *Gur* is made from crushing sugarcanes and gathering the syrup that is poured in a large, shallow, round-bottomed container. It is then boiled at 200° C until all the water content

evaporates and the residue is transferred to another pot to be cooled. It solidifies into *gur*, and is broken into small pieces, ready for consumption. While *gur* is used in making many traditional desserts such as *gur wallay chawal* (rice with *gur*) and *gur papri*, it is also a poor man's main meal, and items like *gur ki roti*, which is *gur* mixed with whole wheat flour and then deep- or shallow-fried offers sustenance at an affordable price.

LAL MAJID

Gur papri. A Gujarati dessert similar to *gundpak* but less sticky, *gur papri* is a rich sweet prepared in winter, as its ingredients have a warming effect on the body. It is basically made of whole wheat flour, almonds, pistachios, poppy seeds, jaggery, and edible gum and shaped into balls, or flattened and cut into diamonds.

Gur roti. A Gujarati casual dessert popular with both children and adults, *gur roti* is broken bits of *chapati* mixed with melted *gur* and eaten warm.

Gushtaba. A Kashmiri speciality, *gushtaba* is a meat loaf of very fresh lamb pounded to a pulp in its own fat and is silky in texture. The meat is shaped into large balls and cooked overnight over a low flame with yoghurt, turnips, and spices. It is eaten with either rice or *roti*. It is often the last entrée served in the traditional Kashmiri feast, *Wazwan*, which often has more than 30 main courses. Considered the *pièce de résistance* of the elaborate menu, the overall quality of the *Wazwan* is often judged by the preparation of *gushtaba*.

H

Habshi halwa. The famous *habshi halwa* of Sindh, also known as the *shehzada* (prince) of all *halway*, is a royal dessert introduced by the Mughals. It is generally believed that it got its name for its dark brown colour—the word *habshi* comes from the Persian *Habashi* which refers to the Habeshi, or Abyssinian, people; in Pakistan the dark-skinned Balochis believed to be of African descent are often called Habshi. This sweetmeat is a combination of wheat, sugar, milk, clarified butter and lots of chopped almonds, pistachios, and cashews. Strangely enough it is known as *sohan halwa* in southern Punjab, which is famous for this dessert, especially Multan, although *sohan halwa* is also a name given to an altogether different dessert popular in Karachi.

Hak. This name is given to a stir-fried spinach dish that is frequently made by Kashmiri Hindus. It also has a hint of asafoetida and sugar.

Halal. All meat (mutton, beef, and chicken are the most popular) cooked in Pakistan is *halal* (permissible for use according to the Islamic law) or kosher—that is slaughtered by cutting the jugular vein while reciting the name of Allah. Swine flesh is prohibited (*haram*), as is blood. Game, which might be thought not to qualify as *halal*, is deemed *halal* if the hunter is a Muslim, the means of death is rapid, without suffering, and the name of Allah is invoked before the animal is killed. While the majority of Pakistanis have no religious problems eating any kind of fish, some, like the Isna Ashri Shias and the Bohras—Muslim sects that are followers of Hazrat Ali (RA)—do not eat fish without scales, while the former does not eat shell fish, either. They regard these fish as 'makrouh'—those food items that are not prohibited by Islam but are frowned upon.

Haleem. Originally a Persian dish, *haleem* is a thick, pasty, high-calorie dish which, it is said, was invented, like many others, by the 6th century Persian king, Khosrow, and when Muslims conquered Persia a century later, it became a firm favourite of the Prophet (PBUH). It later became popular with the Mughal emperors (it is mentioned in the *Ain-i-Akbari*) and subsequently became a renowned delicacy at the hands of Hyderabadi chefs. Although the dish varies in form from region to region, it generally includes cracked grains of wheat, two kinds of pulses—*chana* and *mung*—spices, and meat (usually beef or mutton, though increasingly chicken *haleem* is becoming the rage). It is cooked for seven to eight hours, all the while stirred vigorously so that the lentils and wheat are crushed into a smooth paste, before it is ready to be served. Since it is packed with nutrients it is an instant energy-giver and is particularly popular at meals after breaking a fast. It is associated with the tenth of Muharram (the first month in the Islamic calendar), a day of mourning and usually a day of fasting. *Haleem* is garnished with crispy fried onions, chopped green chillies, julienne ginger, and a touch of lemon. Sister versions of the dish are known as *khichra* and *harisa*. It may be noted that the Bohra *haleem* is different from the Hyderabadi *haleem* as in the Bohra *haleem* no pulses are used, and it is made purely from wheat and mashed meat that has been boiled beforehand. Traditionally, the Bohra *haleem* is eaten with *bharta*, a combination of yoghurt and eggplant, and *kaddi*, a tangy, yoghurt-based curry, and *karak roti*.

SHAHA TARIQ

Half gosht. Unlike most meat curry dishes, *half gosht* is a Khoja community speciality made with mutton and *chanay ki daal*, but the *bhoonna* process takes place after adding the meat rather than at the beginning. Hence, ingredients like onion, that is normally fried brown right in the beginning of the cooking process, remains 'half' cooked as it is only sautéed at the end.

Halwa. The name for a hugely varied range of confections made in the Middle East, Central Asia, Pakistan and India, *halwa* is derived from the Arabic word *hulw*, meaning sweet. In the 7th century Arabia, the word meant a paste of dates kneaded with milk. By the 9th century, possibly by assimilating the ancient Persian sweetmeat *afroshag*, it had acquired the meaning of wheat flour or semolina, cooked by frying or toasting, and worked into a more-or-less stiff paste with a sweetening agent such as sugar syrup, date syrup, or honey by stirring the mass together over a gentle heat. Usually, a flavouring was added such as nuts, rosewater, saffron, or raisins. The finished sweetmeat could be cut into bars or moulded into fanciful shapes. As the popularity of *halwa* spread far and wide, it began to be made with a wide variety of ingredients, methods and flavourings. Brought by Arabs to the subcontinent, *halwa* has many variations; the simplest recipe requires semolina or wheat flour to be fried in *ghee*, mixed with sugar syrup and raisins, and cooked till fluffy or to a dense, pasty consistency (*suji ka halwa/atta ka halwa*). Another popular *halwa* variety is softer and wetter, made basically of a seasonal fruit or vegetable—although gram flours and wheat flour are just as common—ubiquitously served as dessert when the fruit or vegetable is in full season. Popular variations include *lauki ka halwa* (made with Calabash, also known as bottle gourd), *gajar ka halwa* (made with carrots), and *khajoor ka halwa* (made with dates). Another distinct *halwa* is *Gawadari halwa*, a green, jelly-like, chewy *halwa* made with sugar syrup, *nishasta* flour (fermented, sprouted flour) paste, oil and dry fruit, found only on the coastal belt of Balochistan.

Halwa puri. The word *halwa,* originally derived from the Arabic root *hulw* (sweet), is used to describe many distinct types of sweet confection across the Middle East, Central Asia, South Asia, and the Balkans. *Halwa* can take many forms, but the one popularly eaten with *puri* is made with semolina (*suji*). Generally eaten at breakfast, especially on holidays, *halwa puri* basically comprises *suji ka halwa* eaten with deep-fried *puri* made with flour. It is a favourite breakfast item sold at wayside restaurants and *dhaba*s.

Handi. A thick, round-bottomed, deep, and wide-mouthed cooking vessel, *handi* is used specifically for cooking certain Pakistani foods. It is one of the many traditional utensils that will be found in most Pakistani kitchens, without the use of which it would be difficult to muster the right flavour, especially in certain dishes. Since every vessel conducts heat in a different way, the flavour of the final product alters depending on the kind of pan used for cooking a particular dish, even if the ingredients in each case are the same. Therefore, many dishes are only prepared in specific kinds of pots and pans in order to acquire their authentic tastes.

Harappa. The Harappa civilisation flourished in the general area of the Indus Valley from about 3200 BC for 1000 years or a little more. Wheat and barley were the staples and archaeological evidence has recently brought to light the many other foods which were then in common use, as well as the huge granaries built for storage, the ovens, and various cooking utensils. Excavations uncovered peas as well as oilseeds. An 'unmistakable lump of charred sesame' has been discovered at Harappa at a depth of about two metres. Judging from representations of fruits excavated, pomegranates, bananas, coconuts, and lotus were known in Harappan times. Possibly, agriculture was not a complex operation. Agricultural tools have nowhere been found in the valley, though ploughs were known and beautiful clay models of ploughs have been recovered in Harappa. Annual flood inundation along the natural channels was employed for irrigation, as in the Indus Valley system. Flat metal and clay plates resembling modern-day *tawa* have been found at Harappan sites, indicating that baked *chapati* may have been known. Judging from the number of bones excavated, it can be said that animal-based foods such as beef, buffalo, mutton, turtle, tortoise, and river and sea fish were consumed in abundance. Among the nishada types described in the *Yajurveda* are *svanin* (dog keepers), *chandala* (dog eaters), and *punjistha* (fowlers), indicative of the fact that dogs and fowls were domesticated and consumed before the arrival of the Aryans. This is further confirmed by archaeological evidence from Harappa.

Hari mirch aur qeema. Made with minced beef, *hari mirch aur qeema* is a Hyderabadi dish that comprises minced meat marinated in yoghurt and spices and cooked with onions and lots of water. The green chillies (*hari mirch*) are added halfway through the cooking and the dish is allowed to simmer until the water dries up.

Harissa. A Kashmiri speciality, *harissa* comprises beef cooked with green gram into a thick paste. It is served only in winter.

Havan dasta. This is a Sanskrit word implying preparation for rituals which often required herbs and spices to be freshly pounded and thrown into the sacred fire. *Havan* (mortar) is a smooth, deep bowl with a narrow bottom and wide mouth, usually made of copper, stone, metal or wood. *Dasta* from the Persian *dast* meaning hand is a short, stout, pestle made of the same material as the mortar and used upright in a circular motion for pounding or grinding ingredients. Pulverising spices by using a pestle and mortar helps them to retain more of the flavouring elements than when they are blitzed to a powder in a grinder.

SHAHA TARIQ

Hazara. A Persian-speaking people living mainly in Quetta, genetically, the Hazaras are primarily a mixture of eastern Eurasian and western Eurasian peoples. In fact, genetic research suggests that they are closely related to the Mongols and the Uyghurs and are descendants of Changez Khan—a theory supported by the similarities in the language and words that Mongols and Hazaras use even today. Another plausible theory is that Hazaras were Buddhists who actually lived in Afghanistan at least since the time of the Kushan Dynasty some 2,000 years ago. It is believed that they migrated in the 1880s from central Afghanistan into British India and settled to the east of Quetta. Their cuisine is similar to that of Afghan immigrants.

Hindkowan. For Hindkowans, while their food is similar to that eaten in the rest of the Khyber Pakhtunkhwa province, the stress is more on *saag* and *daal* rather than on meat-based dishes. Depending on the availability, *roti* made with *jowar* or *gehon* (wheat) is eaten, while traditionally only *makai ki roti* was popular. Their special bread is called *maani* which is wheat *roti* made with egg and milk, similar to a thin pancake. Depending on preference, it can be made sweet, or saltish. In Ramazan, *ghee* is taken on a daily basis at *sehri* (meal taken before *fajr* [morning] prayers) with *daal* or *qeema* (minced meat). It is eaten with *roti* or *paratha. Chapli kebab* is eaten at every *iftar*.

Hindu cuisine. Although there is a miniscule Hindu population left in Pakistan with most of them primarily located in Sindh—where there are Gujarati Hindus in the cities and Sindhi Hindus in the rural areas—and Kashmir, their cuisine is different from that of the average Pakistani who tends to be a meat eater.

Hindu cuisine has an important place in ancient texts, as a proper diet is considered vital for spiritual development. The concept is that purity of thought depends on the purity of food. Traditionally, rules must be observed before and after eating the food (for instance, greeting the food) and different diets followed in different seasons. All this leads to good health which is necessary to fulfil various aspects of life such as *dharma, arth, kama, moksha*. There are also class-based regulations on what to eat. According to ancient texts, there are three categories of food (based on the effect it has on the body or temperament): *satvic, rajasic,* and *tamasic.*

Over the years the restrictions and rules are no longer as strictly followed as they used to be in ancient times, and Hindus living in the larger cities of Pakistan have adapted themselves to Pakistani culture to such a great extent that many have begun to even eat beef—once considered forbidden owing to religious reasons—what to talk of mutton and other meats.

But, by and large, Hindus do not eat beef; many are semi-vegetarian, avoiding red meat altogether, and only occasionally allowing themselves to eat fish or chicken. However, interestingly enough, in Pakistan, for instance, Kashmiri Pandits, despite being Brahmins, tend to be voracious meat eaters—although a bias for non-vegetarian dishes certainly exists.

Kashmiri Pandit food is very elaborate and is an important part of the local Hindu cultural identity. The food usually uses a lot of yoghurt, oils, and spices such as turmeric, asafoetida, cinnamon, cardamoms, cloves, and dried ginger, which form the base of the curries, but avoids onion, garlic, chicken, eggs, and tomatoes.

Thus, Hindu cuisine remains distinct, and although many of their specialities are made by other communities as well, such as by Muslim Gujaratis, whose cuisine is similar to that of Hindu Gujaratis, some of the ingredients used in Hindu cuisine, like *hing* (asafoetida) are peculiar only to their foods, and rarely used by the other Pakistani communities. Similarly, most Hindu dishes are prepared in green chutney—made with ground mint and coriander leaves—and the use of *garam masala* otherwise common in Pakistani cuisine is minimal. Another peculiarity of Hindu cuisine is that meat items are cooked separately from vegetarian ones and the two are rarely, if ever, combined.

A Sindhi dish cooked by upper-caste Hindus, who avoid onions, ginger, and garlic because they grow underground, is *elaichi gosht*. Among the poorer Hindus, *lapsi karhi, palak paneer,* and soybean are popular dishes. However, in the desert regions of Sindh, Hindu inhabitants known as Tharis have a particularly distinct cuisine. Though the emphasis is more on nutrition than on fuss and ostentation, given the harsh climatic conditions, it is commendable that the Hindus of Thar have produced so much variety from so little. They are strict vegetarians and will not even use garlic and onion in their cuisine. Dried lentils and beans from indigenous plants are the staples of their diet. *Gawar* (green beans) and *chabber* (gherkins) are among the popular vegetables that are boiled and dried and stored for use in later months. Just before serving, they are deep fried for a few seconds, sprinkled with chillies, and, in the case of the former, rock salt.

Millet and maize are used for making various kinds of bread. They use a lot of pulses and gram flour in their cuisine as vegetables are scarce in the desert climate. *Mung daal khilni* (a dry preparation of lentils, tossed in a mixture of spices), *mung godi ki sabzi* (grape-size dumplings of green gram, which have been ground to a paste and sun-dried), and *gatte ki sabzi* (rolls of gram flour, steamed and cooked in buttermilk sauce) are delicacies in this region. Other innovations include the use of mango powder as a substitute for tomatoes, and asafoetida to enhance taste in the absence of garlic and onions. Sweets are also very popular.

ANJALI MALIK AND SHANAZ RAMZI

Hoilo garma. A Hunza speciality, *hoilo garma* is a fresh mustard greens dish cooked with hand-rolled pasta, onions, and potatoes, and crushed almonds and pine nuts. Cooked in a special Hunza apricot or kernel oil, it has an interesting flavour. The pasta is often replaced by un-roasted *chapati* cut into pieces, thus saving on fuel-wood that would have been used for cooking the ingredients separately.

Hunza water. Deceptively called Hunza water, this is a home-made mulberry wine that is served to all guests—in spite of the Islamic prohibition on liquor—by some Hunzakutz and is famous for bestowing long life and youth to its consumers.

Hunzakutz. The people living in Hunza known as Hunzakutz are believed to have descended from five wandering soldiers of Alexander's army—their fair skin and light-coloured eyes lending credence to the legend. Regarded as people who do not age—a myth probably supported by the fact that National Geographic magazine selected Hunza as a kingdom where people lived the longest—Hunzakutz grow maize, wheat, buckwheat, barley, millet, and fruits including apricots, apples, peaches, pears, and pomegranates, as well as certain vegetables and walnuts. Hence, most of their dishes include one or more of these ingredients.

In northern Pakistan, in the high valley of Hunza, food availability has undergone a substantial change in the last five or six decades. Access to Hunza valley, which lies in the heart of the Karakoram Mountains (Western Himalayas), was quite difficult for a long time. But the completion of the international Karakoram Highway, in 1978, became a turning point for Hunza. Traversing the valley, the highway became a thoroughfare between Islamabad and Beijing, opening up Hunza to a variety of extraordinary changes. While earlier, rice, chutneys, curries, processed sweets, and other such delectable items were rare in the area, now they are easily available in local bazaars, and global consumer products are a part of everyday life for the younger generation. Nonetheless, the lifestyles of the scattered mountain tribes have not undergone any radical change over the years and they continue to grow fruits as their staple food. Hunzakutz have an especially high intake of apricots—which is perhaps, the secret to their long and healthy lives. In the summer months, in order to conserve fuel and precious cereals, cooking is forbidden; hence, the Hunzakutz eat nothing other than apricots, and drink juices made from dried apricots. In winter, they eat bread made from apricot kernel flour, and drink soup made from dried apricots, and brandy made from distilled mulberries and wines from the grapes that grow everywhere. They also consume milk products such as buttermilk, yoghurt, butter, and cheese. *Maltash* is the preciously guarded 'aged butter' of the Hunzakutz.

However, the Hunzakuts do have time-honoured, traditional dishes, which, although now largely limited to community celebrations, are still made by households where the elders call the shots. Some of the dishes even have folktales attached to them—for instance, *diram phitti*, a sweet bread which is made from germinated wheat flour, is connected to a folktale about the seed of life. However, the elders feel that even these traditional dishes made today have a different taste from their original versions as the salt sold in the bazaar, either granulated or as chunks of rock, has a different flavour from the salt from local sources. Also, flour which was previously ground at a local water-mill had a different texture from the flour now produced by an electric mill, and this is again different from the flour imported from China.

For the elders, the *bokhari* (steel oven) has itself been an innovation, for they had learned to cook at the *shee* (hearth), using stone pots, when there was no *shuli* (stovepipe) to remove smoke from the single-room farmhouse. All of them know the difference in taste between *phitti* baked in a *tandoor* of sorts, and *phitti* baked in an electric oven.

Huqqa. A single or multi-stemmed instrument for smoking tobacco in which the smoke is cooled and filtered by passing through water, *huqqa* was once popular as much with the nobility as with villagers and was an integral part of many a middleclass household. Today, its usage is almost entirely restricted to villages, and has been replaced in the cities by its close cousin introduced from the Middle East, the *sheesha*, which incorporates fruit flavours.

Hyderabadi achar. *Achar* is an Indo-Aryan word used for pickles in the subcontinent. Hot weather and an intrinsic love for spices have ensured that a huge variety of pickles is always available on any South Asian menu. The *achar* made in Hyderabad Sindh, popularly known as Hyderabadi *achar* is richer than most other *achars* as it is prepared in oil as opposed to water common in other varieties. This allows for the preservation of fruits and vegetables used in the pickle, throughout the year. Typically, raw mangoes, carrots, lime, green chillies, and garlic are tossed together in spices and marinated in vinegar and oil. The pickle does not go bad for years, and particularly complements the patent *daal chawal* or *khichri*, with which it is normally consumed with gusto.

Traditionally, most households used to mix and prepare their own pickles at the beginning of the respective season that the fruit or vegetable was available. While the increasingly fast pace of life in urban centres has made this practice less common, and most households prefer to buy the packaged variety stocked in stores, rather than indulge in the process of cutting and drying the ingredients, they are still made at home in the semi-urban and rural areas.

Hyderabadi *achar* is very much a summer pickle as its main ingredient is raw mango. These days *achar* mixes (spices used to make *achar*) are also available in the market and are often used in curries and may be mixed in *daal* for adding that extra zing to it.

SHAHA TARIQ

Hyderabadi cuisine. The city of Hyderabad was founded in 1589 by Muhammad Quli Qutb Shah, and the Muslim royalty there created a complete distinctive cuisine. However, the history of current Hyderabadi cuisine begins in the 17th century, with the Deccan campaigns.

Over a period of nearly a century, the Mughal armies annexed great areas of southern India to their territories. Over the years, the Mughlai cuisine, brought from the north, slowly evolved, being influenced by the local ingredients, climate, and cuisines encountered along the way. A blend of Mughlai flavours, influenced by the renowned chefs of the royal families or Nizams of Hyderabad Deccan in South India and the cuisine of its Hindu majority population—which commonly used coconut, tamarind, jaggery, peanuts, poppy seeds, sesame seeds, and mustard seeds—gave rise to a distinct rich style of food preparation, which became an identifying feature of the Qutb Shahi Dynasty that believed in promoting the local cuisine. Its singular and most distinguishing feature was the sourness or tanginess of its dishes. With 400 years of history helping it evolve, the cuisine has all Mughlai, Persian, and Telugu strains combined to perfection.

During and after the Partition, Karachi received thousands of Muslim immigrants from Hyderabad Deccan. These people brought with them their traditional dishes and flavours, and over a period of time these delicious delicacies took a permanent place in Pakistani cuisine so much so that today many of the Hyderabadi specialities are cooked by other ethnic groups in Karachi as well.

Pickles and dried meats are quite popular in Hyderabadi cuisine. Among their leavened, oven-baked breads are *kulcha*—a square bread marked with cross-lines—and the sweetish *sheermal*. *Sookha gosht* (dried strips of marinated beef), Bombay duck, sweet and sour green chillies (dried), and *mingoray* (dried crispy lentil dumplings) are part of almost every Hyderabadi meal. The Hyderabadi *kacchi biryani*, a hot favourite with not just the community but with others as well, has a distinct taste with its rice remaining firm and the chunks of meat cooked to almost disintegration. Use of mustard oil instead of other variables gives it a particular edge.

Another Hyderabadi speciality is *haleem*, a finely-ground paste of both wheat and meat, delicately spiced. *Nargisi koftay* (full-boiled eggs cut into halves in a minced-meat coating), *dalcha* (mutton stewed with lentils and tamarind), and *bagharay baingan* (eggplants cooked in a tart, tamarind base) are all Hyderabadi dishes that bear testimony to the imaginative use of local ingredients to create totally new concoctions.

SHANAZ RAMZI AND SHAHA TARIQ

I

Idli. Small, round, greyish white, rice cake, known as *idli*, this is a South Indian speciality. It seems to have been first mentioned in writing in Shivakotiacharya's *Vaddaradhane*, a Kannada work of AD 920, as one of the 18 items offered as refreshment by a lady to a visiting brahmachari. Thereafter, it is frequently mentioned, and in AD 1025 the poet Chavundaraya described it unequivocally as *urad daal* soaked in buttermilk, ground to a fine paste, mixed with the clear water of curd, cumin, coriander, pepper and asafoetida, and then shaped. However, in all mentions, three elements of the modern *idli*—the use of rice grits, grinding and overnight fermentation of the mix, and steaming of the batter—are missing. Literature offers no certain answers as to when in the last few centuries these elements entered the picture. The earliest the origin of the present-day *idli* can be traced to is AD 1129–30 as a book called *Manasollasa*—an early 12th-century Sanskrit text composed by the Kalyani Chalukya king Someshvara III, who ruled in present-day South India—from that period has its recipe. Nonetheless, today, *idli* is made from a dough of ground rice and *urad daal*, fermented overnight. *Idli* is steamed in a special pan which has several smoothly rounded indentations. They are often eaten with coconut chutney or sometimes dipped in a spicy mixture consisting of coarsely ground toasted spices and *daal*. It is not as popular in Pakistan as other South Indian dishes, such as *masala dosa*, and is largely cooked just by the migrant families now settled in Pakistan.

Iftari. This meal is eaten after sunset in Ramazan. Traditionally, a fast is broken at *iftar* time with dates or salt, after which various snack items followed by main meal dishes are consumed. For *iftar* it is the norm to serve *pakoray*, *chaat* items, particularly fruit *chaat*, and *mithai* such as *jalebi* and *halwa*. Sherbet (a refreshing syrup such as Hamdard's Rooh Afza or Qarshi's Jam-e-Shirin) added to water or milk, is another favourite in most households.

Imli aur aaloo bukharay ka sherbet. This is a refreshing drink made of tamarind (*imli*) and dried plum (*aaloo bukhara*), and served in summer months in Sindh, especially by thoroughbred Sindhis.

Imli ke phool. A Dilliwalla speciality, *imli ke phool* consists of tamarind flowers—thus its name—cooked with mutton *qeema* and onions.

Indus Valley Civilisation. Indus Civilisation, also called Indus Valley Civilisation (*c*.3300–1300 BC, flourished from 2600–1900 BC) or Harappan Civilisation so called after the first excavated city of Harappa, is the earliest known urban culture of the subcontinent. The Indus River begins high up in the Himalayan mountains (the tallest mountain range in the world) and flows nearly 3,000 km to the Arabian Sea. As the river moves downstream it carves out a valley. This is where the Indus people settled. The civilisation was first identified in 1921 at Harappa in the Punjab region and then in 1922 at Mohenjo-Daro, near the Indus River in the Sindh region. Subsequently, remains of the civilisation were found as far apart as Sutkagen Dor in south-western Balochistan, near the shore of the Arabian Sea, about 300 miles (480 km) west of Karachi, and in north-western India, making it the most extensive of the world's three earliest civilisations. At its peak, the Indus Civilisation reportedly had a population of more than five million people.

Aside from the two large cities of Harappa and Mohenjo-Daro, the Indus Civilisation is known to have consisted of over 1,052 cities and settlements often of relatively small size mainly in the general region of the Indus River and its tributaries. The two large cities were each originally about one square mile (1.6 sq km) in overall dimensions, and their outstanding magnitude suggests political centralisation, either in two large states or in a single great empire with alternative capitals. It is also possible that Harappa succeeded Mohenjo-Daro, which is known to have been devastated more than once by exceptional floods.

The Indus cities are noted for their urban planning, baked brick houses, elaborate drainage systems, water supply systems, and clusters of large non-residential buildings. These are believed to be large storage structures (granaries) established as a state enterprise in Mohenjo-Daro, Harappa and Lothal, of surprising degrees of sophistication in terms of aeration and rodent control. Adjacent to the granaries were placed grain-pounding platforms. Partly buried pottery jars were used for domestic storage. Grain-pounding cylinders and spice-grinding querns were of designs still in common use, as were hearths and baking ovens. Cooking and dining vessels were made of clay, shell, chert, bronze, and copper. Alcohol was brewed, and apparently even distilled. Trade networks linked this culture with related regional cultures and distant sources of raw materials, including lapis lazuli and other materials for bead-making.

By 2500 BC, irrigation had transformed the region. The Indus Civilisation apparently evolved from the villages of neighbours or predecessors, using the Mesopotamian model of irrigated agriculture with sufficient skill to reap the advantages of the spacious and fertile Indus River valley while controlling the formidable annual flood that simultaneously fertilised and destroyed. The civilisation subsisted primarily by farming, supplemented by an appreciable but often elusive commerce. Wheat and six-row barley were grown; field peas, mustard, sesame, and a few date stones have also been found, as well as some of the earliest known traces of cotton. Domesticated animals included dogs and cats, humped and shorthorn cattle, domestic fowl, and possibly pigs, camels, and buffalo. The Asian elephant probably was also domesticated, and its ivory tusks were freely used. Great numbers of small terracotta figures of animals and humans have been excavated.

Minerals, unavailable from the alluvial plain were sometimes brought in from far afield. The main streets were almost ten metres wide—wide enough for two bullock carts or elephants to pass each other. Drains ran along the edge of the streets to carry the garbage away, and wells were dug for clean water.

How and when the civilisation came to an end remains uncertain. In fact, no uniform ending needs be postulated for a culture so widely distributed. But the end of Mohenjo-Daro is believed to have been dramatic and sudden. One school of thought holds

that Mohenjo-Daro was attacked toward the middle of the 2nd millennium BC by raiders who swept over the city and then passed on, leaving the dead lying where they fell. Who the attackers were, is a matter for conjecture. The episode would appear to be consistent in time and place with the earlier invaders from the north (formerly called Aryans) into the Indus region as reflected in the older books of the *Rigveda*. However, another school holds that the Indus Valley Civilisation did not disappear suddenly, and that many elements of the Indus Civilisation can be found in later cultures. Current archaeological data also suggests that material culture classified as Late Harappan may have persisted until at least *c*.1000–900 BC.

However, one thing is clear: the city was already in an advanced stage of economic and social decline before it received the *coup de grâce*. Deep floods had more than once submerged large tracts of it. Houses had become increasingly inferior in construction and showed signs of overcrowding. The final blow seems to have been sudden, but the city was already dying. As the evidence stands, the civilisation was succeeded in the Indus Valley by poverty-stricken cultures, deriving a little from a sub-Indus heritage but also drawing elements from the direction of Iran and the Caucasus from the general direction, in fact, of the northern invasions. For many centuries urban civilisation was dead in the northwest of the subcontinent.

The names Harappa and Mohenjo-Daro were given to the cities in later times. We do not know what the Indus people called their cities, because nobody has been able to translate their ancient language.

BISMA TIRMIZI

Irani restaurant. In the middle of the 19th century, Iranis, particularly Zoroastrians, settled in Karachi in large numbers, many of whom opened up restaurants, following the footsteps of their predecessors, who had moved to the subcontinent from Iran in the 10th century, and were mostly in business.

With more than a hundred Irani restaurants in Karachi alone by the 1970s, all flourishing, it is no wonder that even today, when there are so few left that they could be counted on the fingers of one hand, they are still regarded as an important part of Karachi's heritage. Most Irani 'hotels' or 'cafes', as they were commonly known, were confined to the older parts of the city, and, with the exception of one or two, such as Café Liberty, none ventured into the relatively newer and more modern areas—which is perhaps one of the reasons why they gradually began to fade out.

Known as much for the quality of their snacks as for their food and tea, these Irani restaurants were particularly popular with the middle-class as they were good value for money. From patties to *chullu kebab*, and from *mahi kebab* to spicy *pulao*, and even succulent beef steak, each of the numerous Iranian joints was famous for one signature food item or the other. With their marble topped tables and bentwood chairs, and large mirrors which give the impression of extra space, these spacious eateries offered basic comfort and décor to its unfussy clients.

Almost invariably located at street corners, these eateries would be open on two sides. Among the more famous Irani restaurants in Karachi there were four in close proximity to one another, namely, Fredrick's Cafeteria, Café George, Eastern Coffee House, and Pioneer Coffee House, all located in Saddar, the downtown commercial hub of the city. Eastern Coffee House, previously known as Zelin's Coffee House before it was bought over by an Irani, was the haunt of writers and student leaders. While most Irani restaurants were only frequented by men, Fredrick's Cafeteria and Eastern Coffee House had sections for families as well.

Irani restaurants may be vanishing but they have left their mark on their city. Proof of this lies in the fact that famous areas in Karachi such as the Tariq Road and Allama Iqbal Road intersection, and the area near Fleet Club, are still called by the names of the Irani restaurants that graced those locations—Café Liberty and Lucky Star, respectively—long after these restaurants pulled down their shutters.

Irrigation. Irrigation from Indus waters has been the basis for successful agriculture in the region since time immemorial. Rising in Tibet, the Indus is one of the longest rivers in the world, with a length of some 2,000 miles (3,200 km) and total drainage area of about 450,000 square miles (1,165,000 sq km), of which 175,000 square miles (453,000 sq km) lie in the ranges and foothills of the Himalayas. It flows down through the Karakoram Mountains that form a part of the northern borders of Pakistan and continues its journey southwards and westwards through the heart of the country, carrying and depositing rich alluvium that accounts for Punjab's highly fertile soil. Prior to Partition, its five tributaries—Jhelum, Chenab, Sutlej, Ravi, and Beas—used to irrigate the Punjab, giving the province its name ('*punj*' means 'five' and '*aab*' means 'water' in Persian).

Modern irrigation engineering work commenced about 1850, and, during the period of British administration, large canal systems were constructed. In many cases, old canals and inundation channels in the Sindh and Punjab regions were revived and modernised. Thus, the greatest system of canal irrigation in the world was created.

However, in 1947, when the subcontinent was partitioned by the British into two independent states—Pakistan and India—a commission was set up to resolve any issue that may emerge as a consequence. The matter of utilisation of water resources of Indus Basin was raised by Pakistan. The boundary commission, chaired by Sir Cyril Radcliffe, awarded control of barrages (situated very close to the border) to India, although 90 per cent of irrigated land lay in Pakistan.

After a protracted negotiation over ten years through facilitation of the World Bank, the Indus Waters Treaty was signed between India and Pakistan in 1960 for distribution of water resources in the Indus Basin. According to the terms of the treaty, India was given the exclusive use of the waters of the eastern rivers namely Ravi, Sutlej, and Beas. Pakistan was not given its full historic share and was allocated only 75 per cent of its legitimate share of the waters in Indus Basin. Consequently, Pakistan decided to embark upon a gigantic project: Indus Basin Replacement Works. The extensive undertaking involved the construction of two major dams, five barrages, and eight link canals.

Today, Pakistan's vast farm lands are sustained by the Indus Basin Irrigation System (IBIS), the largest contiguous irrigation system in the world. The IBIS irrigates 45 million acres of farm land which produces wheat, rice, fruits, vegetables, sugarcane, maize, and cotton in abundance for local use as well as for export.

Pakistan's economy is largely based on its agricultural produce. Water is, therefore, a critical resource for its sustained economic development. The IBIS comprises three large dams, 85 small dams, 19 barrages, 12 inter-river link canals, 45 canal commands and 0.7 million tube wells, and there is still room for the construction of more.

Islam and food. Islam is the faith of nearly 15 per cent of the world's population. It has a certain underlying unity, springing from the simplicity and straightforwardness of Prophet Muhammad's (PBUH) message. The simplicity is evident in Muslim dietary laws and the basic tenets of the faith. The Quran mentions food often and praises it as one of God's gifts to humanity. Islam enjoins that no food be wasted, even leftovers being saved and eaten.

With the advent of Islam in the subcontinent through Arab invasion, the country's cuisine underwent changes since dietary injunctions as prescribed by the Quran and Sunnah had to be taken into consideration. Hence, swine meat became prohibited (*haram*), as also blood, and it became mandatory that animal meat for consumption had to be *halal*, i.e. it is slaughtered by cutting the jugular vein while reciting the name of Allah. Game, which might be thought not to qualify, is deemed *halal* if the hunter is a Muslim, the means of death is rapid, without suffering, and the name of Allah is invoked before the animal is killed.

Alcohol is forbidden in Islam and, therefore, is not sold publicly to Muslims in the country. Seafood is allowed, though certain sects do not patronise all kinds of seafood. *Makrooh* is an intermediate category found in the Shia sect, and indicates food item which is somewhat frowned upon, although not prohibited. Examples are shellfish and some birds.

Fasting is enjoined on all Muslims during Ramazan, the ninth month of the Muslim lunar year, with a meal before sunrise (*sehri*) and one after sunset (*iftar*), which should preferably commence by eating some dates.

J

Jaggery. Gritty, brown sugar of the subcontinent, jaggery is called *gur* in Urdu. Though the sugarcane itself is mentioned even in the *Rigveda*, the mention of solid *guda*, made by boiling sugarcane juice, first occurs a millennium later in Sutra literature. All through history, jaggery has been the low-cost sweetener with a distinctive flavour. While health conscious people in the cities are beginning to replace sugar with jaggery in their diet, it has always been a popular sweetener in the villages and smaller towns. In the northern areas of Pakistan, *masala gur* which has spices added to it, is served as *hors d'oeuvres* rather than a sweetener.

Jalebi. The '*jil-abi*' is first mentioned by this name in AD 1600 in Kannada literature, and as *jilebi* later. According to Hobson-Jobson, *jilebi* is 'apparently a corruption of the Arabic *zalabiya* or Persian *zalibiya*'. A Jain scripture penned in AD 1450, by Jinasura, has a reference to a feast which includes the *jalebi*. It has been described 'like a creeper, tasty as nectar' made of *chana* flour. According to Hobson-Jobson, *jalebi* is saffron and sugar-drenched, deep fried, pretzel-shaped sweetmeat with a Persian influence. Later it became as popular in Mughal courts as it is today in Pakistan.

Essentially, the *jalebi* is a flat, spiral of fermented batter, about 8 cm wide, which is crisp fried and, while still hot, soaked in sugar syrup (scented with saffron and rosewater) of medium consistency and then taken out after a while. The spirals are formed by piping the batter into hot oil with a cone of sorts.

The batter varies in different areas. It usually comprises plain flour, baking powder, and water but may include other ingredients such as ground white lentils with a little rice flour as a binder, or ground chickpeas and flour; both the mixtures are sometimes slightly fermented with curd. A crisp texture and golden colour are sought, for which colouring is used.

Jalebi is a must in practically every affording household in the month of Ramazan, when it forms a regular feature at the *iftar* table, and is often also partaken of, dabbed in milk, at *sehri*, as it is believed to quench thirst.

Jardaloo salli murgha. Basically, this is a Parsi chicken dish, but its variation, *jardaloo salli gosht* could also be made with boneless pieces of meat instead of chicken. This recipe, incorporating dried apricot, red vinegar, and sugar along with a blend of mouth-watering local spices has strong Persian touches. Topped with fried potato shoestrings, this dish is served on auspicious occasions. *Jardaloo* (dry apricots) are soaked in water for a few hours, par-boiled, and gently folded in the dish before serving. To make the *salli*, grated potatoes are soaked in water and then strained and deep-fried till golden and crispy. They are then added to the half-cooked mutton and simmered until the meat becomes tender.

ZARNAK SIDHWA

Jat. In ancient times, Jats inhabited the whole valley of the Indus down to Sindh. They now form a vast and important section of the agricultural population of the Punjab. In fact, Punjab's population basically comprises indigenous Punjabis who trace their ancestry to pre-Islamic Jat and Rajput castes that arrived from Rajputana and Jaisalmer, later inter-marrying with other ethnic groups, which came to the area. In southwest Punjab, the name Jat covers various tribes. The name's significance tends to be occupational: to denote a body of cultivators or agriculturists.

Jhal frezi. An Anglo-Indian dish that became popular with aristocratic locals during the British Raj, *jhal frezi* is meat and vegetables stir-fried in thick, spicy, red-sauce, generally served with toasted bread triangles. It continued to feature as an important dish on the menus of all clubs and most restaurants till a few years ago and is still popular with the older generation in urban centres, who have associations and memories attached with the dish.

Kaak/kurnu. Similar to the Rajasthani speciality, *batti*, *kaak* is a rock-hard bread; though not easily digestible, it is popular among the nomadic Baloch. A blow on the stone breaks open the *kaak*. It is made by wrapping dough round a smooth, blazing hot stone and putting it on embers inside the ground. Most people eat their bread plain and without relish, but *krut* (yoghurt pressed in cloth and dried) is sometimes poured over the pieces of bread, to which boiling *ghee* is added. It is also often eaten with *sajji*, cooked in the same fire that is used for preparing *kaak*. Flock owners and camel breeders use milk and its preparations, generally buttermilk, as accompaniments with *kaak*.

Kabuli pulao. A dish of Middle Eastern/Central Asian origin, *pulao* or 'palav' is often considered to be one of the oldest preparations of rice which has Persian roots. In fact, Persian culinary terms referring to rice preparations are numerous and have found their way into the languages of neighbouring areas. *Kabuli pulao* is a rice and chickpeas dish in which the rice is cooked in seasoned broth and then brewed. It was known to have been served to Alexander the Great after he captured modern Samarkand. Alexander's army took the recipe back to Macedonia and spread it throughout Eastern Europe. *Kabuli pulao*, which has come to be regarded as the national dish of Afghanistan and has made its way to Khyber Pakhtunkhwa, is made with chopped nuts such as pistachios and almonds, and dried orange peel, and topped with fried, sliced carrots, and raisins. The dish could be made with lamb, chicken, or beef, and could incorporate other vegetables as well, like cabbage and cauliflower. It is served to special guests and on special occasions like weddings. A similar version known as *jhalla pulao* or *chana mewa* in Peshawar comprises chick peas, meat, rice, and raisins.

Kachaloo (*Colocasia esculenta*). This is a tropical plant grown primarily as a root vegetable for its edible corms, commonly known as taro. It is the most widely cultivated species of several plants in the family Araceae, which are used as vegetables for their corms, leaves and petioles. In Pakistan, taro (*arvi*) is used to make a tangy snack, *kachaloo*, although often people substitute sweet potatoes and even potatoes to make it if taro is unavailable.

Kachcha papita. Raw papaya, *kachcha papita*, is a natural meat tenderiser which contains anti-bacterial properties as an added advantage and promotes good digestion. In fact, the highest concentrations of the beneficial digestive enzyme papain are found in raw papaya. It is often used to tenderise kebabs, such as *Bihari kebab*.

Kachchay gosht ki biryani. A variant of the famous Mughal dish *biryani*, it is essentially layering of Basmati rice and meat (preferably mutton) curry, steam-cooked, and garnished with coriander and chillies. A Hyderabadi speciality, this light, dry *biryani* is prepared by boiling the meat with *garam masala* and yoghurt, as opposed to cooking with tomatoes and in oil. Once the meat is tender, it is added in layers to the almost-boiled rice with an additional layer of browned onions in hot oil. The cooking pot is then made air-tight with a dough sealant to keep the aroma of spices locked in and put on *dum* (the process of simmering on low heat) till the rice is tender, but firm. A complete dish in itself it is traditionally served with cold yoghurt *raita*.

ZUBAIDA TARIQ

Kachchi lassi. A Punjabi, refreshing summer drink, *kachchi lassi* is different from the *lassi* otherwise available everywhere in the country, the basic ingredient for which is yoghurt, while *kachchi lassi* is made with cold milk. A refreshing local sherbet made with rose syrup and extracts of cooling herbal ingredients is generally added to it, though if the sherbet is not available, then any rose syrup, or even rose essence mixed with red food colour suffices. In Khyber

Pakhtunkhwa, however, *kachchi lassi* denotes a drink popular with the Pakhtuns, which is a combination of fresh yoghurt and water, that is neither sweet nor salty.

Kachnar. This is a local name in Pakistan for the edible buds collected from *Bauhinia variegata*, a species of flowering plants in the legume family Fabaceae, that bloom only in spring. It is native to the subcontinent and is widely used as an ingredient in many recipes, particularly in the Punjab, where the terrain is mountainous. Traditional *kachnar* curry is prepared with *kachnar* buds, yoghurt, onions, and spices. *Kachnar* buds are also eaten as a stir-fried vegetable and are also used to make *achar*. It is also cooked with minced beef.

Kachori. A Gujarati *farsan* (salty snack) item, which is eaten either as a snack or with a main meal, *kachori* can be traced to ancient times. Lentil-stuffed, deep fried circular puffs made out of dough, usually based on wheat flour, these are normally accompanied by potato curry and *achar*. A favourite side item at weddings these days, *kachori* is a popular snack sold at wayside stalls also, and often serves as the poor man's main course.

Many different forms of *kachori* exist. Gujaratis generally make it as thick round balls of flour filled with a stuffing of *mung daal*, black pepper, red chilli powder, and ginger paste. Other versions commonly found include thin *puri* stuffed with *mung daal* or *urad daal*, *besan*, ginger paste, and red chilli powder, and served with *aaloo bhurta* (potato curry). The Chakwali (in north Punjab) version comprises stuffed vegetables in deep-fried, square pockets of rolled-out flour dough.

Kachri ka qeema. A small, wild, brown melon found in desert areas, *kachri* is a common ingredient in Rajasthani and Thari cuisine, where it is used as a food tenderiser and is incorporated fresh, although it is available in powder form as well. *Kachri* spoils easily on contact with moisture and should be stored in airtight containers when not in use. Whole *kachri* stays better, and it is best to crush them as and when needed. A speciality of the region, *kachri qeema* is a delicious mutton *qeema* (minced meat) dish, made by marinating the minced meat with grated raw papaya, *kachri*, and spices and then cooking it in yoghurt. The dish is smoked in the end to give it an added flavour.

Kachumar/kachumber. A raw vegetable accompaniment, inspired by the Turkish yoghurt with cucumber side dish, the Pakistani version, *kachumber* usually includes both onion and cucumber and can be served with or without yoghurt. Instead of yoghurt, vinegar is often used. Generally, *kachumber* is a mixture of chopped onions, tomatoes, green chillies, freshly chopped coriander, salt, vinegar or lemon juice or yoghurt, and a sprinkling of red chilli powder.

Kakori kebab. The immense popularity of the Lucknawi *seekh kebab* led to further refinements and improvements, and one *bawarchi* (cook) from Kakori—the small hamlet on the outskirts of Lucknow whose *galavat kebab* are famous—found much acclaim for his efforts in this direction. During the British rule, it was customary in this region for the rich rajas and nawabs to entertain senior British officers and ply them with the best hospitality they could offer. Legend has it that at one such party in Kakori, the host, Nawab Syed Mohammad Haider Kazmi, stung by the remark of a British officer regarding the coarse texture of *seekh kebab*, summoned his cooks and asked them to evolve a more refined version of it. The result was the now famous *Kakori kebab* which was as close to perfection as possible. Of course, the nawab invited the same officer again and presented him with the new version. Needless to say, it met with great applause. Since then, the *seekh kebabs* of Kakori have become famous and have acquired the universal name of *Kakori kebabs*.

Kalakand. The origin of this sweetmeat can perhaps be traced to the period between AD 1000–1500 during which a wheat preparation called *suhali* had become popular. It consists of hard cakes of wheat flour fried in piping hot oil and coated with sugar.

Kalash/Kalasha. Spread over three valleys in the Chitral region, namely, Bumburet, Rumbur, and Birir, the Kalasha or *Kafir* Kalash are the smallest ethno-religious community in Pakistan. They have a distinct lifestyle that is reflected in their cuisine as well. Their ancestry is enveloped in mystery and is the subject of much controversy. The Kalash, believed to have arrived in the Chitral area in the 10th century, came from Bashgal valley, now in Afghanistan. They had been pushed out by other *Kafir* tribes who in turn were being pursued by invading Muslim armies from the west. According to another school of thought, the Kalash descended from the Greeks after the invasion of the subcontinent by Alexander the Great. Even today, the Greeks continue to support the Kalash valley's cultural heritage. During the 7th century AD, much of this area was invaded by the Arab forces and converted to Islam. These valleys are the last enclaves to withstand conversion to Islam. Kalash grow wheat, which constitutes their staple diet, as well as corn and millet. For breakfast they eat cheese, butter, milk, and yoghurt. Their cuisine, like that of the Khows (an ethnic community living in Khyber Pakhtunkhwa), consists mainly of soups and breads of various kinds. Aside from the traditional wheat bread, *tasili*; thin pancake-like wheat bread; bread made of corn or crushed walnuts; and soup made of tomatoes, onions, potatoes, and boiled vegetables are eaten. However, if they cannot afford to eat bread in winter, they stock on fruits such as dried mulberries, apricots, and their kernels from summer to autumn to meet their winter requirements. Their traditional foods also include buttermilk, milk, butter, herbal green tea prepared from herbs and grasses from the high passes, wine, *daal*, rice, walnuts, and kidney beans. Beans are an important source of protein. Kalash sacrifice goats, although they are not primarily meat-eaters. They only eat it at festivals or when it is sacrificed. A sort of porridge is made with the meat's soup and wheat flour. Billy-goats are eaten only by men; however, women may eat the meat if it has been slaughtered in the Islamic way during funerals or at other major festivals. Goat cheese is an essential source of protein produced in the summer, though most of the cheese is eaten by men. A number of festivals are held through the year, connected one way or the other to the crops sown or harvested. Like in other parts of Pakistan, food plays a major role at these events. Eggs and chicken are regarded as forbidden foods by the Kalash though now many tend to eat them; they consider onions to be a blessing sent from the heavens. In olden days, fish from the rivers too, were not eaten. Local wine is prepared during autumn and partaken of especially at festivals.

Kaleji (liver). This is a delicacy in Pakistan, as indeed are other organs like brain and kidneys. Calf's liver is generally considered the best among animals, because of the smooth texture and delicate flavour. Lamb's liver is smaller but also delicate as is chicken liver, which is widely eaten too, and is popularly cooked as a curry, barbecued, or lightly fried in masala. The trick is not so much in the way it is cooked as in the time taken to cook it, as it hardens if cooked for too long. Liver is a rich source of vitamin A and B-12, as well as iron so has health benefits as well, in spite of being high in cholesterol.

Kali. A Khow (an ethnic community living in Khyber Pakhtunkhwa) speciality, *kali* is a soup made with pieces of bread boiled in water and then mixed in a broth made from *ghee*, onions, tomatoes, red pepper, and milk or water left over from the preparation of cheese. Meat can also be added to the soup.

Kalmi bara. A Dilliwallay speciality, *kalmi bara* are *daal bhajia* (fried whole *mung* lentil dumplings) cut in wedges and then re-fried to a crisp brown.

Kalmi shora (potassium nitrate). Also known as saltpetre, this is crystallised salt used in many recipes such as hunter beef. It is used for food preservation and colour retention, particularly in cured meats, and helps to tenderise meat and reduce cooking time.

Kanji. This is a Punjabi beverage made from black carrots that sprout very briefly in the season. The carrots used to make *kanji* are peeled, dried, cut lengthwise, and put in an earthenware pot along with mustard seeds, salt, and water. The pot is then kept out in the sun to ferment for five to seven days before it is ready for consumption and is considered to be very cooling. It is regarded to be beneficial for the liver and digestive system.

On the other hand, the Gujaratis use the term *kanji* for residual starchy water (derived from the Sanskrit *kanjika*) in which rice has been boiled, or even for a weak suspension of boiled rice in its water. It is used as food for invalids, or nursing mothers, with milk substituting water. Frequently, the product is left to sour overnight and drunk as a morning beverage, either hot or cold.

Kantra. In the Gujarati community, *kantra* is served to the nursing mother daily, for the first few months after childbirth, as it is believed to increase milk flow and strengthen the back. Comprising dry fruit, herbs, and gum cooked together, *kantra* is a nourishing source of energy normally consumed more in winter, when it is easier to digest this oil-rich food.

Karachi. Pakistan's largest and most cosmopolitan city, Karachi's recorded history goes back to the 18th century, when it was a small trading post known as Kalachi-jo-Ghote (village of Kalachi). With the development of its harbour, it gradually grew into a large city and an important centre of trade and industry. Its selection as capital of Pakistan, in 1947, added to its importance and boosted the rate of its growth and development. Although the seat of government later shifted to

Islamabad, Karachi continued to be the epicentre of commerce and industry. Today, with Karachi reportedly boasting a population of over 16 million there is hardly an ethnic community that does not exist in this megapolis. In fact, thanks to the lure of big business and industry, this commercial hub has attracted such large numbers of people from all over the country that the original residents of Karachi have become a small minority.

A salad bowl of people from all parts of Pakistan and beyond, Karachi is home to Makranis; Sheedis; Balochs; Pakhtuns, Punjabis; Sindhis; Parsis; Memons; Bohras; Khojas; Urdu-speaking communities from India; Hindus; Bengalis; and Afghan refugees. Goanese and Anglo-Indian Christians, who were once present in sizable numbers, have now mostly migrated and have been largely replaced by Punjabi Christians. Although the Chinese community too, had shrunk considerably, it is still mainly concentrated in Karachi and has been responsible for influencing the cuisine of the city, perhaps as much as any of the other communities located here.

Karachi halwa. A Karachi speciality, *Karachi halwa* is popular in certain communities and is especially served on special occasions. In the Ismaili Khoja community of Karachi, it was traditionally served on engagement or Nikah (signing of wedding contract) ceremony, while in the Hindu community it is a popular Diwali sweet. A chewy, rubbery textured dessert, it is garnished with dry fruit, such as pistachios and cashews, and comes in a variety of bright colours such as orange and green.

Karhai. Very similar to a wok, a *karhai* is slightly heavier and with a ring-shaped handle on either side. Food is not only prepared in it, but often also served in it. Gourmands insist that certain foods can only be cooked in a *karhai* as the utensil affects the flavour of the food, and so will not taste the same if cooked in a normal pot or *degchi*. In fact, so associated has a certain meat or chicken dish become with this utensil, in which it is always prepared, that it is often just referred to as *karhai*, rather than its full name, *karhai gosht* or *karhai chicken*.

Karhai Namak Mandi. While *karhai* is a popular dish throughout the country, the one made in Namak Mandi in Peshawar stands apart. Representing the traditional food of the Afridis—a Pakhtun tribe which many historians believe inhabited this terrain even during prehistoric times, while others think they are descended

from the Jews, and still others feel they are the original inhabitants of the Gandhara area, *karhai namak mandi* comprises tiny lamb pieces tossed with fat, salt and ginger. Unlike its counterpart made in other parts of the country, no tomatoes are added to this dish. It is usually eaten with long *kandhari naan*.

Karhi chawal. Similar to the Khoja's *gosht ki kari*—it probably has the same roots as both communities tend to have links to Gujarat—*karhi chawal* is a typical Parsi thick, spicy, and sour curry served with boiled rice. It is usually accompanied by *kachumber*. The secret to a good *karhi* is the fineness and smooth grinding of its curry masala. The main ingredients include peanuts and grams, roasted and ground with coconut, spices and red chillies. Poppy seeds give it a unique taste and hence it is no surprise that a siesta is required after indulging in *karhi chawal* the Parsi way! Many variations of this *karhi* exist in Parsi cuisine. Boiled whole eggs are added in the gravy right at the end before serving the egg *karhi* version. Prawns and fish cook quickly and so are added at simmering time for the seafood *karhi*. For mutton *karhi*, the meat is boiled separately and then added to the gravy, as is the case with chicken *karhi*. A boneless chicken *karhi* is unheard of in Parsi cuisine. Potatoes are a must in *karhi* in some households. A 100-almond *karhi*, and a pistachio and almond *karhi* were once popular as well, though seldom made nowadays because these ingredients have become too expensive.

ZARNAK SIDHWA

Karmo. Made of boiled and mashed rice, jaggery and yoghurt, *karmo* is a simple Bohra dessert that is garnished with crushed almonds and pistachios.

Karri. A Baloch speciality, *karri* is made by drying *lassi* and storing the dried pieces for a few days. Its basic ingredients are yoghurt and spices.

Kashmir. Azad Kashmir is the southern-most political entity within the former princely state of Jammu and Kashmir. It borders the present-day Indian illegally occupied Jammu and Kashmir to the east (separated from it by the Line of Control); Khyber Pakhtunkhwa to the west; Gilgit-Baltistan to the north; and the Punjab to the south. With its capital at Muzaffarabad, Azad Kashmir covers an area of 13,297 sq km and has an estimated population of about 4 million. Among the major ethnic groups inhabiting Azad Kashmir are Hindkowans and Hindus.

Kashmir's climate and fertility of the soil make it uniquely blessed in the subcontinent, with food resources of the sort associated with the temperate regions of the world. It has been said that Kashmir is a land of milk and honey, and it is true that Kashmiris enjoy both, sometimes adding to milk or yoghurt a sprinkling of saffron. The quality of saffron grown there is regarded by some experts as equal to the best available in Iran or Spain. Kashmir's rich agricultural areas boast rice plantations, and yellow fields of mustard; in fact, mustard oil is the standard cooking medium in the valley.

Salt tea is served in abundance—a special leaf is boiled together with water, milk, salt, and cooking soda until an almost pink colour permeates through the tea. Lotus roots are also prominent in Kashmiri cuisine, which is not surprising considering the large number of pink water lilies—which spring up from the rhizomes of lotus roots—covering the lakes that Kashmir is famous for.

Kashmiri chai/nun chai. Gita Samtani (1995) observes about Kashmir, 'It is here on the fields that salt tea is served in abundance. A special leaf is boiled together with water, milk, salt and bicarbonate of soda until an almost pink colour permeates through the tea.' Pink tea or Kashmiri *chai* popular in Azad Kashmir is flavoured only with salt and desiccated coconut and is quite different from the tea by the same name that has become popular in other parts of the country. It entails a time-consuming cooking process, which if compromised, affects the taste of the tea. Kashmiris normally have it for breakfast with fresh *bakarkhani*.

The tweaked version served in cities like Karachi and Lahore incorporate crushed almonds, cocoa, and pistachio nuts; this version has become so popular, especially in the winter months, that the original Kashmiri *chai* pales in comparison. This tea is served primarily at weddings and formal occasions, as it requires too long a preparation time for daily cooking and consumption.

Kashmiri chilli. Many subcontinental spicy and savoury dishes are made using Kashmiri red chillies; though green chillies and black pepper powder may also be part of the ingredients, the long Kashmiri *lal mirch* (chillies) are used more for their colour than their spice content. The signature ingredient of all Kashmiri dishes, Kashmiri *mirch* is vibrant in colour, much like paprika, and is also mild and distinct in flavour. It is especially used to add crimson-coloured hues to chicken and the Kashmiri *roghan josh* dishes.

Kashmiri cuisine. Kashmiri cuisine has evolved over hundreds of years. The first major influence was the food of the Kashmiri Buddhists, and Pandits (the Brahmin Hindus who lived in the valley in the Middle Ages). Kashmiri cooking developed initially as two great schools of culinary craftsmanship, viz. Kashmiri 'Pandit' and 'Muslim'. While both ate meat, the basic difference between the two was that the Hindus used *hing*, fennel seeds, mint, ginger, and yoghurt in their cuisine, and the Muslims used onions and garlic, two ingredients that orthodox Hindus avoided. The Muslim version of the cuisine also incorporates the dried flower of the coxcomb plant (*maval*). Indigenous to Kashmir, the plant produces a furry red flower, similar in shape to a cockscomb, and is extremely popular with Kashmiri Muslims. The herb imparts a bright red colour to the food. In the cuisine of the former, no meat delicacy—except certain kebabs—was cooked without yoghurt. Even vegetarian dishes often incorporated it.

The cuisine was, subsequently, heavily influenced by later cultures which arrived, beginning with the invasion of Kashmir by Taimur (aka Tamerlane) in the 15th century from what is now Uzbekistan, and the migration of 1,700 skilled woodcarvers, weavers, architects, calligraphers, and cooks from Samarkand to the valley of Kashmir. The descendants of these cooks, the *wazas*, are the master chefs of Kashmir. Other strong influences included that of Central Asian, Persian, Afghan, and Punjabi cultures.

In fact, Kashmiri cuisine today is a unique blend of Indian, Iranian, and Afghani cuisines. It is essentially meat-based—so much so that unlike most Brahmins, Kashmiri Brahmins are also non-vegetarian and centred on a main course of rice, the staple food, cooked in many ways. Not surprisingly, Kashmir excels in the preparation of non-vegetarian cuisine and more so in meat-based dishes, with lamb preferred over others. A special *Mishani* dinner is served, say, at a wedding, in which exactly seven dishes, all made from lamb, are served. Kashmiris are also liberal in the use of spices, condiments, and yoghurt. The medium of cooking is chiefly mustard oil. Another characteristic of the Kashmiri cuisine is the generous use of saffron or *kesar*, produced locally. Kashmiri chillies, which give an intense red colour and a tart rather than spicy flavour, are also liberally used. Wheat breads include *kulcha*, *sheermal*, and the soft *bakarkhani*, all eaten for breakfast with tea. Kashmiri *paratha*, roasted in the *tandoor*, instead of fried in a pan, and sprinkled with poppy seeds, is a quintessentially Kashmiri breakfast item. Tea is made in metal samovars and brewed either green or with cardamoms and almonds to yield the richer *kahva*, both of which are sipped all day long.

The ubiquitous *daal*, popular almost throughout the country, is, surprisingly, not favoured in Kashmir, where *maash daal* (white lentils), is the only lentil to be eaten. However, black-eyed beans are a popular substitute and constitute a common side dish to a main meat course. A local spinach-like green called *haak* is popular in summer, as are lotus roots, which are used as a meat substitute. In fact, fresh vegetables are abundant in the summer, including a prized variety of mushrooms called *guchhi*, used only for special occasions. Vegetables grown in summer are dried for winter use in large quantities. Fresh fish is also favoured in the summer, while smoked meat, dried fish, and sun-dried vegetables are used in the winter. The abundance of dry fruit and nuts (walnuts, dates, and apricots) in the region has inspired their use in desserts, curries, and snacks. Chutneys are made from fresh walnuts, sour cherries, yellow pumpkins, and white radishes. Sauces for curries are also made from dairy-rich products. Fruits such as cherries, apples, peaches, pears, and plums serve as dessert.

The ultimate formal banquet in Kashmir is the royal *Wazwan* brought to the region about 500 years ago from Central Asia. It is a blend of the culinary styles of the Mughals and Persians who were Muslims, and the Kashmiri Pandits who were Hindu Brahmins. As many as 40 courses may be served during *Wazwan*, with at least 12 and up to 30 courses being non-vegetarian, cooked overnight by the *vasta waza* (master chef), and his retinue of *wazas*. *Wazwan* is regarded as the pride of Kashmiri culture and identity.

Guests are seated in groups of four and share the meal out of a large metal platter called the *trami*. The meal begins with a ritual washing of hands in a basin called the *tasht-e-naari*, which is taken round the guests by attendants. Then the *tramis* arrive, heaped with rice, quartered by four *seekh kebabs*, and containing four servings of *methi qorma*, two *tabak maaz*, white *murgh* or saffron *murgh*, and much more. Yoghurt garnished with Kashmiri saffron, salads, Kashmiri pickle and chutney are served separately in small earthen pots. Every time a *trami* gets polished off, it is removed and replaced by a new one until the dinner runs its course.

Seven dishes that are a must in such banquets, all made from lamb, are *rista* (meat balls), *roghan josh* (literally red meat), *tabak maaz* (rib chops), *daniwal qorma* (light yoghurt-based curry), *aab gosht* (lamb cooked in thickened milk), *marchwangan qorma* (lamb mince), and *gushtaba* (meat loaf of minced mutton). Other Kashmiri specialties which could be included in the feast are *Kashmiri gobi*, *nalagarh* eggplant, and *narangi pulao*. The former is cauliflower cooked with cashew nuts and cayenne pepper, together with an aromatic tomato sauce. *Nalagarh* eggplant comprises eggplants served in yoghurt, while *narangi pulao* is traditionally served with a layer of fried potatoes and yoghurt mixture sandwiched between rice, which makes it a wholesome meal. The feast ends with an elder leading the thanksgiving to Allah, which is heard with rapt attention by everyone.

Kata-kat. Also known as *taka-tak*, this is a very popular street food, originally from Karachi, but now very common throughout the Punjab. Comprising organs of lamb or goat—heart, kidney, liver, testicles—*kata-kat* is prepared on a large *tawa* by pounding the organs into very tiny pieces with a putty knife-like meat cleavers. *Kata-kat* is the sound that emanates from the pounding. Preparation of *kata-kat* is a familiar sight on food streets in both Karachi and Lahore, and outside Pakistani food restaurants abroad.

Kataway. This is a beef curry dish that is especially served at weddings in the Pakhtun community. It is made with large pieces of meat that are cooked slowly overnight, which makes the meat extremely tender.

Katlama. Similar to the spicy pizza by the same name, served in Central Asia, *katlama* is Pakistan's take on it and has become a popular street food in Lahore, as well as in Peshawar. Its name is derived from *katlamba*, which means a foot long. Variations exist for its toppings even in Pakistan, so that no one specific recipe can be used to describe it. Basically, it is a large, layered *paratha* (fried bread), the size varying from 2 ft in diameter to 4 ft—the larger ones are normally prepared on special occasions and sold at festivals in rural Punjab. They are even sold by weight. The topping could vary from vegetarian—green *mung daal* mixed with spices or spiced *besan* coating—to a minced meat coating. It is normally relished on its own, without requiring any accompanying dish.

Kebab. The kebab has been an evolving term. Although the dish has been mentioned in Sanskrit and Tamil literature where they describe roasting marinated meat on skewers while basting with fat, it is regarded as native to the Near East and East Mediterranean, especially Greece, since ancient times. It is believed that the first kebab introduced to our part of the world was during the times of Changez Khan, when the horseback riders would kill an animal, clean it, cut it into pieces, thread the pieces over their daggers or swords, and cook it over open fire.

However, in the 14th century dictionary *Lisan al'Arab*, kebab is defined to be synonymous with *tabahajah*, a Persian word for a dish of fried meat pieces. Persian, in the olden days, was considered to be a more sophisticated language, hence, the term kebab was used infrequently in Arabic books of that time. Then in the Turkish period, with the appearance of the phrase *sheesh* kebab (skewer with grilled meat), kebab gained its current meaning, whereas, earlier *shiwa* had been the Arabic word for grilled meat. With time, kebab has evolved from whole muscle meats to minced meats, and even non-meats. Ibn Battuta records chicken being served by royal houses during the Sultanate period. Even common folk ate kebab and *paratha* for breakfast, and in the Mughal reign a few centuries later, it was still *naan* and kebab. In *Ain-i-Akbari*, kebab is listed as one of a class of foods in which meat is cooked with accompaniments.

Today, kebabs have become a highly popular dish in Pakistani cuisine. They come in a vast variety of forms and range from barbecued to fried kebabs. Depending on which type of kebab it is, they could be partaken of at any meal, be it breakfast, lunch, tea, or dinner. Among the fried variety the most common are *shami* and *kachche qeemay ke kebab*. Barbecued kebabs include *reshmi*, *Bihari*, and *seekh*. Steamed and baked variety include *dum ke kebab* and *galawat ke kebab*.

Kebabs in Khyber Pakhtunkhwa and Balochistan tend to be identical to the style of barbecue popular in neighbouring Afghanistan, with salt and coriander being the only seasoning used. While beef is generally the most preferred form of meat in Khyber Pakhtunkhwa, in other provinces, kebabs could also be of mutton or chicken, and seasoned with various masalas, tend to be spicy.

SHANAZ RAMZI AND SHAHA TARIQ

Kebab roll. A local fast-food that was introduced in Karachi in the 1970s by an enterprising entrepreneur, kebab rolls started off as a simple *paratha* roll with chunks of barbecued beef or chicken wrapped in it along with onions and brown chutney. Silver Spoon, the founder of the ubiquitous kebab roll enjoyed monopoly over this delectable and economical fare for many years, till others joined the bandwagon, and reintroduced the kebab roll with a twist, to suit modern, Western tastes. The *paratha* became crispier, the simple chutney replaced by cheese and garlic-mayo spreads, and what have you. In fact, up to 72 different types of rolls are now on offer by most take-away joints in operation—from chicken or beef cooked in *reshmi*, *Bihari*, or *malai* style to fish kebab rolls served with cheese, ketchup, or garlic-mayo dip. Even the *paratha* now has variety—from low-fat to *chapati*, to the regular fried offerings.

Kewra (screw pine/pandanus). The many plants of the genus *Pandanus*, often called *pandanus*, of which there are hundreds of species, these grow in the tropics from the subcontinent through South East Asia to North Australia. Classification of the species is still uncertain. The principal species is *Pandanus tectorius*, the 'fragrant screw pine'. A clear, delicately scented liquid, *kewra* essence is made from the exquisitely scented flowers of the screw pine. It is used for flavouring many sweet dishes in Pakistan, such as, *kheer* and some poultry as well as exotic rice dishes, such as *biryani*.

Khadda/khaddi kebab. In the northern parts of Pakistan and Balochistan, particularly in the mountainous regions, a dish that is popular for an entire meal, made either with whole sheep or goat, is *khada kebab*. After the animal is slaughtered and skinned, the meat is marinated in vinegar, salt, and spices. The goat is stuffed with rice and dry fruit. A ditch is dug (thus the name *khadda*, meaning hole) in which the marinated and stuffed sheep or goat is placed, and then tightly covered with a lid that is sealed with clay. The meat is cooked in its own juices and fat over slow-burning coals placed inside the pit. After about two hours, it is ready to be consumed, crispy from outside, and tender from inside.

Khagina. The literal meaning of *khagina* in Persian is fried eggs cooked like minced meat. It is a dish made with eggs, tomatoes, onions, green chillies, coriander leaves, and butter/oil. It is regarded as comfort food, easy to make, and consumed at any time of the day with *roti* or bread slices. A Pakistani version of scrambled eggs, it is also called *anda bhurji* or *anda ghutala*. It is a very popular weekend breakfast dish served with *paratha*.

NAYYER RUBAB

Khaja. The etymology of *khaja* could be traced to *khajjaka*, a Gujarati wheat flour preparation, plain or sweet, fried in clarified butter, made as way back as around AD 1130. Believed to have originated from Kutch, this crisp layered dough dessert, with or without dry fruit or other stuffing—most popular being fresh cream, and *khoya*—and lightly fried in oil, is still a favourite with the Gujarati community. *Khaja* is also the name for a crisp, wafer-like, fried, savoury, disc-shaped item, normally made by confectioners in Ramazan, and partaken of at *Sehri*. It is also known by the name of *khajla*.

Khakra. A tea-time snack *khakra* is a dry, crisp, roasted, crunchy paper-thin *chapati* made of whole wheat flour kneaded with milk, oil, and water, popular among Gujaratis. Added to it are different supporting ingredients such as *methi* and masala to make the *khakra* chunky. They stay well for long and are, therefore, carried on long travels.

Khameeri roti. Heavier, richer and crustier than the normal *tandoori roti* that was once regarded as being exclusively Afghani and Balochi, the dough of the *khameeri roti*, which used to be a staple in Balochistan, has to be mixed with some stale dough—generally leftover from the day before—so that it works as a raising agent and makes the bread fluffy. The *tandoor* is traditionally, also different—it is a special clay oven called *daash* which is built inside a wall. The dough is placed on a metal plate at the end of an eight-foot long stoke and baked in the *daash*. In the days of yore there used to be a *daash* in every area. The dough would be prepared at home and then taken to the *daash* to be cooked. Nowadays, they are rarely eaten because of the elaborate preparation process.

SHANAZ RAMZI AND SHAHA TARIQ

Khamuloot pie. A Hunzakutz speciality, *khamuloot pie* is a thick bread, almost like the Western pie, filled with onion and meat and cooked on wood fire, although nowadays it is also baked in the oven. Once ready, the upper crust is removed and used to scoop out the filling just like a *naan* would be used to eat curry.

Khandvi. A tender, rolled-up pancake, *khandvi* is a Gujarati speciality made from ground chickpea batter rolled out extremely thin, and sprinkled with mustard seeds and green coriander sprigs. It is regarded as a snack item. A paste is made with *besan* and spices and allowed to set; it is cut into squares after it becomes hard and cooked in curry made with spices and yoghurt.

Khara papeta ma gosht. Similar to the *gosht ka salan* or *aaloo gosht* normally consumed all over the country, the difference is that *khara papeta ma gosht*, a Parsi mutton dish, is cooked only in onions and whole spices, with no tomatoes or yoghurt added to it.

Khara prashad. Food that has first been offered in a temple to the presiding deities by Hindu worshippers and then given to the devotees, is termed *prashad*. It is believed to maintain an individual's spirituality. Each temple has its own form or forms of *prashad*. This special sweet prepared as a holy offering is made from wheat flour, sugar, butter, and water. It is generally served to visitors at gurdwaras (Sikh place of worship) and at funerals. It is similar to *attay ka halwa* made by some Gujaratis.

Kharak. Made by Bohra community especially on Eid to serve guests, *kharak* is a dried date slit lengthwise from the centre, de-seeded, and soaked in sugar syrup for a couple of hours. It is then filled with a rich mixture of powdered dry fruit and sugar and served to all visiting guests on Eidul Fitr.

Kharia. Mostly served in winter, *kharia* is a must-have Parsi speciality, so much so that special *kharia* parties are held once a year to relish this delicacy. *Kharia* is the Parsi version of *paya*, made with trotters, *lobia* (black-eyed beans), and bong meat (optional) cooked for hours over a slow flame. They are served with *gur* and *imli kachumber* (onions with tamarind and jaggery). The proof of good *kharia* is in the lips and fingers becoming sticky after eating it. A day before serving the *kharia*, the trotters are cleaned well and cooked in a pressure-cooker or a deep, wide pan for a few hours till very sticky and soft. Most Parsis leave this overnight on a very low flame, making it gluey soft and sticky. Then the soup is cooled and refrigerated so as to congeal the fat. The following day, the fat is skimmed off, which is not discarded but melted again. Ground masala of red chillies, ginger, garlic, cumin seeds, and green chillies is sautéed in this fat. Black-eyed beans are soaked overnight separately in water, and boiled the next day, till they are tender yet retain their shape. A stiff dough is made and used to seal the rim of the pan the trotters are cooked in, so as to ensure that the steam stays within.

Crisp *pao* or crusty bread (also known as *kark roti*) is served with *kharia* to mop up the sauce.

ZARNAK SIDHWA

Khashkhash ka salan (poppy seeds curry). A Hyderabadi speciality, *khashkhash ka salan* is a side-dish made with poppy seeds, and often used as a savoury dip served with papadams but is also eaten with rice or *roti*. Poppy seeds, quite frequently used in Hyderabadi cuisine for their graininess and delectable taste, are used in this curry dish as its base. Washed and cleaned poppy seeds, garlic/ginger paste, cumin powder, crushed green chillies, turmeric, red chilli powder and salt are combined to onions in hot oil and cooked to a blend.

SHAHA TARIQ

Khatia. This Bohra version of shepherd's pie, *khatia* is made of leftover *biryani*, yoghurt, and masala cooked into a paste.

Khatti daal. An iconic Hyderabadi dish and greatly loved for its simple yet unique flavour, *khatti daal* is usually cooked with *masoor daal*. It is actually a tangy variation of regular *daal* as it combines the sweet and sour flavour of tamarind with the garnish of roasted whole chillies, curry leaves, and onion seeds.

To make *khatti daal*, tamarind paste mixed with basic spices is added to boiled lentils and allowed to blend in on slow heat. Once the lentil dish is ready to serve it is garnished with a tempering of curry leaves and whole red chillies. Served with boiled white rice and usually accompanied by fried beef/mince, it makes a delicious, economical meal.

SHAHA TARIQ

Kheer. The Urdu word *kheer* derives from the Sanskrit *ksheer* for milk and *kshirik*a for any dish prepared with milk. One of Pakistan's most loved and commonly made desserts, *kheer* probably originated in Persia where a similar dessert is known as *sheer birinj* (rice pudding). *Kheer* is traditionally served at festivities, providing that extra finish to any meal. It is a must-serve item at *koonday ki niaz* held in many homes in the Islamic month of Rajab where it is traditionally served in large earthenware pots.

A pudding made with rice, milk, sugar, and nuts, it is prepared by boiling the ingredients to somewhat thickish consistency. The consistency varies from household to household. There are many variations in the flavourings which can include raisin, cardamom, cinnamon, almond, pistachio, saffron, *kewra*, or rosewater. For special occasions it is customary to decorate the *kheer* with silver leaf.

SHAHA TARIQ

Khichra. A dish made by the Khoja community, *khichra* is prepared with ground wheat, four kinds of lentils, rice, meat, and spices. The wheat and lentils are cooked on low heat for seven to eight hours, all the while rigorously stirred, till it acquires a paste-like consistency and is ready to be served. The meat is cooked like a *qorma* and then mixed into the paste. A high-energy provider, it used to be cooked in *deghs* in the days of yore, to feed army camps.

SHANAZ RAMZI AND SHAHA TARIQ

Khichri. Various versions of this simple Khoja rice and lentil combination, called *khichri*, exist: from a dry version made with rice and *mung daal* without skin, clarified butter, and some spices, relished with fish or yoghurt curry and eaten with papadams, to an over-cooked, porridge-like version normally made with rice and *mung daal* with the skin on, and eaten with plain yoghurt, milk, or *achar*. If none of these accompaniments are available, then it is eaten with green chutney or even *ghee*. This dish has been in existence from at least the 15th century and has been described in the writings of a Russian adventurer, Afanasy Nikitin, who travelled to the subcontinent at the time. In fact, the Mughal Emperor Jehangir is believed to have sampled this Hindu-Gujarati favourite while travelling through the province of Gujarat, and finding that it suited him a lot, had ordered his people to serve it to him on his vegetarian days, thus integrating it into the Mughlai repertoire.

Khista shapik. As the name suggests, *khista shapik* (*khista* means yeast and *shapik* means *phulka*) is a thin *chapati* or *phulka* prepared on an iron griddle. It is popular in the Khow culture and is normally eaten with cottage cheese and herbs (coriander, chives, etc.) sandwiched between the *phulka*, and as per tradition served with butter; the dish is known as *khista ghalmandi*.

NAYYER RUBAB

Khobani ka meetha. Apricot or *khobani* is thought to have been introduced by Central Asians to the subcontinent. *Khobani ka meetha* is essentially a Hyderabadi dessert which has now become a popular and much-loved sweet dish in Pakistan owing to its simple and wholesome recipe. Instead of fresh, dried apricots are used for this signature dish. Typically, dried apricots are boiled with sugar/brown sugar into a pulp. Seeds are removed and the mushy pulp is served chilled with cream/custard topping and sprinkling of nuts. Nuts are usually blanched for the perfect soft, nutty crunch. Variations of this dish are now also popular, varying from household to household.

SHAHA TARIQ

Khoja. Hailing originally from Kutch and Kathiawar in Gujarat, Khojas are a mainly Nizari Ismaili Shia community that converted to Islam from Hinduism some 500 years ago. The etymology of the term Khoja can be traced to Khwaja (New Persian Khaje), a Persian title of honour for pious individuals, used in Turco-Persian influenced regions of the Muslim world. The specific term Khoja in the Gujarati and Sindhi languages was first bestowed by the Persianate Nizari Ismaili Sadardin (d. *c*.15th century) upon his followers during the lifetime of the Nizari Ismaili Imam Islam Shah (1368–1423 CE). The term was used then for the many Lohana Rajputs of Gujarat who converted to Nizari Ismailism due to the efforts of Pir Sadardin.

Though mainly engaged in business, Khojas are well known for producing professionals from several walks of life. The founder of Pakistan, M.A. Jinnah himself was a Khoja.

Today, Khojas are spread all over the world—East Africa, Madagascar, Pakistan, India, the Persian Gulf, the Caribbean, Europe, the USA, Canada, and Australia—and their cuisine differs substantially because of the varied influences of the countries in which they have settled. In Pakistan, for instance, there is a strong Mughal influence on many Khoja dishes. An exotic mixture of culinary styles, Pakistani Khoja cuisine includes delicately flavoured meat, fish, and chicken dishes cooked with locally grown herbs and piquant home-ground *masalas*.

Khoja specialities. Many food experts believe that Khoja cuisine is the best Mughlai food of all, for it combines the flavoursome meaty dishes of the Mughals with some interesting Gujarati influences. An exotic mixture of culinary styles, Pakistani Khoja cuisine includes delicately flavoured meat, fish, and chicken dishes cooked with locally grown herbs and piquant home-ground masalas. There are some specialities that are typically associated with the Khoja community

universally, no matter which part of the world they are settled in, and which have become popular in other communities as well. These include *khichra, samosay, khichri, daal gosht aur methay chawal, ghatia salan, anday ka qeema, anday wala khana, methi anda, gosht ki kari, Bombay biryani, dahi ki kari, lassan, masoor pulao, aaloo chaap, naan chaap,* and *half gosht.* Desserts include *malpuray, ghas ka halwa and aam ka ras aur puri* (in mango season).

Khow. The Khow are believed to be the backwash of the second wave of Aryan immigrants from about one millennium BC. The mountainous extreme north regions of Khyber Pakhtunkhwa—particularly the Chitral region, an area that supposedly boasts the greatest linguistic diversity in the world—are home to these diverse ethnic groups that are nomadic in nature, generally referred to as Khow. Since then, hundreds of clans and tribes belonging to different ethnic groups have come to Chitral from the northern, southern, eastern, and western passes, settled there and mingled with the Khow by intermarrying and adopting their culture.

Later, when Islam reached Chitral, they all embraced the religion and became one people collectively called Khow or Khowistanis as they are now generally known.

The main crops of Chitral are barley, wheat, and millet, followed by rice, vegetables, fruit, and pulses if the land is arid, hence, the diet of the Khows revolves around these basic ingredients. Although Khow diet is simple, focusing on dairy products like cheese, and wheat, especially different types of breads, it is rich in variety. Lunch generally comprises bread and tea, while rice is consumed for dinner with vegetables, and occasionally meat. Specialities include *shushp*, similar to the soft *halwa* popular throughout Pakistan, but made from fermented wheat grain ground into flour and vigorously stirred and fried for nearly four hours; and *lajek* which is similar to wheat porridge and simmered for quite a few hours on a wood-burning stove. It is made on special occasions.

Khow Suey. A Burmese speciality, *khow suey* is an elaborate dish comprising boiled noodles, coconut-based curry, meat curry (made with bite-sized undercut pieces), and condiments including boiled eggs, lime, fried noodles, fried garlic and onions. Variations of this dish are made using chicken instead of undercut, and by combining the two curries into one. Even the condiments vary depending on taste.

Khoya. The ultimate thickened milk product, *khoya* is the solids of milk, obtained by boiling it in a large metal wok, stirring the liquid at first, and constantly scraping it when most of the water has evaporated, with a flat ladle to prevent caramelisation. The resulting mass is finally shaped into a large ball or small parts. While *khoya* itself is a sweet concoction, it is sometimes further sweetened with sugar weighing a quarter of its weight of sugar to yield *barfi* and flavoured with cardamoms to yield *peray*. It also forms the base of the frozen dessert, *kulfi*, and has a high content of all the three major nutrients, protein, fat and sugar.

Khurood. Essentially a Balochi summer dish because of its cooling effect, *khurood* is made in the same way as cottage cheese—by putting curdled milk in a muslin cloth and letting the water content drain out. When the milk ferments, it is cooked with salt and made into balls, which are left to dry and harden, in much the same way as the *quroot* is made in Afghanistan. To eat them, the balls have to be ground—traditionally they were ground over wood, with water sprinkled on the board, though nowadays blenders are also used for the process. Mixed with water, it acquires a soup-like consistency. It is often consumed with pieces of bread soaked in the soup. Variations are now made with chicken pieces added to the balls.

Khyber Pakhtunkhwa. Situated in the northwest of Pakistan, the province of Khyber Pakhtunkhwa is bound by Afghanistan to the west and north, Azad Kashmir to the northeast, the Punjab to the southeast, and Balochistan to the southwest. Dubbed as 'the land where the mountains meet'—both the ancient Silk and Spice routes run through it—this is a land of scenic beauty; the terrain of this province consisting of rugged mountain ranges, undulating hills, and lush plains. In the north, the mountain ranges generally run north to south, and boast five rivers flowing roughly parallel: Chitral, Dir, Swat, Indus, and Kunhar. South of the Kabul River, which bisects the province from east to west, the mountain ranges also generally run east to west. Khyber Pakhtunkhwa is accessible by land through natural mountain passes, the best known of which is the 56-km long Khyber Pass. Since time immemorial, the Pass has served as an entry point for numerous invading armies and formed an important route for trade.

Khyber Pakhtunkhwa's economy is essentially agrarian, even though the largely mountainous terrain is not favourable to extensive cultivation. Irrigation is carried out on about one-third of the cultivated land and the principal crops grown are wheat, corn (maize), sugarcane, and tobacco, while barley and millet are also harvested. Rice and spinach are also grown in the province. Fruits are grown in abundance here, not to speak of dry fruit, and are in great demand all over the country. Khyber Pakhtunkhwa, like Afghanistan, is notorious for its poppy crop.

A single community, the Pakhtuns who are among the most numerous tribal people in the world—they account for over 15 per cent of the population of Pakistan, making them the second largest ethnic group in the country—predominantly inhabit Khyber Pakhtunkhwa. The racial composition of the Pakhtuns (also known as Pashtuns) is less than clear, to say the very least. By and large, it is believed that the tribes which dwelt in the region, including Afghanistan, in the days of the Greek historians, were part of the great Aryan migration from Central Asia a millennium earlier, a belief that is given credence by the fact that their language is similar to that of the Aryans. The Greek historian, Herodotus, also spoke of a group called the Pactyans living in the area around 1000 BC, while there is a description of the Pakthas in the region in the *Rigveda*. It is also believed that the Pakhtuns may be related to the Bactrians, Scythians, and/or Kushans. Still others suggest that they were first seen in the Kandahar area and could have been Jews, Zoroastrians, Buddhists, or members of other religions prior to the Islamic invasion in the 7th century AD. Over the course of centuries, inter-marriages with the Persian, Greek, Turk, and Mongol invaders who passed through the frontier enriched their ethnic composition greatly.

While various divisions exist within the Pakhtuns, suffice it to say that the one trait that seems common to all the Pakhtun tribes is that through the centuries they have managed to retain their cultural integrity. Their eating habits, too, remain broadly the same. A Pakhtun community located to the south of Khyber Pakhtunkhwa that needs to be specifically singled out, though it exists basically in Bannu district is the Bannuchi. Ethnologically, the Bannuchis are believed to be Aryans with a mixture of Mongolian and Semitic blood, and their cuisine is distinct.

A non-Pakhtun community of Khyber Pakhtunkhwa that cannot be ignored is Hindkowans, an Indo-Aryan ethno-linguistic group native to Khyber Pakhtunkhwa but also found in substantial numbers in the Punjab and Kashmir. According to a survey conducted in 2008, they number nearly 4 million in Pakistan. Also, there are now anywhere between 2 million and 5 million Afghan refugees settled in Pakistan—census figures regarding their number are varied—with their greatest concentration in Khyber Pakhtunkhwa.

To the north of Khyber Pakhtunkhwa is the Chitral region, an area that supposedly boasts the greatest linguistic diversity in the world. The mountainous extreme northern regions of the province are home to diverse ethnic groups that are nomadic in nature, generally referred to as Khow. (*See* Khow).

The lower part of Chitral was once home to the indigenous Kalash—meaning black, referring to the black clothing made of goat hair worn by their womenfolk—believed to be the descendants of Alexander the Great's army, and now confined to three small valleys in Chitral, namely, Bumburet, Rumbur, and Birir. Numbering a few thousand, their way of life is rooted in the worship of ancestral spirits and trees, and they have managed to retain their unique culture and lifestyle. Two sets of crops are harvested in the Kalash villages—wheat as a winter crop, and maize, beans, and vegetables as summer crops. Apples, grapes (generally used for wine which the Kalash are permitted to produce and drink), mulberry, pears, apricots, and walnuts are among the many foods grown in the area. Millet and barley used to be the vital crops, but they seem to be vanishing.

Close to the Khyber Pass, at the head of the fertile Indus Valley lies the verdant Peshawar, the capital of Khyber Pakhtunkhwa. Peshawar represents an urban city of Pakistan where people still closely adhere to their local customs and traditions. It is a city where residents have not incorporated changes in lifestyle at the same rate as residents of the larger cities of Pakistan, and consequently follow a slower pace of life. Interestingly enough, the largest urban population of Pakhtuns is not concentrated in Peshawar but in Karachi. A number of Sikhs, on the other hand, are settled here, as in the erstwhile tribal areas, though their largest concentration is in the Punjab.

The seven tribal districts once known as agencies that constituted FATA and are now part of Khyber Pakhtunkhwa, lying north to south are Bajaur, Mohmand, Khyber, Orakzai, Kurram, North Waziristan, and South Waziristan. They were the most impoverished regions of the nation, chiefly pastoral with some agriculture practiced in the region's few fertile valleys. Wheat and maize are the two principal crops here but paddy, barley, mustard and even poppy are grown as alternative crops. Fruits are found in abundance and vegetables are also grown.

Khyber Pass. Pakistan's northern and western borders with China and Afghanistan are marked by rugged hills and mountains ranging in height from 2,000 feet in the southwest to over 28,000 feet in the far north. The gateways through this otherwise unbroken barrier are occasional natural passes. By far the best known of these is the Khyber Pass, which is 56 km long; of which 48 km are in Pakistan and the remainder in Afghanistan. Since ancient times, the Khyber Pass formed a vital route for overland trade between Pakistan and Afghanistan, and a point of entry for invading armies. Its military importance is easily explained. It is wide enough to allow troops and cavalry to march through it in disciplined ranks at its highest point.

In the 4th century BC when Alexander the Great of Macedon invaded the Punjab, one of his divisions came through the Khyber. In the 10th century AD, Sabuktigin, who founded the Ghaznavid Dynasty, and his more famous son Mahmud, brought their armies through this Pass on their way to the conquest of much of Pakistan and northern India. There is evidence that Changez Khan and Timur/Tamerlane made use of the Pass in the 13th and 14th centuries. Babur, the first of the Mughals, marched down to the subcontinent from Afghanistan in 1525 taking the same route. And the Turk, Nadir Shah, also took this way when he entered the subcontinent during the waning days of the Mughal Empire.

There are even many commonalities between Indo-Persian cookbooks used at the Mughal court and contemporary culinary works from Safavid Iran; this literature, manuals and cookbooks passed through the Khyber Pass with conquerors.

Mughlai cuisine is renowned for its richness and aroma of meals owing to extensive use of spices, such as saffron, cardamom and black pepper, dry fruit as well as rich cream, milk, and butter in preparation of curry bases. This has influenced the development of the region's cuisine.

What may at first be surprising is that many of the subcontinent's invaders did not use the Khyber Pass and those who used it once rarely did so again. The explanation may be found in the war-like nature of the Afridi tribesmen who lived there in the past for a millennium and often fought with or extracted tolls from those who tried to use it as a thoroughfare. Historically speaking, lamb and goat meat has always been a favoured meat of South Asia, the Middle East, Central Asia, and the Mediterranean, and primarily of the people living in the Pakhtun region, partly because of the influence of these areas on their cuisine.

It is believed that the ruling Mughal's hearty appetite for beef, lamb and goat clashed with the dietary habits of many of their subjects in the subcontinent, who were Hindus. But the mountain people of the Khyber were used to the hearty meat-based diet of the nomadic shepherds of the region. The warrior nature of Pakhtuns, Mongols (the ancestors of the Mughals), and others in the mountainous region emphasised the consumption of the undomesticated animal, and vegetarianism was considered the diet of the people of the plains.

BISMA TIRMIZI

Kisir. A flatbread or traditional fried pancake made from buckwheat and ground walnut, milk and eggs paste, *kisir* is a popular bread among Baltis as it is economical, since both walnuts and buckwheat grow abundantly in Baltistan.

Koftay ka salan. Margaret Shaida (1992) says that the word *kofta* is derived from the Persian *koofteh*, meaning pounded meat, and that the first evidence of Persian meatballs appeared in one of the early Arabic cookery books. They then consisted of finely minced, well-seasoned lamb, made into orange-sized balls, which were cooked and glazed in saffron and egg yolk three times. From Persia the *kofta* migrated to the subcontinent with the Mughal emperors and was perfected by the Lucknawis. These now took on the form of balls of minced or ground meat, usually beef or mutton, and generally cooked with gravy, though they are also occasionally baked or charcoal-grilled on skewers. With growing health-consciousness, variations made with minced chicken or fish have also become popular. Herbs such as mint and coriander are often mixed in along with the commonly used spices such as coriander and cumin seeds, and red chillies, and either soaked slice/s of bread or roasted gram flour to bind the balls. For *koftay ka salan* the balls are immersed in yoghurt-based curry.

SHAHA TARIQ

Kokum. The botanical name of *kokum* is *Garcinia indica choisy*. Belonging to Guttiferae family, it is a fruit which is native to certain regions of the subcontinent. The trees of *kokum* are found growing widely in tropical rain forests of western ghats in Konkan, Goa, South Karnataka, and Kerala. They also flourish in the evergreen forests of Assam, Khasi and Jayantia Hills, West Bengal, and Surat district of Gujarat. As such, it is a popular ingredient in Gujarati recipes prepared in Pakistan and used almost exclusively by the Gujarati communities settled in Karachi. The evergreen trees are 16 to 20 metres high, slender, pyramid-shaped with dropping branches and oblong leaves. The trees yield fruits annually in the summer season during the months of March to May. The round fruits of *kokum* are around 2.5 cm in diameter. They are green when raw and red to dark purple when fully ripe. The fruits contain about eight large seeds.

Kokum is used in food as a flavouring agent. It is sour in taste and can be substituted for tamarind in cooking. That is why it is also called Malabar tamarind. After the fruit is picked, the rind is removed and then soaked in the juice of the pulp and sun-dried. It is this rind that is used to flavour the curries. From the culinary perspective, one of the most popular preparations is *solkadi*, a Goan speciality in which coconut milk and *kokum* are used. It is also a common ingredient in fish curries made by Gujaratis and is used to make delightful chutney served with *pakoray*. A very cooling summer drink is also made with it. It can be consumed as a drink after meals to aid digestion or along with rice and vegetables. The seeds of *kokum* contain 23 to 26 per cent oil which remains solid at room temperature. That is why it is also used in cosmetics and confectionary.

Kokum has multiple health and medicinal benefits. The dried rind of the fruit has garcinol which is anti-oxidative, anti-inflammatory and has anti-cancer properties. It helps to minimise the impact of many diseases. *Kokum* is used in case of piles, flatulence, constipation, heatstroke, pain, allergies, and tumour.

ANJALI MALIK

Koonday ki niaz. The seventh month of the Islamic year, Rajab, is a month of *niaz*. Traditionally, friends and relatives are invited to partake of *kheer* and *puri* that have been cooked as a dedication to Imam Jaffer Sadiq, the sixth imam—a direct descendent of Prophet Muhammad (PBUH). The *kheer* is served in earthenware pots (*koonday*), thus its name, and often silver rings are mixed into the *kheer*. It is believed that those who find them when pouring out the *kheer* into their bowls will have a lucky year.

Kulcha. A square *roti* often marked with criss-cross lines, *kulcha* is among the popular Hyderabadi leavened, white-flour dough, oven-baked breads. According to one belief, the Nizam of Hyderabad, Mir Qamaruddin, adopted the symbol of the *kulcha* bread on his flag. Today, *kulcha* is a favourite at weddings within other communities as well. A variation of the *roti*, it incorporates more clarified butter in the dough, making the bread more elastic. Stuffed versions also exist.

In Quetta, *kulcha* takes on a different connotation from the more common version seen in the other cities. Inspired by the Afghani *kulcha*, it is usually enjoyed with black or green tea, and is particularly popular on Eid and Navroze. It is believed that this version was invented by the Mongols during the time of Changez Khan, from where it was taken to a few parts of Afghanistan. Up to six varieties are sold here which include sweet, savoury, and a mixture of both. The basic ingredients in most of them are flour, sugar or salt, baking powder, and oil. Cinnamon and nuts are added for variation in flavour, while sesame seeds are used for garnishing.

Kulfi/kulfa. Rich and creamy, made with condensed/evaporated milk, saffron, almonds and cashew nuts, *kulfi/kulfa* is a frozen milk dessert that has come to be regarded as a *desi* version of un-churned ice-cream and is normally served with *falooda*. The latter are arrowroot noodles that are boiled and then simmered in milk and cooled over ice.

Originating in Persia, *kulfi* is believed to have been introduced in the subcontinent to please the palate of the great Mughal Emperor Akbar and developed further by later Mughals. The Mughals brought ice to Delhi from a mountain near Kasauli called *Choori Chandni ka Dhar* which is perennially covered with snow. The method of making *kulfi* has remained unchanged to the present day. Thickened milk is put into special conical metal moulds (from which this dessert derives its name) and frozen by putting the moulds in a large pot filled with a mixture of ice and salt, which is shaken gently till the *kulfi* freezes.

The *Ain-i-Akbari* (*c.*1590) describes its preparation in Emperor Akbar's royal kitchens by freezing (probably in an ice-salt mixture) a mass of *khoya*, pistachio nuts, and *kesar* essence in conical metal receptacles after sealing the open top with dough, exactly as it is made today.

Kunna. A Chiniot speciality, *kunna* is a mutton dish that is similar to the *nihari* made by Dilliwallay except that *kunna* is made with mutton while *nihari* is a beef speciality. Also, while *nihari* is best made in a *degh*, *kunna* is at its authentic best when cooked in an earthenware pot (*matka*). An important flavouring in *kunna* is cumin seeds. In northern Punjab, especially in Chakwal, *kunna* is known as *katwa*, deriving its name from the earthenware pot in which it is cooked.

Kurutz. A salty, sour, rock-hard, home-made goat cheese prepared by Hunzakutz, *kurutz* is eaten both on its own, and as a flavouring in a soup. It is made by condensing buttermilk for a whole day, pressing it, and then sun-drying it on the roofs of the huts. Cheese is made using a similar method, all the way from Mongolia to Tibet.

Kushan. Sharing borders with China, India, and Afghanistan, Gilgit-Baltistan was part of the Kushan Empire during the 1st and 3rd century AD, and was occupied by Tibet, areas of China, and Afghanistan. Some areas of Kashmir and Xinjiang were also part of the Kushan Empire during the 1st and 2nd century AD. Kushans under whom the country became a centre of Buddhism, left their mark on the culture and cuisine of the country, wherever its influence was felt. Pockets of Greek populations in the region probably remained for several centuries longer under the Kushans. Some people think that the Pakhtuns may be descendants of the Kushans.

L

Labsi. A delicious Gujarati dessert of fried, coarsely-ground or broken wheat, *labsi* is cooked with milk, butter and sugar.

Lachha paratha. A layered, shallow fried flaky bread, *lachha paratha* is different from the plain *paratha* in that it is rolled out differently, making it richer than the regular *paratha*. Whether the dough is of whole wheat flour, or refined flour, or a combination of both—all are popular—the style of rolling out the dough is the same. After kneading and dividing the dough into soft balls, the ball is rolled out into a disc, and then folded into strips like a fan; the strips are then further rolled into a Swiss-roll. The roll is pressed gently and rolled out lightly, so that the layers remain intact, and fried on an iron griddle. An equally popular and usually commercially-made variety is deep-fried until it is almost golden in colour.

Laddu. A sweet confection popular practically all over Pakistan, *laddu* takes the form of a ball of varied ingredients held together with thick jaggery or sugar syrup. The base ingredients could consist of roasted sesame seeds, wheat semolina, or fried globules (*boondi*) of the batter of various pulses, especially *besan*. The origin of the present day *laddu* can be traced to ancient times, mention of which (*laddukas*) has been made way back in AD 1129–30 in the book called *Manasolla* written by King Someshwara, where it has been described as sweet balls prepared with rice or pulse flours and sugar. Among other things, *boondi* grains made using pulse flour of *chana* were shaped with sugar syrup into *laddu*. Traditionally, *laddu* is distributed and eaten on festive occasions, particularly at weddings and at the birth of a child, more so if it is a male child.

Lagan nu custard. A Parsi custard, it is a creamy, sweet dessert made with milk, condensed milk, eggs and pistachios, flavoured with vanilla essence and garnished with almonds. It is an intrinsic part of the cuisine at the Parsi festival Gahambar.

Lagan seekh. A Bohra community speciality, *lagan seekh* is basically meat loaf, made with mince meat, eggs, potatoes, and onions mixed together, patted into a tray, and baked in an oven.

Lahori fried fish. A batter-coated, spicy fish dish, the Lahori fried fish, popular in the Punjab and Sindh, is generally made with fillet pieces of *rohu*. It is deep fried in a huge *karhai* and eaten with chutney and finely cut radish.

Lai. A paper-thin *chikki*—a brittle, caramelised sweet made with peanuts, mixed nuts or sesame seeds—*lai* is a Hindu desert normally made on Diwali, a Hindu festival.

Langar. The word *langar* means communal feast. Not surprisingly, this Sindhi community dish is served at deaths to all and sundry who come to offer their condolences after the burial services. It is a simple dish prepared with *chana daal*, rice and *gur*.

Lassan. Made with *hara lehsan* (garlic chives) and *bajray ki roti* (pearl millet bread) mashed together, lightly seasoned, smoked, and then made into balls with lots of *desi ghee*, *lassan* is a Khoja community winter favourite when garlic chives are in season. It is eaten normally for breakfast. *Bhurta* made with yoghurt and smoked eggplant is generally served as an accompaniment.

Lassi. A refreshing Punjabi beverage, as popular in the rest of the country as in its place of origin, *lassi* is made by whisking yoghurt with water, salt, or sugar. It is a popular, cooling drink, especially in summer, and is partaken of in accompaniment to a meal, or just on its own.

Lazhek. A Khow speciality, *lazhek* is made of crushed wheat cooked with meat and eaten with a spoon. It is generally served on the fourth day following a death to formally denote the end of the mourning period.

Leganu. A specialty of Chitrali cuisine, this is a soup made with tiny balls of pulse flour boiled in water and then mixed in a broth made from *ghee*, onions, tomatoes, red pepper, and milk or water leftover from the preparation of cheese. Meat can also be added to the soup. A variation made with wheat is called *chira leganu*, while wheat balls boiled in milk is called *rishiki*.

Lentil (*Lens culinaris*). This is a legume which originated in the Near East. The subcontinent is the chief producer, followed closely by Canada. The plant is an annual, around 40 cm tall, whose edible seeds develop in short pods, each typically containing two seeds. The seeds come in various sizes, from tiny to small. They also vary in colour in both the husked and unhusked state. Pink lentils are among the popular lentils in Pakistan. The best-known cultivar is Red—also known as *masoor*—salmon in colour when husked. However, attempts to list lentils run up against a fundamental difficulty; the use of the word in a Pakistani context is much looser, spilling over from *Lens culinaris* into other species, as though lentil had much the same meaning as *daal* (split pulse). So, to take but one example, the seeds of *Cajanus cajan*, pigeon pea, may be called 'yellow lentils'. Next to soya beans, lentils have the highest protein content of all vegetables (just on 25 per cent). They are valued for this reason in Pakistan and regarded as the poor man's protein.

Lettuce (*Lactuca sativa*). By far the most popular of the leafy salad vegetables, the lettuce belongs to the very large family Compositae, which includes cultivated species and various wild plants with edible leaves, all more or less tough and bitter. The original reason for cultivating lettuce was probably medicinal. Wild lettuce and, to a lesser extent, its cultivated descendant contain a latex with a mildly soporific effect. The subcontinental lettuce belongs to a different species, *Lactuca indica*, and has been developed separately from *Lactuca sativa* varieties. It is rather coarse, and has reddish leaves, or leaves with a red midrib. In recent years, Pakistan has begun to grow iceberg lettuce, with an increasing demand for it by high-end restaurants serving continental cuisine. Crisp firm leaves growing in compact, medium-sized heads, the iceberg lettuce is light green, fringed, and has heavily ruffled outer leaves with hearts that blanch to silvery white. It grows best in cool weather.

Lime. This is an important citrus fruit which seems to have originated in Malaysia. While lemons are the major acidic citrus fruits in the subtropics, limes are the most prominent in the tropical regions. The fruits of *Citrus aurantifolia*, the archetypal species, have seeds, and propagation is usually from these seeds. It is this fruit which is known as the *kaghzi nimbu* of Pakistan. The use of fresh lime in beverages and as an ingredient to flavour both sweet and savoury items, is common in Pakistan, as is their incorporation in relishes such as *achars*. They are also frequently served as an accompaniment to a meal, to add a pungent flavouring to an entrée, such as *nihari*, *haleem*, kebabs and much more.

Long chiray. These are basically, mince and *besan kebabs* made by Dilliwallay which, like *seekh kebabs*, are grilled on skewers. They are particularly popular in Ramazan.

Lucknawi cuisine. Awadhi or Lucknawi cuisine has its origin in the city of Lucknow, the capital of the state of Uttar Pradesh located in northern India. The cooking patterns of the people hailing from there are similar to that of people belonging to Central Asia, the Middle East, and other parts of northern India. Greatly influenced by Mughal cooking techniques, Lucknawi cuisine particularly bears similarities to the cuisines of Kashmir and Hyderabad, and is famous for its 'nawabi' foods particularly kebabs made with minced meat or meat paste as opposed to skewered kebabs. While drawing on exotic spices and creams to enrich their dishes, the *bawarchis* (chefs) of Awadh concentrated on the *dum* style of cooking or the art of cooking over very low heat, so much so that it has become synonymous with Lucknawi cuisine today. The Lucknawis of the 18th century particularly prided themselves in having perfected the Mughlai *qorma* and the Central Asian inspired *pulao*.

Lukhmi/lukmiya. A variation of *samosa*, *lukhmi* is flat and square, the pastry filled with mince. Best when eaten hot, it is served at festive occasions as a starter. The pastry dough has flour, semolina, and cumin seeds combined to give it its grainy, aromatic texture. It is kneaded and cut into flat squares that are sealed with the filling inside and then deep fried. The mince may be mutton, beef, or chicken. It is an iconic part of Hyderabadi cuisine and known for its crisp, spicy flavour.

SHAHA TARIQ

Lychee (*Litchi chinensis*). The best-known of a group of tropical fruits native to southern China and South East Asia, lychee was introduced to the area by the Portuguese residents of Bengal at the end of the 18th century AD. Pakistan began to cultivate the fruit after the separation of East Pakistan, as till then it was being grown in abundance in Bengal which was meeting the market demand. Lychees are borne by a large evergreen tree that will fruit only in a subtropical or tropical climate where there is a distinct dry season. The round fruit is about three cm in diameter, with a tough knobbly skin which is red when the fruit ripens but turns brown a few days after being harvested. Inside, is a delicate, whitish sweet pulp surrounding a single, large, shiny, dark brown, oval seed. Only the pulp is edible.

Maash daal (urad daal/white lentils). One of the three pulses—the other two being *mung* and *masoor*—*maash* is constantly mentioned from *Yajurveda* onwards as the most commonly used grain legumes. *Mung* and *maash* are believed to be indigenous, and to have arisen from the same basic form: this gave rise to two forms of *Vigna sublobata*, from one of which came *maash*, and from the other *mung*, through adaptive variations.

Skinned and split *maash daal* is creamy white and somewhat bland and sticky. *Maash* is considered to be a kind of delicacy as its grainy texture and chewable quality sets it apart from other pulses. Traditionally, mixed with milk, garlic, and ginger, it is steamed till it is tender, and garnished with fried onions, ginger strips, fresh coriander, and mint leaves. Unlike other pulses, this one is never served in a liquid form, and cooked with masalas to be eaten with *chapati*. Thanks to its high content of the phosphorus compound, phytin, *maash* is popularly used in a paste form to prepare *baray* for a popular *chaat* item, *dahi baray*, and is also the favoured grain for making *papars*.

SHAHA TARIQ AND SHANAZ RAMZI

Mace (javitri). This is one of the two spices produced by the nutmeg tree *Myristica fragrans*, a tree originating in the Mluccas, yielding a fruit bearing a single nut-like seed. Nutmeg is the kernel of the seed. This is surrounded by a scarlet aril, mace, which becomes visible when the fruit ripens and bursts open. The mace is pressed flat, dried to a translucent red-brown, and cut into strips for sale. Simply dried, it retains most of its natural red colour. Like nutmeg, mace is used for both sweet and savoury dishes such as *kheer* and *biryani*, respectively. The properties of nutmeg and mace are not dissimilar, since they derive from the same essential oils, but mace is considered to have finer flavour. If used in excess, both products give rise to nausea and hallucinations.

Machli ke kebab. A Sindhi speciality, *machli ke kebab*, as the name denotes is fillet of fish marinated in rich spices and shaped into kebabs. They are skewered and char-grilled in the *tandoor*.

Machli kofta. A Sindhi speciality, *machli kofta* comprises fish balls gently poached in an aromatic curry.

Maggio. Made with boiled rice layered over boiled *mung daal* that has been cooked with yoghurt, onions, tomatoes, and spices, *maggio* is a Bohra speciality prepared through the *dum* technique of cooking.

Maghaz (brain). *Maghaz* especially that of calf and goat is regarded as a delicacy, valued mainly for its creamy texture. It is often cooked on its own after boiling with turmeric and going through a laborious process of removing any membrane or nerves that appear on the top. The boiled *maghaz* is broken into little pieces and fried with tomatoes and onion to yield a delicious dish, or incorporated in meat dishes like *nihari*, or flattened into cutlets and deep fried with a coating of breadcrumbs and eggs. Generally, *maghaz* is a very rich food, of which a little goes a long way.

Main dish. While staples can constitute a meal by themselves, in Pakistan the main course is never eaten on its own. For breakfast, a large number of households prefer to eat eggs as the main dish, which are normally either fried or prepared as omelettes—frequently with green chillies, onions, coriander leaves, and tomatoes—normally partaken of with a staple such as bread, *paratha* or *naan*, while many eat leftovers of the night before. In semi-urban areas such as Hyderabad, Peshawar and Multan, a variety of vegetarian dishes, such as *aaloo baingan* (potato and eggplant), *aaloo bhujia* (potato curry), and *chanay/cholay* (chickpeas curry) are also popular for breakfast. As a norm, meat dishes are not consumed at breakfast, but when they are, the ones preferred, especially on special occasions, include *shami kebab* (minced beef patty), *qeema*, *kaleji* (liver), *maghaz* (brain), *paya* (goat trotters), and *nihari*. For lunch and dinner, a choice of a wide variety of curries, *daal*, and vegetable dishes comprise the traditional cuisine, and many affluent households serve at least two dishes at a meal—generally one meat dish, either wet or dry, which becomes the main dish, and one vegetable or *daal* platter, which is treated as a side dish. However, while the majority of Pakistani dishes contain meat in one form or another (whether beef, mutton, chicken, or fish) there are a large number of homes that cannot afford or do not cook meat, especially in the rural areas. In such cases the *daal* and vegetable dish alone serves as the main course, eaten with the desired staple. Normally, the drier the item, the greater the likelihood of eating it with bread, while the curries are eaten with rice. The ubiquitous *daal* has probably been around since the mid-third millennium BC, as lentils were cultivated on the fertile basin surrounding the Indus. Simple to cook, all it requires is the split lentils to be boiled and simmered before giving it a *tarka* of one's choice—generally with either a combination of whole red chillies, sliced onions, curry leaves, garlic, and spices, or any of these. The *daals* most commonly used are golden yellow lentils or split peas, split moong beans (*mung*), split pink lentils (*masoor*), white lentils (*maash* or *urad*) and deep yellow lentils (*arhar*). There are tons of *daal* recipes around, using different spices, lemon juice, tamarind, raw mango, or mangosteen (*kokum*) to add to their flavour. Meat or vegetables are also added, if they can be afforded, to make mouth-watering dishes that can be eaten with either *roti* or rice. Vegetables such as potato, pumpkin, eggplant, bitter gourd, okra, and spinach which are available throughout the year, or seasonal veggies such as cauliflower, peas, and carrots are also abundantly eaten throughout the country. Single vegetables are more popular than mixed vegetables and include the popular okra and potato. A mixed vegetable dish often contains potatoes combined with other vegetables such as pumpkin, cauliflower, and peas. The most common form of meat dish cooked with a vegetable is *aaloo gosht* (meat with potatoes). Popular variations include *palak gosht* (meat with spinach), *kaddu gosht* (meat with pumpkin), and *aaloo qeema* (minced meat with potatoes), while combinations with eggplant, bitter gourd, okra, rutabaga, or mustard greens are not uncommon.

Maize (makai). *Zea mays* or maize, one of the most important cereal crops in the world, also goes by the name of corn. Like millet and sorghum, maize is a kind of grass, but it is readily distinguished from its relations by the large seed heads (cobs), and by the relatively short time which it takes to mature. No present form of maize is capable of self-propagation; wherever it grows it is grown by humans. Maize plants bear seed heads ('ears') which are larger than those of any other kind of grass. In all modern varieties, the whole ear is covered by a few modified leaves which form the husk, which prevents the grains from falling off when they are ripe. This feature is what prevents the plant from reproducing itself naturally; if left on the plant, the ears simply rot away. There is some evidence that maize or corn was grown in the subcontinent before the inflow of New World plants in the 16th century AD. Pollen grains, from sites in the Kashmir Valley, of a very early period have been identified with those of maize. The rise in the production and cultivation of maize in Pakistan is recent though, as for the longest time it was the ignored cereal crop of the country. But the advent of hybrid corn seeds in the Punjab some 25 years ago instigated unexpected growth. Hence, moving forward, newer and improved germplasm was introduced by seed companies accompanied by investment in farmers' education and agronomic research. Today, an extremely important crop in Pakistan, maize is placed behind only wheat and rice, and since the crop turned a corner in the 1990s, it is attracting multitudes of farmers towards harvesting it, especially in the Punjab where over 95 per cent of the maize cropping area has now adopted hybrid seeds. Today, almost 59 per cent of the overall cultivated maize area is in the Punjab, while Khyber Pakhtunkhwa contributes 40 per cent of national maize crop acreage; the combined production output is in excess of 5 million metric tons. However, realistically speaking, maize is mostly labelled as, what economists refer to, an inferior food. The grain is readily abandoned for other choicest cereals such as rice and wheat as income levels rise, and international market rate for maize is an indication of that. However, farmers in Pakistan do harvest maize over other crops simply because of value addition. Poultry industry, in recent years, has emerged as the foremost source of cheap and accessible animal protein for the people, because the abundant availability of maize grain is used in poultry feed. This contribution is also evidenced in Food and Agriculture Organisation's (FAO) nutrition indicators for Pakistan, showing 20 per cent increase in daily per capita consumption of animal protein across the country since 2001. Based on Global Agriculture Information Network's Pakistan Crop Report, poultry feed accounts for 65 per cent of the total grain consumption, 15 per cent is used in the wet milling industry, another 10 per cent goes to livestock feed and silage making, while the remaining, a very small percentage, is consumed directly as flour. Hence, it can be rightly assumed that maize has limited traditional culinary uses, and *makai ki roti* (maize *roti*) seems to be the only mainstay food in mainstream subcontinental cookery. It is gluten-free and has a unique, sturdy texture when cooked. In fact, *roti* made with the flour of freshly harvested corn was always available in the winter in the Punjab, since corn is vastly cultivated there, and remains popular to date, especially eaten with butter and *sarson ka saag* (greens).

BISMA TIRMIZI

Makai ki roti. *Roti* or bread made from the rather coarsely ground flour of maize, *makai ki roti* is particularly popular in the Punjab in winter months, when it is especially eaten with butter and *sarson ka saag*. This unleavened flatbread is gluten-free and is roasted on the *tawa* like the ubiquitous *chapati*. It contains vitamin B-Complex and is a good source of Vitamin A, C, K, beta-carotene and selenium. It is also good for the skin, hair, heart, brain, and digestion.

Makrani. A distinct ethnic group in Balochistan is the Makranis, so called, according to one theory, because they live on the Makran coast that stretches from Karachi to the Iranian border. The Makranis are a fishing community and, according to a folk-tale, their ancestors were fishermen from Ethiopia who were blown far off-course by a storm and ended up in Balochistan. However, according to some historians they could be the genetic legacy of the African slaves that were brought to the Indo-Pakistan subcontinent by the Arab and European invaders. Bilge Sener feels that there is also the possibility that Makranis are the descendants of the earliest humans who arrived in Pakistan along the coastal route out of Africa.

Malai khaja. This is a Bohra dessert comprising rich puff-pastry filled with *malai* (full cream), dry fruit and cottage cheese. *Malai khaja* is often distributed on special occasions like engagements and weddings. It has become popular with other communities as well, especially the Gujaratis.

Malai tikka. Also known as *malai tikka kebab*, this is a type of kebab made of beef or chicken that has been marinated in cream and yoghurt and, hence, is soft and juicy. They are often served on skewers, though they are also served as *boti* (cubes or chunks) pieces.

Malida. Similar to the Parsi *malido*, *malida* is a typical Afghani dessert popular in communities with Persian roots. It is made with flatbread (made from all-purpose flour and whole wheat flour) ground to a fine powder, oil, sugar, and cardamom powder.

Malido. Made from whole wheat flour, flour, and semolina, *malido* is traditionally served along with *daran* and *papri* as part of the tray of food on which prayers are offered for the soul of a deceased Parsi. Traditionally, the priest and his wife would undertake the tedious task of preparing this delicious Parsi sweet dish. Cooked in *ghee* and milk, and then mixed with sugar syrup, eggs, almonds, cashew nuts, and lots of pistachios, the secret of a great *malido* lies in its texture, which is grainy rather than smooth. This Parsi sweet dish can be stored in the refrigerator for a month. It is eaten hot or at room temperature. The Bohra community also makes *malido*, but it is a different dish altogether. Made with fried and crushed whole wheat flour, butter, edible gum, jaggery, almonds and pistachios, it is a rich dessert popular in winter.

ZARNAK SIDHWA

Malpua/malpura. Barley, the major grain eaten by Aryans, was fried in clarified butter and consumed in the form of cakes dipped in honey called *apupa*. The modern-day Bengali sweets *pua* and *malpua* (known as *malpura* in Pakistan) preserve both the name and the method of preparing *apupa*. These sweet pancakes made with flour, milk, sugar, eggs, and orange food colour, are fried and served with full cream. While it was once popular only among the migrant Bengalis and Gujarati communities settled in Karachi, over the last decade its popularity has spread to other communities in Karachi as well, and it has become a regular feature at weddings and dinners where *malpuray* are fried live at the site. They are also particularly popular in Ramazan.

Maltash. Aged butter prepared from milk that is scalded before churning, *maltash*'s strong taste is so valued by the Hunzakutz community that it is often given as a gift at the birth of a son, weddings, and funerals. The older the *maltash*, the more valuable it is. Wrapped in birch bark and buried in the ground, it may lay there for years or even decades before the head of the family decides it is time to dig it out. Even the arrival and availability of modern factory-made butter has not been able to replace the popularity of the labour-intensive tradition of making *maltash*.

Maltashta. A special dessert prepared at weddings by the Baloch community, *maltashta* is made with small pieces of bread mixed with sugar and butter.

Mamtu/mantou/mantu. A name which, in one form or the other, is found all the way from Turkey to Japan, *mamtu* denotes a whole family of items which fall in the category of dumplings. Varying from boat-shaped to fist-shaped pastas that are either open at the top or nearly closed but are almost always poached, the meat dumplings popular in Gilgit-Baltistan and Hazara region, are closer to the *mantu* made in Central Asia, and are filled with onion and ground beef or chicken marinated with local spices. *Mamtu* is steamed and usually topped or accompanied with a tomato-based sauce and a yoghurt-based sauce, and garnished with dried mint.

Mandazi. Typically, an East African street food from the Swahili coastal areas, *mandazi* is a popular snack item that was adopted by Gujaratis settled there and brought to the places they later made their homeland. Similar to doughnuts, it is also eaten at breakfast, and often at lunch and dinner as a side item.

Mango. One of the finest and most popular tropical summer fruits, mango (*Mangifera indica L.*, family Anacardiaceae) is much loved wherever it is found. Known as 'king of all fruits' mainly owing to its delicious taste, sweet scent and high nutritional value, mangoes are low in saturated fat, cholesterol, and sodium; they are also an excellent source of dietary fibre and vitamin B6, as well as a good source of vitamin A and vitamin C. Held in high esteem all over the world, the mango is considered to be native to South Asia. According to the book, *Mango: Botany, Production and Uses*, the mango has been cultivated in the South Asian region for over 4,000 years. In the book *Historical Geography of Crop Plants*, Jonathan Sauer writes that the mango was first domesticated in the subcontinent in 2000 BC. From here it made its way to East Asia, as mentioned by the Chinese traveller Xuanzang, who visited India in the first century

AD. In the 16th century, it was introduced to various African and South American regions by European traders, travelling from the subcontinent, making its way into North America by 1860. The so-called, 'King of Fruit' played an important role in cultivation activities during the Mughal Empire, as is apparent by the fact that Akbar the Great (1556–1605) planted an orchard of 100,000 mango trees. Mughal kings, during their reign between the 16th and mid-19th centuries, greatly encouraged the plantation of mango trees across the country. Often used as tools of diplomacy, nobles and growers would gift Mughal kings crates of mangoes and expect favours in return. By the 1930s, Muslim and Hindu growers, maharajas and nawabs, were shipping mangoes as gifts to countries such as Sweden and Holland. Nature has blessed Pakistan with favourable agro-climatic conditions, which are conducive to the production of high-quality mangoes. Over 250 varieties of mangoes are grown in Pakistan. The average yield of mangoes is 11.20 tonnes/hectre and Pakistan ranks fifth among the mango-producing countries of the world. The main mango growing areas are in the Punjab province and include Multan, Bahawalpur, Muzaffargarh, and Rahimyar Khan. In the province of Sindh, home to some of the best varieties of Pakistani mangoes, it is primarily harvested in Mirpur Khas, Hyderabad, and Thatta, while in the province of Khyber Pakhtunkhwa it is grown in Peshawar and Mardan. There are many varieties which are grown in Pakistan, including: Sindhri, Langra, Chaunsa, Fajri, Samar Bahist, Anwar Ratole, Dasehri, Saroli, Tuta Pari, Neelam, Maldah, Collector and Bengan Phalli. Each variety has its own unique taste, and rating one kind superior to the other is purely a matter of personal choice.

Some of these mangoes have interesting stories surrounding their etymology. According to Kusum Budhwar's book *Romance of the Mango: The Complete Book of the King of Fruits* (Penguin, 2002), the delicious Chaunsa or Chausa, which is mostly grown in Pakistan's southern Punjab area, was named by the founder of Suri Dynasty, Sher Shah Suri, after he defeated Mughal Emperor Humayun, at Chausa Bihar, in 1539. Sindh's most popular mango, the large Sindhri, is believed to have been named by the father of the country's tenth prime minister (1985–88), Mohammad Khan Junejo. According to the organisers of the 2018 Sindh Mango Festival held in Mirpur Khas, the former prime minister's father had brought back some mango seeds from Bombay in the 1920s. He cross-bred the mangoes from these seeds with some other mango species from Sindh's Tharparkar region and named the mangoes Sindhri. Then, there is the curiously named Langra (meaning lame in Urdu/Hindi), grown in both Pakistan and India. According to an essay by Indian food journalist Sarika Rana, the Langra originated two to three hundred years ago in the Indian region of Banaras, from a tree planted by a lame farmer. The Anwar Ratol is another popular mango of Pakistan. Its roots lie in the Indian village of Rataul, though it is not so widely grown in India. According to a legend, a Muslim from Rataul migrated to what is now Pakistan's Punjab, with the seeds of an obscure mango species. He named the mangoes he grew after his father, Anwar. Another source, however, claims that Pakistan Agricultural Research Department actually developed the species from a graft of a Rataul tree, and named it Anwar, meaning 'better'. Aside from being eaten on its own as a summer fruit—or even 'drunk' by making a hole at the top of the mango and sucking the juice—mango is widely used in Pakistani cuisine. Sour and unripe mangoes are used in making chutneys and pickles, including a spicy mustard oil and vinegar pickle, especially popular in the province of Sindh. Mango shake is popular practically throughout Pakistan in summer and is prepared by mixing ripe mangoes or mango pulp with milk and sugar. Mangoes are also used to make *murabba* (fruit preserves), *amchoor* (dried and powdered unripe mango), ice creams, and various desserts. Mango juice is dried in thin layers to make the chewy *aamsath*, popular as a snack. Semi-ripe mangoes, boiled, pulped, strained, and sugared make the refreshing *keri ka sherbet*, the perfect antidote to beat the heat.

LAL MAJID

Mangro qeema. A Sindhi speciality, *mangro qeema* is a unique dish made of shark mince, cooked with spices.

Marchwangan qorma. This dish has the honour of being one of the seven permanent dishes in the 36-course or so *Wazwan*. It is made using either lamb or goat meat and incorporates the quintessential Kashmiri chillies after they have been roasted and ground, yoghurt, jaggery, and lemon, aside from the usual flavour enhancers and aromatics.

BISMA TIRMIZI

Marzan. *Mar* means oil, while *zan* means food, so *marzan* literally means 'food with oil'. This Balti dish is normally cooked at weddings and funerals, and is made with wheat flour that has been boiled in water for 15 minutes and then pounded into dough with two wooden ladles. The cooked dough is then eaten with *shorba* or soup.

Masala. Spice mix, whether wet or dry, is called masala. The blending of spices is the essence of Pakistani cookery and there are many different types and combinations of spices which suit particular dishes, regional specialities, and taste preferences. Masala can be ground or whole spices, mild or strong, bland or sharp, and dry or wet. Every version imparts its own distinctive flavour. The combination selected depends on the kind of dish that is being prepared. The best-known masala is *garam masala*. *Garam* comes from the Persian word *garm*, meaning hot. A classic *garam masala* will, therefore include some of the spices that are 'hot', viz. cinnamon, cloves, black pepper, and black cardamom. Nowadays, however, *garam masala* may also include some 'cooling' or more aromatic spices such as coriander and cumin.

Masala dosa. The *masala dosa* is traditionally made of a thin, large crispy crepe, slightly spongy on the inside, stuffed with spicy potatoes and served with spicy coconut chutney and tangy *sambhar* made of lentils. *Dosa*'s origin can be traced to the 6th century AD; Tamil Sangam literature mentions it, while there is a recipe of it in a book called *Manasollasa* from AD 1129–30. A shallow, pan-fried snack based on rice, known as *dosai* then, it is now made by fermenting overnight a mixture basically of rice and *urad daal*, before grinding it to a batter the next day and pan-frying lightly. The origin in Pakistan, of present day *dosa* though, can be traced to the South Indian speciality being brought to the country by its migrant community settled in Karachi—perhaps the only dish of the community to have gained popularity with other ethnic groups residing in Karachi as well. However, unlike in South India, where it is mostly eaten for breakfast, in Karachi it is mostly eaten at dinner or high tea. According to a legend, *masala dosa* was introduced when the king of Mysore hosted a big festival and ordered his cook to re-use the leftovers to avoid wastage. The chef came up with the brilliant idea of stuffing a plain *dosa* with potatoes and spices, thus the arrival of this delectable dish on the culinary scene. Since Pakistanis are basically meat eaters, over time, local variations of this delicacy, such as chicken *dosa* have also come into existence and have become highly popular.

Masalay wallay aaloo. A Gujarati snack, *masalay wallay aaloo*, is a delectable, tangy dish made with small boiled potatoes marinated in tamarind pulp, lots of crushed garlic, coriander, and cumin seeds, and soaked and crushed Kashmiri red chillies. It is tempered with curry leaves.

Masalaydar gur. Jaggery is mixed with black pepper, ginger, and coconut to make *masalaydar gur*, which is served at the end of a meal as a dessert in Khyber Pakhtunkhwa. It is also often presented as a gift.

Masoor daal. Among the three pulses mentioned in Aryan literature *masoor daal* (*Lens culinaris*) or pink gram is one of the oldest of cultivated grains and has even been found at many sites from the 7th and 6th millennia BC. It is regarded as one of the three Ms of Aryan literature—along with *mung*, the green gram, and *maash* or *urad*, the black gram. A quick-cook, protein-rich lentil, it is gluten-free and pairs well with both rice and *roti*. Power-packed with nutrients, it is also flavourful as it has a tinge of natural sweetness. It is not surprising that it is regarded as the most delicious among all the lentils eaten in the country, so much so that there is even a popular idiom, '*Yeh moonh aur masoor ki daal!*' signifying a person aiming for a lot more than they deserve!

Masoor pulao. This is a Khoja community speciality made with Basmati rice, and *masoor daal* (with the skin on) which has been pre-soaked in water, boiled eggs, and potatoes. Often minced meat is also added to the dish.

Matar pulao. Especially prepared when peas are in season, *matar pulao* features rice and peas with fried onions and aromatic spices. It is served to guests with a main course, generally a curry, instead of serving the entrée with plain boiled rice, as the *pulao* looks dressy. Often, it is even served on its own as a main course, with yoghurt or chutney.

Matschgand. A Kashmiri specialty, *matschgand* is minced meat balls cooked in their signature red gravy, with Kashmiri chillies giving the dish its rich colour.

Meetha paratha. Extremely popular in the rainy season among the Baloch community, *meetha paratha* is made with dough kneaded with whole wheat flour. *Gur* is added to the dough before it is kneaded, and the rolled-out dough is either fried or cooked on a *tawa* depending on whether a *paratha* or *roti* is to be made.

Meethay chawal. Similar to the ubiquitous *zarda* served as a sweet dish in many communities, *meethay chawal* is Basmati rice cooked in sugar syrup and whole spices, and mixed with dry fruits such as almonds, pistachios, and currants. Doused in yellow or orange food colour *meethay chawal* is served with *daal gosht* instead of as a dessert in the Gujarati community, which often mixes its savoury and sweet foods. In Khyber Pakhtunkhwa, *meethay chawal* is made with rice and *gur* and is served white, unlike the *meethay chawal* served everywhere else in Pakistan. At weddings, it is served with apricot chutney as this fruit grows in abundance in Khyber Pakhtunkhwa.

Meethi dahi (in Bengali: Mishti doi). Made and served in clay containers (*kulyas*), *meethi dahi*/*mishti doi* is a popular Bengali dessert. Basically, sweetened yoghurt, it is made by boiling and fermenting milk and sugar overnight and adding curd.

Mehrgarh. The oldest civilisation of South Asia, Mehrgarh is a large Neolithic and Chalcolithic area located at the foot of the Bolan Pass on the Kachi plain of Balochistan. Continuously occupied between 7000 to 2600 BC, Mehrgarh is the earliest known Neolithic site in the northwest of the subcontinent, with early evidence of farming (wheat and barley) and herding (cattle, sheep, and goats). Linking what is now Afghanistan and the Indus Valley, Mehrgarh is believed to be a part of the trading connection established in the early period between the near east and the subcontinent. Archaeological evidence from Mehrgarh provides a keen insight into the kind of life people led before the initial stages of the Indus Valley Civilisation, which is thought to be one of the earliest sites of human civilisation. Archaeologists have been trying to ascertain what life may have been like at Mehrgarh by evaluating the finds such as pottery, mud-brick ruins, tools, as well as human and animal bones, discovered at the ancient site. In 2004, the Department of Archaeology and Museums in Pakistan submitted the Archaeological Site of Mehrgarh to UNESCO for consideration as a World Heritage Site. Plant foods used during this period included domesticated and wild six-rowed barley, domestic einkorn and emmer wheat, and wild Indian jujube and date palms. Sheep, goats, and cattle were herded at Mehrgarh during this early period.

Hunted animals included gazelle, swamp deer, nilgai, blackbuck, onager, chital, water buffalo, wild boar, and elephant. The earliest living quarters at Mehrgarh were freestanding, multi-roomed rectangular houses built with long, cigar-shaped and mortared mud bricks. They were without doors with no signs of having been in residential use, suggesting that at least some may have been storage facilities for grains or other commodities which were communally shared. The presence of large storage jars in rooms and courtyards of unearthed residential quarters also confirms that grains were in use and stored even in that early period.

BISMA TIRMIZI

Melmastya. Central to their identity as a Pakhtun is adherence to the male-centred code of conduct, known as the *Pakhtunwali*. A major dimension of *Pakhtunwali* is hospitality or *melmastya*, a trait common among the Pakhtuns, whether rich or poor. The Pakhtuns serve their guests often beyond their means. They also overspend on food on festive occasions, when goats and sheep are generally slaughtered to celebrate. During the harvesting season, for instance, a farm owner whose land is due for harvesting hosts a special dinner. After the neighbours turn up in large numbers and help their fellow farmer, the landowner's family serves them meat or chicken *yakhni* with *naan* broken into pieces. The guests sit around large earthenware bowls in groups of fours or fives and eat directly out of the pot. A complex etiquette surrounds the serving of guests, in which the host and his sons do not sit with those they entertain, as a mark of courtesy.

Melon. The wild ancestors of *Cucumis melo*, melons seem to have been native to the region stretching from Egypt to Iran and the subcontinent. Trailing or climbing plants, whose fruits are characterised by a hard skin, soft body, and numerous seeds, these are commonly called melons, gourds, and pumpkins. The melon group serves both as vegetable and fruit. The Cucumis family also includes some melons. Of these *C. melo*, the popular *kharbuza* or musk melon, probably originated in Africa, but 'exploded in terms of variety' when it came to the subcontinent. Other melons belong to the Citrullus family, the best known being the luscious watermelon or *tarbuz*, *Citrullus lunatus*, of Indo-African origin. The delicate vegetable is *C. lunatus* var. *fistulosus*.

LAL MAJID

Memon. Majority of Memons in Pakistan trace their roots either to Kutch or Kathiawar. However, one school of thought believes that they originated from the Hindu community settled in Thatta, Sindh. Those who converted to Islam were first called 'Momins' and the term subsequently evolved into 'Memons'.

Memon specialities. There are some dishes that are associated specifically with the Memon community, although over the years some of them, like the *dhokray*, have become popular in other communities, particularly in Gujarati speaking communities in Karachi, as well. Aside from *dhokray*, Memon specialities include *akhni*, *dhokri wali kari*, *daal baray*, and *monthal*.

Methi anda. This is a delicious egg curry consisting of boiled eggs simmered in yoghurt, spices, and fresh fenugreek leaves.

Methi maaz. A Kashmiri speciality that is often served in the traditional Kashmiri feast, *Wazwan*, *methi maaz* is a lamb dish with a dominant aroma of fenugreek. It is made with boiled meat and fenugreek, and few spices. This dish is also cooked in milk.

Mewawalla gur. Made of dry fruits and *desi ghee* (organic clarified butterfat), *mewawalla gur* is a soft *mithai*, eaten all year round in the Punjab.

Milk. This is the most versatile of all foods. Fresh milk and products made from it—cream, butter, buttermilk, whey, all kinds of cheese and soured milk products such as yoghurt—are widely used in Pakistani cuisine, as in many parts of the world. Milk has long been held in high esteem for its nutritious value, which even in pre-scientific days was apparent from the fact that it provided complete nourishment for young animals and humans. The Aryans had a strong association with cows and dairy farming. However, there is indirect evidence of the prevalence of dairy farming, even before the Aryans arrived in the subcontinent, in the form of magnificent bull and cattle seals of the Indus Valley Civilisation (2500–1500 BC). Today, while cow milk is the most popular, buffalo, goat and camel milk are also consumed in Pakistan. Historical literature contains various uses of milk for medicinal and health purposes. As an ingredient in cooking, it is used to prepare large varieties of both sweet and savoury dishes. Milk can be thickened to various degrees by boiling—to half, one-third, one-sixth, and one-eighth. The product of each stage has its special use. This last is the present-day *khoya* or *mawa*, a base for sweetmeats. The boiling and cooling of milk causes a thick, creamy layer to form on the surface; when skimmed off, this constitutes *malai* or cream, usually eaten as such. If the milk is not stirred while it is being boiled down, films of coagulated milk form on the surface, which are set aside using bamboo splints. This constitutes the delicacy *rabri* (usually sweetened). Solids obtained either by dewatering curds, or by the acid precipitation of milk, are pressed under a weight into a flat slab, and then cut into cubes, to make *paneer*; this can be used as such, or fried to chewiness, or cooked in curries (say with spinach). Milk, in the course of time, turns sour by fermentation and sets to a curd. Controlled fermentation yields a quality product, called *dahi* in Urdu and yoghurt in English. When diluted and churned, curd yields buttermilk, called *chaas* and butter; the latter, on boiling, yields *ghee*.

Millet. The general name used for many similar cereals, notably of the genus *Panicum*, millet bear small grains, yielding a coarse flour. Extensively grown around the world in arid and semi-arid, tropical environments, as crop or grains for both human food and fodder, millet plants may grow up to 2m tall with big seed heads bearing many small seeds. It is an important coarse grain crop and essential source of fodder in Pakistan, especially in areas where drought is common. Despite its economic importance, this crop has received little attention compared to wheat, rice, and maize. It is grown in Gujrat, Gujranwala, Chakwal, Mianwali, Bahawalnagar, Bahawalpur, Rawalpindi, Attock, and Jhelum in the Punjab; Hyderabad, Khairpur, Dadu, Nawabshah, and Sanghar in Sindh; Loralai, Khuzdar and Sibi in Balochistan; and Bannu, Karak and Dera Ismail Khan in Khyber Pakhtunkhwa. About 90 per cent of the grain produced is used on the farm as food and as seed. The little surplus is sold mainly as seed for the fodder crop in the irrigated areas where farmers do not keep their own seed.

BISMA TIRMIZI

Mint (*Mentha* spp.; podina). The common name of most plants of the genus *Mentha*, there are about two dozen species of mint, and many hundreds of varieties. Mint is a pungent herb that is widely found in multiple environments throughout the year. Mint prefers a wet environment and rich, moist soil with a slightly acidic pH between 6.5 and 7.0 for its growth. Mint is a genus of about twenty-five species of flowering plants in the

family of Lamiaceae, six species of which are cultivated as well as grow wild in various agro-ecological zones of Pakistan. The leaves have a pleasant, warm, fresh, aromatic, and sweet flavour with a cool after-taste. The fresh taste of mint leaves makes it a popular ingredient in many Pakistani dishes, particularly in *raitas* and chutneys. It gels well with coriander and the two are often used together. Mint or *podina* is commonly used in daily cooking in a number of dishes prepared across the country. *Podina* and *dhania* chutney is a common accompaniment to a number of main courses in many households of Pakistan, while in the lower income groups it often serves as the main course eaten with a staple such as *roti*. Mint leaves are also used to provide flavour in tea, beverages, jellies, syrups, candies and ice creams, not to mention *chaats*.

LAL MAJID

Mirchon ka salan. A Hyderabadi speciality, *mirchon ka salan* is a vegetarian dish that consists of long green chillies—normally used as a flavouring in dishes—as its prime ingredient. Cooked in a paste of onions, sesame seeds, chillies, peanuts, desiccated coconut, coriander seeds, poppy seeds, cumin seeds, ginger/garlic paste and tamarind pulp, it is seasoned with salt, crushed red chillies, fenugreek, and curry leaves. However, the most prominent flavours in this thick curry are that of sesame and peanuts. Slightly spicy, it makes for a delicious accompaniment and is an essential part of the meal on festive occasions. Served often as an accompaniment to the *Hyderabadi kache gosht ki biryani*, the dish is also eaten with *roti* or *daal chawal*.

ZUBAIDA TARIQ

Mithai. A term used to define *desi* desserts—the local alternate to pastries and confectioneries—*mithai* by and large constitutes *halway* of various kinds. They are popular at any time of the day, more so after meals or as part of tea-time snacks. The history of these delectable delights dates back to the Vedic era, when the first recipes emerged incorporating ingredients such as fruits, vegetables, grains, dairy products, and honey. Later, as more and more people from different parts of the world travelled to the region, they introduced many new ingredients which became a part of the local *halway* and *mithai*. However, it wasn't until the Mughal era that *mithai* such as *laddu* (a sweet that is often prepared to celebrate festivals or household events such as weddings) evolved and became popular practically throughout the country. *Laddu* is made of flour and other varied ingredients formed into balls, which are dipped in sugar syrup. Variations include *motichoor laddu*, *besan ke laddu*, and *boondi ke laddu*. Other popular *mithai* include *gulab jaman* (deep fried, milk-based balls dipped in sugar syrup), *qalakand* (made with cheese and milk) and *jalebi*.

Bengali sweets also occupy an important role in the evolution of *mithai*—and in fact, most *mithai* can trace their origin to Bengali sweets—and are especially a part of social ceremonies. Since it is an ancient custom in this part of the world to distribute sweetmeats during various festivities, the confectionery industry has particularly flourished because of its close association with social and religious ceremonies. In fact, with *mithai* being an important part of the Pakistani lifestyle—there is rarely a happy or sad occasion when it is not served—it is not surprising that sweetmeat shops catering mind-boggling varieties have sprung up practically throughout the country. Competition and changing tastes have helped to evolve many new sweets, but the traditional *mithai* will always hold its own, and is undoubtedly there to stay.

Mixed chaat. A concoction of boiled chickpeas, potatoes, finely sliced green chillies, onions, coriander, and tomatoes topped with tamarind chutney, sweet chutney, spicy yoghurt, lentil dumplings, and *chaat masala*, and garnished with crispy fried dough wafers made from refined white flour and oil, *mixed chaat* is a universal favourite with Pakistanis practically across the country.

Modur pulao. A Kashmiri sweet *pulao* prepared using dry fruits, *modur pulao* is a delicious, aromatic rice preparation using a surplus amount of *ghee*.

Mohajir. The migration of 1947 is considered to be one of the largest exoduses in human history, as millions of people moved from both sides of the border of the recently liberated British colony, India. The Arabic/Urdu word for an immigrant, *mohajir*'s etymology can be traced to the verb *hijrat* meaning migration. The term is traditionally used to identify people who came and settled in Pakistan after Partition. They were not the indigenous inhabitants of Pakistan like the Punjabis, Balochis, Sindhis, and Pakhtuns but were Urdu speaking people hailing from various parts of India, in particular, Delhi, Bihar, Hyderabad Deccan, and Lucknow, where they had been settled prior to Partition. They brought with them intrinsic parts of their culture and traditions

and emerged as a new diaspora in Pakistan. As such, the cuisine of this community varies, depending on the roots of their people, as each set boasts their own signature foods and specialities. Over the years, these diverse specialities have made a place for themselves in general Pakistani households as well as in their festivities.

SHAHA TARIQ

Momo. Steamed, meat-filled dumplings, *momo*'s origin can be traced to neighbouring Tibet, and are very popular in the northern areas of Pakistan. They are remarkably similar to *mantou* also eaten in the region, introduced through Iran, Afghanistan and Central Asia. They are folded in various shapes to suit the many occasions they may be served at, some plain and some fancy, and some 'with a tiny hole left in the top so the juice can be sucked out before the *momo* is eaten'.

Mongol. Mongolian cuisine primarily consists of dairy products, meat, and animal fats. Use of vegetables and spices is limited. Owing to geographic proximity and deep historic ties with China and Russia, Mongolian cuisine is also influenced by Chinese and Russian cuisine. Meat is cooked; used as an ingredient for soups or dumplings; or dried for winter. Milk and cream are used to make a variety of beverages, as well as cheese and similar products.

Monthal. This is a gram-flour dessert made in the Memon community. It is prepared with condensed milk, sugar syrup and milk, and garnished with pistachios and almonds. It is allowed to set in a greased pan and cut into squares before serving.

Muchki. A variety of bread made in a *daash* but with sugar added to the dough, *muchki* is normally consumed at breakfast by the Baloch community.

Mughal cuisine. The last Afghan king of India, Ibrahim Lodhi (Delhi Sultanate) was defeated in the Battle of Panipat in 1526 by Babar (1526–1530), a Central Asian/Mongolian/Turkic nomadic invader who declared himself emperor of India, thus becoming the first Mughal emperor of the subcontinent. The Mughals brought with them a unique cuisine, which formed the foundation of Mughal cuisine reflecting the strong Persian, Mongol, and Turkic influences of their homelands. The popularity of this cuisine increased, mainly in the royal kitchens, and over the next two centuries mingled with the classic flavours of subcontinental food and spices. A new Mughal cuisine evolved which was quite different from the traditional Persian or Central Asian style, owing to the presence of highly aromatic Indian spices. Dishes ranging from creamy, nutty, buttery curries and *qormay* to richly marinated grilled meats, and floral, nutty, milky, and heavy desserts became widespread. Mughal kitchens boasted a preference for spices such as cardamom and saffron and used these liberally in both savoury and sweet dishes.

It was particularly during the reign of Akbar (1556–1605) when the real integration of subcontinental flavours permeated into the royal kitchens. Akbar allowed local princes to join the Mughal royal courts, leading to a fusion of both culture and cuisine. Apart from the influences of the local princes, intermarriage between Indian and Mughal aristocrats took place, with Akbar himself marrying a local Hindu princess. A love for lavish banquets in both the cultures led to an explosion of recipes in the royal kitchens where chefs from all over the Islamic world and the subcontinent brought their own regional techniques and experiences. Many of the chefs learned from one another, giving rise to the rich blend of cooking styles that created the new Mughal cuisine. For instance, since the use of *makhan* (butter) was widespread in Mughal kitchens, many vegetable, chicken, and lentil dishes made in a creamy style became part of the subcontinental cuisine. The Mughal kitchens, courts and culture flourished further in the reign of Akbar's successors, Jahangir (1605–1628) and Shahjahan (1628–1658).

However, feasts were held not just for the entertainment of guests, but also, sometimes, to be rid of them! The region's history is replete with stories of how rulers would sometimes invite their adversaries to a banquet and then murder them by offering them poisoned food!

Mughal cuisine has influenced Pakistani food as it exists today in many ways, particularly the cuisines of the northern parts of Pakistan, the Punjab and Sindh. Many of the Mughal cooking techniques are an important part of Pakistani cooking such as *bhoonna* and *dum*.

Most of Pakistan's celebratory and lavish festive food that include dishes such as *biryani*, *shahi tukra* (sweet saffron bread pudding), *pulao*, *qorma*, *koftay* and *murgh mussalam* are also heavily influenced by Mughal cuisine.

SUMMAYA USMANI

Muji gaad. Served on festivals and special occasions, Kashmiri *muji gaad* is a dish of fish, prepared generally with radish or *nadur*. An amalgamation of vegetarian and non-vegetarian items, the taste of fish and lotus stem blend to give it a unique flavour, while a variety of spices and herbs—such as dry ginger, Kashmiri red chillies, fennel, curd, tamarind, cumin, cloves, turmeric—add to its amazing taste and aroma. The fish and radish are fried separately, and then boiled with all the herbs and spices. This dish is usually served during Kashmiri festivals like 'Gaada Bata' in the month of December.

Mulberry. *Shehtoot* or mulberry are large, deciduous trees found in Khyber Pakhtunkhwa and the northern parts of the Punjab. Technically, the mulberry fruit is an aggregation of small fruits arranged longitudinally around the central axis. In most species, these berries are purple-red when ripe; however, they can be white, red, purple, or multiple colours in the same fruit. Black mulberry is the tastiest and the juiciest among the available varieties. Pakistani mulberry is a peculiar looking, long, slender, purplish, snake-like fruit, anywhere from one to five inches long, with three inches being archetypal. Though still not very common, they are not nearly as rare as they used to be a few years ago. They are not appealing to look at, but they are quite scrumptious, with a mild, fruity flavour and the right balance of sweetness and acidity. A major advantage of the Pakistani mulberry, compared with the more celebrated Persian ones, is that it is firmer and has stronger skin, so that it remains reasonably dry during picking, packing and sale, and thus has a longer storage life. It is also popular in its dried form and sold throughout Khyber Pakhtunkhwa when not in season, which is from April to May.

Mulidah. A Khow speciality, *mulidah* are pieces of *phulka* (roasted bread) cooked in milk.

Mulligatawny soup. A thick chicken and lentil soup, *mulligatawny*'s basic ingredients today comprise pink lentils, rice, coconut milk, stock, lemon juice and local spices. Although it is made in many different ways now, it usually has rice and chicken pieces floating in it. An Anglo-Indian invention of Tamil origin, *mulligatawny* soup is believed to have been created for the British Raj which demanded a soup course from a cuisine that had never produced one. The nearest dish to a soup that South Indian cooks knew was a watery broth made from black pepper, tamarind and water called *molo tunny* or *milagu-tannir* in Tamil, or pepper water. The South Indian cooks inventively added some rice, lentils, a few vegetables and little meat to the broth and transformed it into *mulligatawny* soup, one of the earliest dishes to emerge from the new hybrid cuisine.

According to a popular legend though, a district officer in the Punjab went for dinner to Malik Tiwana's house where he was served *daal chawal* and thoroughly enjoyed it. He returned home and asked his cook to conjure a similar dish. The concoction created was corrupted from Malik Tiwana's to *mulligatawny*. Sadly, the soup is now not as popular as it used to be till the early 2000s, and only restaurants of five-star hotels or elitist clubs, mostly existing from the time of the Raj, continue to offer it.

Mung (green or golden gram). *Mung* bean or *mung*, the seed of the plant *Vigna radiaa*, is a native of the subcontinent where it has, for long, been under cultivation. *Mung* is one of the three pulses—the other two being *urad* and *masoor*—constantly mentioned from *Yajurveda* onwards as the most commonly used grain legumes. *Mung* and *urad* are believed to be indigenous, and to have arisen from the same basic form: this gave rise to two forms of *Vigna sublobata*, from one of which came *urad*, and from the other *mung*, through adaptive variations. Split and peeled, all kinds reveal a pale-yellow inside. Used as a dried pulse, *mung* beans need no soaking, cook relatively quickly, have a good flavour, and are easily digestible: a collection of merits which few other legumes can match. Consumption of *mung* causes the least flatulence among common pulses. While *mung* is commonly eaten as a *daal* it is also widely consumed in a *khichri* with rice. It is also used in a number of dishes including *chaats*, salads and rice dishes.

Mung chaat. A Gujarati dish which is served as a delectable snack, *mung chaat* is made with *mung* sprouts, capsicum, tomato, green mango, carrot, sev, and a mix of spices. This nutritious *chaat* is actually relished anytime during the day. It is light on the stomach and rich in protein. Strangely enough it hasn't caught on in popularity in other communities.

Mung salad. Rarely made by any other community, this *mung* bean salad is a speciality of the Bohra community. It is made with roasted *mung* beans, boiled and cubed potatoes and shredded cabbage, mixed with tamarind chutney and yoghurt and topped with a *baghar*.

Murgh cholay. Chicken cooked with boiled chickpeas, *murgh cholay* is a quintessentially Punjabi dish that has recently become popular in other parts of the country as well.

Murgh mussalam. A special dish of Persian origin *murgh mussalam* is a classic royal dish basically comprising stuffed chicken in a creamy sauce. The spices are fried or dry-roasted, ground into a paste made rich with cashew nuts, almonds and raisins, and stuffed into the chicken. It is generally simmered in milk and then finally thickened with natural yoghurt. It is as popular now as a festive dish in Pakistan, as it was in the royal courts of the Mughals.

Murgh sajji. Unlike the Balochi *sajji* made of lamb, this Sindhi version is made with spiced whole chicken slow roasted over a wood fire.

Murgh wardh (salt steamed chicken). A Balochi speciality, *murgh wardh* is a chicken dish made with the addition of just salt. A thick layer of the local salt is used to layer the base of the pot and is then covered with newspaper in which holes have been made. The chicken pieces are arranged over the paper and then the pot is covered tightly with a lid. It is allowed to cook for three hours, while the salt filters through the holes.

Muri/murmuray. Parched, puffed, and parboiled or soaked rice that have been tossed on very hot sand so that the grains expand and burst, *muri* go back to ancient times when they were known as *dhanah* (mentioned in *Rigveda*) and were made of beaten or parched barley. Charaka lists not only parched barley but also parched pulses like *mung*, *masoor*, and *matar* under the generic name *bhrstadhanya*. There are other Sanskrit words for parched grains as well, including *chipita* which survives in *chewra*—the spiced snack made from parched rice— even today. While *muri* are an essential part of *chewra* and many other snacks like *bhel puri*, they are eaten on their own as well, dressed with a little salt, and are particularly delightful when mixed with lemon, chopped onions and red chillies, while Bengalis like to add pungent mustard oil to them. They are also popular as a dessert when they take on the form of *murmuray kay laddu* (caramelised *muri* shaped into balls).

Murree Brewery. One of the oldest breweries in South Asia, established in 1860 in the north of Punjab, to meet the growing demands for beer by British personnel (mainly army), Murree Brewery is thriving to-date. A branch of the Rawalpindi Murree Brewery was established in a suburb of Quetta soon after the arrival of the British in Quetta in 1877, but it was destroyed by the earthquake of 1935. The original brewery is located in Pir Panjal Range of the Western Himalayas at an elevation of 6,000 feet above sea level, near the resort town of Murree. The brew became quite popular among the British troops stationed there, and virtues of the barley malt and hops as a light alcoholic beverage were not lost on the local populace as they too became fans of it. With the turn of the 20th century the name 'Murree' became synonymous with refreshing beers in kegs and bottles at bars, beer halls and messes across the subcontinent. Since its inception the beer has earned numerous awards in its illustrious 140-year history. Beyond beers, Murree Brewery boasts a wide range of vodkas, whiskeys, tequilas, lagers and ales. One of the reasons for the success of the products of Murree Brewery is believed to be the water that flows in that region. Despite the public ban on alcohol, Murree Brewery remains a well-known brand and its products are sold at legal shops and served discreetly at high-end restaurants across the country.

Mushroom. A term of uncertain derivation, first recorded as an English word in the 9th century, mushroom seems likely to have come from *mousseron*, a French term which now applies only to various small mushrooms. Scientists now use 'mushroom' in the strict sense to denote the fruiting body of a fungus of either the order *Agaricales* or the order *Boletales*. But in everyday usage, the word can be used very generally, applying to any edible fungi, and is certainly taken to include any edible fungus of the same general shape as a proper mushroom, having a round cap and usually a stalk. Most mushrooms are edible, but only a small proportion are worth eating; the rest are tasteless or unpleasant. A few are indigestible enough to cause stomach aches, especially if eaten raw. And a very few are toxic, even fatally so. Mushrooms are not very nutritious in terms of energy value, since they are about 90 per cent water, very low in fat, and have most of their carbohydrates in the form of indigestible chitin. In Pakistan, oyster, button, and straw mushrooms are commercially cultivated. Grown in the Punjab and Balochistan, mushrooms are not used in typical Pakistani cooking. It is generally used for topping pizzas, in exotic omelettes, Chinese soups, and in continental dishes that are served in most high-end restaurants in the country.

Mustard seed (*Brasica nigra, b. juncea*; rai dana). Several species of the plant in the cabbage family are known as mustard. The seeds of three of them provide the condiment mustard. Several species also have edible leaves; some yield a culinary oil. The seeds were discovered at an Indus Valley site from 1500 BC. Though these are mostly from the *Brassica species* (*rai*), brown *sarson*, which is *B. napus* var. *glauca* followed by reddish-brown *toria, B. napus* var. *napus* are also widely found. There is also a minor crop of yellow *sarson*. All these are oil-bearing seeds; however, they are never crushed singularly for oil, but always in a judicious admixture so as to yield a 'mustard' oil of unique taste and flavour, to which each seed type contributes something distinctive. Regardless of the colour, these seeds are round in shape and sharp in flavour. Used for flavouring curries and pickles, they develop a delicious nutty taste when first fried in oil. Often, the initial *baghar* operation begin with the frying of mustard seeds in hot oil till they cease to splutter, followed by the frying in the same oil of other spices and flavourings. The *baghar* can also be used to top a finished dish. Mustard seeds stimulate the appetite and are said to be good for the skin.

Mutanjan. Similar to *biryani* eaten in the rest of the country, *mutanjan* is a sweetish, Kashmiri meat and rice dish made by boiling whole spices and onions placed in a bag, and lamb meat. When cooked, sugar and lemon is added to the meat, and then it is sandwiched between layers of par-boiled rice. The rice is topped with saffron milk and lots of nuts. This royal dish of Kashmir and Mughal courts is believed to have been introduced during Shahjahan's reign when Mughlai cuisine was at its peak.

NAYYER RUBAB

Muthia. This is a Gujarati winter speciality that includes assorted seasonal vegetables, such as carrots, peas, greens, along with potatoes, and mutton, and flavoured with anise and fenugreek. It has been given this name because the millet dumplings in this dish are shaped like a fist (*muthi* in Urdu). A winter favourite, when a vast variety of vegetables are available, this dish is a complete meal and needs no staple to eat it with. The Gujarati *muthia* is inspired by the Hindu *dhokri* except that this version also includes meat.

Mutton. While for the rest of the world mutton is the meat of domestic sheep over one-year-old, in Pakistan, goat meat is referred to as mutton which is the meat of choice in Sindh and the Punjab. Goat meat is taken from the adults of the species *Capra hircus*, closely related to sheep. Adapted to mountain habitats, goats are sure-footed, able to climb steep cliffs to find food, surviving on tree bark and thorny scrub. There is evidence of goats and sheep being eaten by people of Indus Valley civilisation. Although goat meat and mutton are terms used interchangeably in Pakistan, it is goat meat that is popular almost throughout the country, and mutton (sheep meat) is popular only in Gilgit–Baltistan and Khyber Pakhtunkhwa. Sheep meat has a stronger flavour and deeper colour than goat meat and for those not accustomed to its taste, it is difficult to replace the latter with the former.

Mutton vindaloo. According to Madhur Jaffrey (1995), the correct spelling *vindalho*, gives away the main seasonings of the original dish which was once a kind of Portuguese pork stew seasoned with garlic (*alhos*) and wine (*vinho*) vinegar. It probably included some black peppercorns as well, especially at the tables of affluent families. The vinegar acted as a preservative, allowing the stew to be eaten over several days. It was first brought to Goa by the Portuguese and became a Goan meal often served on special occasions. It evolved into the *vindaloo* curry dish eaten in the subcontinent when the Goans added plentiful spices to it: ginger, cumin, cloves, cardamom, mustard seeds, and an enormous number of dried red chillies (with more colour than bite) and the souring agent which became not the usual tamarind or vinegar, but the dried rind of the *kokum* fruit. In Pakistan, however, lots of vinegar has again replaced *kokum* as many communities are not familiar with this souring agent. This speciality underwent further transformation with pork being replaced by mutton.

N

Naan. The Persian word for bread, *naan*, is in common use in the subcontinent, and, indeed, in several other countries. *Naan's* popularity can be traced as far back as the ubiquitous *chapati*, as remnants of a *tandoor* have been discovered from excavations at the Indus Valley sites. However, the Persian-speaking central Asian nations—particularly the regions around Afghanistan, Uzbekistan, Iran, and Tajikistan—have also, for centuries, been consuming *naan* the way Pakistanis know it, and it is believed that through conquests and trade, the basic recipe of the *naan* found its way to the subcontinent.

Thicker and spongier than the *chapati* and usually made of white flour, though whole wheat or rice flour could also be used, the dough of which the *naan* is made contains yeast. The dough is kneaded for a few minutes, then set aside to rise for a few hours. Once risen, the dough is divided into balls, patted into shape, flat, round or tear-shaped, and pushed through a *tandoor*. About four feet deep, a bed of charcoal heats it. The dough, plastered to the oven wall, is removed with a pair of long metal spikes when ready. The ensuing bread is flattish and has a crisp crust.

Interestingly, *tandoors* started out in the Punjab not just as a means of cooking but also as social institutions. Since not all homes could accommodate them, communal *tandoors* were used by people to cook bread from flour kneaded at home, offering them the opportunity to meet neighbours and catch up with news and gossip at the same time.

Rarely made at home other than in Peshawar, *tandoori naan* is normally bought as an alternate to homemade *chapati*. Eaten for breakfast only in Peshawar, it is widely consumed at other meals all over the country.

The most common derivatives of *naan* are the Peshawari and Kashmiri *naan*. These are filled with a mixture of nuts and raisins and are much broader and thicker than the normal *naans*. With variations in the original recipe, in the form of flavourings or fillings, the *naan* can offer exotic dimensions. Hence, there are varieties of stuffed *naans* such as those with mince meat, chicken, or potato; and flavoured *naan* such as those with garlic or butter. Popular sprinklings on *naan* include cumin, sesame, and nigella seeds.

Other bread varieties include *sheermal*, *taftan* (soft rice flour bread), *Kandahari naan*, *kulcha* (square roti with sesame seeds), *roghni naan* (sprinkled with sesame seeds and covered with minute amounts of oil), and *Bumbaiya naan*. *Bakarkhani* (crisp layered bread) is another favourite.

Naan chaap. Quite deceptively named, various versions exist *of naan chaap*, but traditionally this Khoja speciality is a cutlet made with mashed potatoes with a minced meat filling.

Nadur palak. A Kashmiri vegetarian speciality, *nadur palak* (*nadur* are lotus roots and *palak* is spinach) is made of stir-fried lotus roots and spinach. A variation of *nadur palak*, *nadur yakhni* comprises boiled lotus roots made by simmering the boiled lotus in sautéed yoghurt instead of stir-frying it.

Namkeen gosht. A Pakhtun favourite, *namkeen gosht* is a meat delight hailing from Pakhtunkhwa and its adjoining regions where meat fare is a favourite among mountain people. The consumption of meat is a way of combating the rigorous terrain of the region, staying strong, warm, and warrior-like. The small cubes of meat that *namkeen gosht* is made of, have a tender, melt-in-the mouth texture, because of slow cooking and minimum use of ingredients such as salt, ginger, pepper, and animal fat. The fresh meat provides the fat base for the cooking, and it is most delicious when served with a side of hot *naan* and chopped onions.

Namkeen gosht is believed to be the ancestor of the *karhai gosht* since tomato and green chillies are not indigenous to the region, but black pepper has been indigenous to the subcontinent for thousands of years and travelled to the mountains of the Pakhtuns with conquerors, explorers and travellers, making it the spice of choice in *namkeen gosht*. From the north, the delicious *namkeen gosht* travelled to the Punjab, where the people of the plains started adding green chillies to it.

BISMA TIRMIZI

Namkeen tikka. Introduced by the Turks, *tikka* is lamb pieces prepared over *seekhs*, while *namkeen tikka* is salty, barbecued lamb pieces. As in the case of kebabs, the use of spices other than salt is negligible in the *tikkas* eaten in Khyber Pakhtunkhwa. In fact, a variety of *tikka*—mostly served as a starter, known locally as *patay tikka* (concealed *tikka*)—is made of liver pieces wrapped in fat, cooked over coals only with salt.

Nankhatai. A modified form of *khand kulcha*, *nankhatai* is a local biscuit that used to be initially baked in a wooden *tandoor*. Allegedly, a bakery set up in Surat by two Dutchmen introduced this biscuit to cater to Surat's Dutch population. When the Dutch left the subcontinent, this bakery was taken over by a Parsi, Faramji Pestonji Dotivala, and eventually it was introduced in the areas that now constitute Pakistan by a Parsi bakery set up in Karachi after Partition.

Narangi pulao. This is an orange-flavoured Awadhi-style rice, made by using freshly squeezed orange juice, and flavoured with whole spices such as fennel seeds, cinnamon, star anise, and cardamom. The saffron added in the end to the *narangi pulao*, gives it a lovely colour and rich flavour as well. Since it has a slightly sweet tinge it tastes excellent when paired with a spicy gravy dish or just served with a simple *raita*.

Nargisi koftay. Full-boiled eggs wrapped in minced meat, *nargisi koftay* derive their name from the 'nargis' flower (narcissus) as once these meat-and-egg balls are cut from the centre, the golden yolk surrounded by the egg white against an earth-brown meat background resembles the *nargis* flower sprouting from the earth. This Mughlai dish which came to the subcontinent all the way from Persia with the Mughal emperors, became a Hyderabadi favourite and is now popular practically throughout the country where it is consumed on special occasions, as a dry gravy-based dish, with the balls prepared separately and placed in the gravy once it is ready. It is believed that Scotch eggs, a traditional British dish made with hard-boiled eggs wrapped in mince, coated with breadcrumbs, and deep-fried, are inspired by *nargisi koftay*.

Nashasta ka meetha. This is a Pakhtun sweet dish made by soaking wheat for a fortnight in water that is changed daily. It is then mashed into a thick paste, which is then left to dry in the sun for several days until it turns into powder, after which it is fried in *ghee*. *Nashasta ka meetha* is especially served to mothers for forty days after the birth of the child as it is regarded to enhance lactation. It is also believed to be a cooling agent and is added to sherbets during summer.

Navroze. Jamshed Peshdadiyan, one of the most illustrious kings of the Peshdadiyan Dynasty of ancient Iran, founded the festival of Navroze (hence the term Jamshedi Navroze, pronounced *nauroze*, meaning new day in Persian) to be celebrated on 21 March, heralding the bounties of spring after the barrenness of winter. Today, Navroze is celebrated by people influenced by Iranian culture, notably the Zarathushtrians, the Bahais, the Ismailis, and the Kurds. In fact, Navroze is unique in the sense that it is the only holiday celebrated by more than one religious community.

The highlight of this festival is the laying of *sofreh haft seen* or Navroze tablecloth. Each of the items on the table is symbolic. Seven items beginning with 's' or 'sh' in the Persian language, and symbolising new beginnings are placed on the table, hence the term *haft seen* (or *sheen*) table. These are generally: *samanu*—a sweet pudding made from wheat germ, representing wealth; *seer*—garlic, symbolising health; *saib*—apple, representing beauty; *somaq*—special berries symbolising the colour of the sunrise; *serkeh*—vinegar, representing maturity and patience; *sumbul*—the hyacinth flower with its strong fragrance, heralding the coming of spring; and *sekkeh*—coins symbolising prosperity and wealth.

A variety of vegetables and nuts, fruits, sweetmeats, grains, and cereals also form part of the goodies arranged on the table to herald a plentiful year. Flowers, a mirror and candles, a photograph of Zarathustra, and a copy of the *Avesta* (the holy book of the Zoroastrians), are also included in the setting. A few days before the Navroze, raw wheat and lentils are soaked in water placed in bowls to sprout into a mass of greens, signifying growth and the roots of the person's life. Goldfish in a bowl, and a basket of coloured eggs kept replenished for thirteen days, signifying new life, are also placed on the table. Among the many items served on this day, *falooda*, a rich drink, is a must.

Custom dictates that visitors on Navroze should be sprinkled with rosewater, have a red dot (*tilli*) placed on their forehead, and be asked to look into a mirror to make a wish. Some say that these rituals signify 'smelling as sweet as roses' and 'shining as bright as a mirror' throughout the New Year.

ZARNAK SIDHWA AND SHANAZ RAMZI

Nimco. A classic example of how the widespread popularity of a product has turned its brand name into a generic one, *nimco* is a term widely used to describe a large variety of munchies, including chilli and plain crisps, chilli and salted peanuts, *chewra* (a parched rice spiced snack), crispy *mung daal, daal chana, ghatia* (besan-based snack) and much more. The first outlet to sell these delicious snacks by the name of 'Nimco' was established by Haji Muhammad Jan in the early 1950s. Gujarati cuisine has mastered the art of *nimco*-making and *nimco* mix and is often referred to as Bombay mix as well. It is one of the most popular items bought by the expat community visiting Pakistan, to take back with them for their own consumption as well as for gifts.

Nutmeg (*Mystica fragrants*; jaifal). Nutmeg is one of the two spices obtained from the nutmeg tree, *Myristica fragrans*; the other is mace. Nutmeg is the dried kernel of the fruit of the flowering evergreen tree native to the Moluccas. The trees thrive in tropical conditions near the sea. They start to bear fruit between ten and 15 years of age and continue to do so for another 30 or 40 years. Its rich, sweet, warm, and aromatic flavour is at its best if the whole nutmeg is crushed and grated as and when needed. Nutmeg is traditionally thought to have general tonic properties, especially for the digestive system, heart, brain, and reproductive organs.

Offal. Those parts of an animal which are used as food, but which are not skeletal muscle, are given the name offal. The term literally means 'off fall' or the pieces which fall from a carcass when it is butchered. Originally, the word was applied to the entrails and now covers insides including the heart, liver, and lungs, all abdominal organs and extremities, tails, feet, and head, including the brains and tongue. Offal is a good source of protein, and some organs, notably the liver and kidneys, are very valuable nutritionally.

In Pakistan, feet, brains, liver, and kidneys are popular organs, cooked with masala, though kidneys are often barbecued as well. The Parsi community has a special fascination for offal in their food. Their favourites are *kharia* or *paya*, *gurda kapura* (kidney and testicles), *gurday* (kidneys), and *maghaz*. *Leti Paleti* is a traditional Parsi breakfast made with chicken liver, chicken heart, and chicken gizzard. It is also made with goat liver and offals and cooked during Parsi weddings with the offal from the mutton used for *pulao*, etc., and served for breakfast. It is eaten with *paya* or *roti*. A dish called *khurchan* using goat liver, lungs, and heart is also prepared and served at breakfast. It has a unique taste as *dhansak masala* powder is added to it.

ZARNAK SIDHWA

Ogra. This is a porridge made of crushed wheat, millet or maize, rice, white lentils, or other food grains that are boiled in water with the addition of buttermilk or *ghee*. Sometimes it is made of crushed wild almond fruit (*zarga*). *Ogra* is particularly popular among the Kakar tribe of Balochistan.

Okra (bhindi). *Hibiscus esculentus*, commonly known as okra, is an annual plant of tropical and subtropical regions which bears pods that are eaten as a vegetable. It is the only member of the mallow family, Malvaceae, to be used in this way. The pods, which are typically ridged and tapering, but may be almost round, contain many small seeds and a gummy substance which gives okra its special character. The general appearance of the pods has given them the name ladies' fingers. The immature seed pods of a small bush related to the cotton plant, when fresh, they have a wonderful rich flavour and are filled with edible seeds in mucilaginous juices which act as a natural thickening agent for any dish in which they are used. No matter how it is cooked, okra remains slippery unless the pods have first been thoroughly dried. Cooked in wet or dry form, okra is highly nutritious, rich in vegetable protein and folic acid, and the juices are believed to soothe the gut. Okra is an extremely popular vegetable in Pakistan and loved for its soft texture and nutty flavour. It is also often combined with meat and cooked in a curry. *Tali hui bhindi* (fried okra) are also a favourite, especially with the Sindhi community. The dried, shrunken pods are cut into short sections and then fried and drained, after which they have the appearance of small croutons and taste quite different from okra in its usual forms. They are often combined with diced and fried potatoes and seasoned with red chilli powder and salt.

Onion (*Allium cepa*). The onion belongs to the same family as the garlic (*Allium sativum*) and both are believed to be native to Afghanistan region. Onions have been eaten and cultivated since prehistoric times. Muslim royalty consumed onions extensively. An early 12th century AD Sanskrit text, *Manasollasa*, written by King Someshwara, describes numerous meat dishes in which onions were fried in the initial *baghar*. Ibn Battuta describes *samosa* stuffed with (fried) onions served in the Sultanate court in the 13th century AD. The cultivated onion was introduced to the New World by Christopher Columbus on his second voyage to Haiti (1493–4). Over the millennia since onion cultivation began, many different types of round onion have been bred. The size varies from small pickling onions to large ones. Colours may be white, brown, yellow, or red, although Pakistani onions are usually white or purplish in colour. The flavour ranges from very mild to strong, whether harshly biting or simply with a pronounced flavour. While onion may serve as a main course in many a family which cannot afford anything more lavish to consume with a staple, generally *roti*, it is by and large used as a base ingredient for most curries prepared in the country. Often, it is fried crisp and red to be used as a garnish, with *haleem*, *paya*, *biryani*, and much more.

Onion seed (*Allium cepa*; kalonji). Black in colour and triangular in shape, onion seeds are tangy seeds used both in pickles and as a condiment when making vegetable curries. They are supposed to enhance the secretion of milk in expecting mothers. Scientific studies have shown that they contain potent sexual hormones, stimulants, urine and bile diuretics, digestive enzymes, antacids and sedatives, among other useful compounds.

P

Paan. An amalgamation of many items, *paan* is derived from the Sanskrit word *parna*, meaning leaf. An important component of *paan* is betel nut, a popular stimulant in the subcontinent, which is the fruit of the areca palm, Areca catechu, and, therefore, also known as areca nut. The nut contains a stimulating alkaloid (arecoline) and tannins which give it a pleasantly astringent taste.

The nuts are gathered either green or ripe, according to taste. Green nuts are shelled, boiled to mellow the flavour, and sun-dried. Ripe nuts are simply dried. The nuts are then crushed and along with slaked lime and a smear of catechu (a scarlet and astringent extract made by boiling chips of wood from the areca palm [known as *kattha* paste]) are wrapped in a betel leaf to make a *paan*, usually in triangular shape. The betel leaf comes from a different tree, viz. *Piper betle.*

While chewing *paan* was a South Indian practice, recognised even in Sanskrit literature, it was once considered a royal item and only served to rajas and maharajas. Mughal Empress Nur Jahan is credited with making it popular among the masses as an after-meal item and something to be served to guests. At that time, betel leaves were soaked in rose water and filled with *gulqand*, cinnamon, cardamom seeds, and clove, and wrapped in silver or gold foil.

A traditional mouth-freshener and digestive aid usually eaten after meals, *paan* was such a regular feature in olden days that practically every house boasted the paraphernalia that goes with the culture of eating *paan*.

In fact, whole technology has developed around the practice of chewing *paan*. Beginning with sectioned containers of brass, copper, or silver, called *paandan*, to hold the various ingredients in one place, to nutcrackers and spittoons, there is as much attention paid to the paraphernalia that goes with serving *paan* to one's guests as to the quality of the *paan* itself. Till today, *paan* is served at traditional ceremonies, weddings, receptions, and religious festivals. Among the popular versions of *paan* available in Pakistan are *Saada, Saada Khushboo, Meetha, Tambaku, Qiwami,* and *Raja Sahib.*

SHANAZ RAMZI AND NAYYER RUBAB

Packaged spice. Traditionally, spices were ground at home, often pulverised through the age-old method of grinding on stone or with a pestle and mortar. However, with the passage of time and changing lifestyles, urbanites have come to rely more and more on purchasing ground spices, and now there is hardly a home that prepares its own, particularly for day-to-day meals. While many households buy unbranded loose spices as they are relatively cheaper, even if their quality is dubious, many prefer to rely on known brands that guarantee quality at a premium price. The first few packaged spices to be introduced by National Foods way back in the 1970s were red chillies, coriander, turmeric, black pepper, and *garam masala.* After that there was a speedy growth in the marketing of mixed and recipe-based spices. Practically every popular dish, be it a curry, rice, snack, or dessert can now be made by the most inexperienced chef by merely following the instructions on the package and using the prepared spices. They are particularly popular with students living abroad on their own and with newlywed housewives. In fact, they are exported in large quantities to the West where the expatriate community eagerly pays a hefty price for them so that they may conjure up the dishes that remind them of home. Although a vast variety is now available, the most popular spice mixes tend to be *Biryani Masala, Tikka Masala, Karhai Gosht Masala, Qorma Masala,* and *Nihari Masala.*

NAYYER RUBAB

Paddy. A paddy field is a flooded parcel of arable land used for growing semiaquatic crops, most notably rice and taro. Originating from the Neolithic rice-farming cultures of the Yangtze River basin in southern China, it spread widely in prehistoric times and to date paddy field farming is practiced extensively in a number of

South Asian countries, including Pakistan, where it remains the dominant form of growing rice in modern times. Fields can be built into steep hillsides as terraces and adjacent to depressed or steeply sloped features such as rivers or marshes. They can require a great deal of labour and materials to create and need large quantities of water for irrigation. Oxen and water buffalo, adapted for life in wetlands, are important working animals used extensively in paddy field farming.

Pakhtun. The Pakhtuns of Khyber Pakhtunkhwa generally take two main meals a day, one at forenoon and the other at night or late evening. Breakfast, if taken, generally comprises a cup of tea and *roti* or *paratha* fried in *desi ghee*, depending on the family's financial status. Eggs, if the family can afford, are also consumed. *Naan* is baked in a *tandoor*, especially in Peshawar—where, traditionally, practically every house has its own *tandoor*—and is consumed even for breakfast, or large thin *chapati* is prepared on the *tawa* or on the *tabai*—a special kind of *tawa* intrinsic to many households in Peshawar. This is deeper than the regular *tawa*, has a lid, and the *naan* is baked in it on low heat for a longer period of time than the *chapati*.

Food in Peshawar is almost similar to the neighbouring Afghanistan's fare—with the ethnic composition of the dominant communities in both areas being the same—than to the Punjabi cuisine. The staple food at lunch and dinner consists of bread made of wheat flour, substituted by *makai ki roti* on some days, as corn is grown in abundance in the province. Other popular variations of bread include *til walay naan* (sesame seed *naan*), *Afghani roti* (very long and thick *naan*); Peshawari *naan* (stuffed with a mixture of nuts and raisins), *khameeri roti* (bread with yeast), and *gunzakhi* (a small *roti* or roll prepared with milk, pure fat, and *gur*. The last is a speciality commonly made in Khyber Pakhtunkhwa when a girl visits her parents' house for the first time after marriage.

Among the street food specialities that Peshawar is famous for are its *chapli kebab*, *charsi tikka*, *namak mandi seekh kebab*, pink tea, green tea, cottage cheese and fish *pakoray*.

Makai ki roti is usually taken with *saag* (indigenous green plants), *lassi* and yoghurt, while wheat bread is consumed with cooked vegetables, *daal* or *achar*. When *khameeri roti* is eaten at dinner, it is a common practice to save at least one, which is kept overnight in the smouldering *tandoor* normally found in every household, and then eaten the following day with the

evening tea. It is so popular, that family members normally make a beeline to get to it first.

Fresh water and river fish are popular with the fishermen residing in the Swat region. Local river fish include *rohu* (carp), *mahseer* (tor species), trout, and silva. Accompaniments include raw onions and green chillies, though, traditionally, the Pakhtuns are not in the habit of consuming spicy food which is more common in central and southern regions of the country. Chilli is consumed mostly in its fresh form and that too, generally by the women folk, green chillies being their favourite. There is, however, liberal use of certain spices in the urban areas of Khyber Pakhtunkhwa.

The poor eat barley or millet—both grown in the region—while dates are often used to supplement food requirements. However, the Pakhtuns are very fond of beef and would prefer to partake of it at both meals, if they can afford it. Their fondness for meat is more than amply reflected in the Pushto proverb, which says that even burnt meat is better than pulses. Food of the Pakhtuns in the erstwhile tribal areas is normally cooked in lamb fat as most of them rear sheep. *Turai gosht* (ribbed gourd and meat) is a popular dish.

A quintessentially Peshawari meal known as *khauncha roti* comprises a *thaal* (a large, round steel platter) with food enough to serve four people. It is always served to groups of four people sitting together and the meal normally contains *roti*, a rice dish, and one or two meat items.

In the absence of meat, milk or milk products and/or vegetables are consumed with bread or rice. Potatoes are the most widely used vegetables. *Gur* is commonly used to prepare sweet dishes, as there is an abundance of sugarcane in the area; it is normally served at the end of a meal. As with the Pakhtuns of Afghanistan, green tea with lots of sugar is popular among the Pakhtuns here, and is usually taken after meals. When guests are served green tea, the hosts keep refilling their cups until the guests turn their cup over which indicates that they have had enough.

Central to their identity as a Pakhtun is adherence to the male-centred code of conduct, *Pakhtunwali*.

Pakhtunwali. The Pakhtuns living in Afghanistan, Pakistan, and other parts of the world have a male-centred code of conduct, *Pakhtunwali*, which is strictly practised by every proud Pakhtun and is central to their identity. *Pakhtunwali* literally means 'the way of the Pakhtuns'—an unwritten tribal honour code that has governed the male Pakhtun way of life for centuries.

One of the key components of *Pakhtunwali* is *melmastya*, a trait common among the Pakhtuns, whether rich or poor. The Pakhtuns serve their guests often beyond their means. They also overspend on food on festive occasions, when goats and sheep are generally slaughtered. During the harvesting season, for instance, a farm owner whose land is due for harvesting hosts a special dinner. After the neighbours turn up in large numbers to help their fellow farmer, the family of the landowner serves them meat or chicken *yakhni* (soup) with *naan* broken into pieces. The guests sit around large earthenware bowls in groups of fours and fives and eat directly out of the pot. A complex etiquette surrounds the serving of guests, in which the host and his sons do not sit with those they entertain, as a mark of courtesy.

Another key component of *Pakhtunwali* is *nanawatai* (sanctuary), protection of guests. Pakhtuns will never allow anybody to harm or surrender their guest. If a person seeks refuge in the house of a Pakhtun, even if it is an enemy, the host is honour-bound to offer him protection, even at the cost of his own family.

Yet another component is *badal* (revenge), seeking justice or taking revenge against the wrongdoer. There is no time limit as to when the injustice can be avenged. If *badal* is not exercised, the offended man or his family would be considered stripped of honour, hence this practice sometime leads to generations of blood feud.

Pakistan Administered Jammu and Kashmir. Azad Jammu and Kashmir, abbreviated as AJK and commonly known as Azad Kashmir, is a region administered by Pakistan as a nominally self-governing jurisdiction. It constitutes the western portion of the larger Kashmir region which has been the subject of dispute between India and Pakistan since 1947, and between India and China since 1962. The territory shares a border with Gilgit–Baltistan, together with which it is referred to by the United Nations and other international organisations as 'Pakistan administered Kashmir'. Azad Kashmir is one-sixth the size of Gilgit–Baltistan. The territory also borders Pakistan's Punjab province to the south and Khyber Pakhtunkhwa province to the west. To the east, Azad Kashmir is separated from the Indian occupied Kashmir by the Line of Control—the *de facto* border between India and Pakistan. Azad Kashmir has a total area of 13,297 sq. km. (5,134 sq miles), and a total population of 4,045,366 as per the 2017 census. Nearly 87 per cent of households own farms in Azad Kashmir, while the region has a literacy rate of approximately 72 per cent and the highest school enrolment in Pakistan.

The territory has a parliamentary form of government with its capital located at Muzaffarabad. The president is the constitutional head of state, while the prime minister, supported by a council of ministers, is the chief executive. The state has its own Supreme Court and a High Court, while the government of Pakistan's Ministry of Kashmir Affairs and Gilgit–Baltistan serves as a link with Azad Kashmir's government, although Azad Kashmir is not represented in the parliament of Pakistan.

Interestingly enough, in Azad Kashmir, one would be hard pressed to find authentic Kashmiri fare served at restaurants and hotels. The most common dishes available on their menus are the ubiquitous *karhai*, and *biryani* whereas in vegetarian fare *lobia* and a local *saag* are abundantly consumed.

Pakora. The origin of the pakora can be traced to the Gujarati *bhajiya*, a term now only used among Gujaratis themselves, and has been widely replaced by the more popular *pakora*. An ancient snack, and among the *farsan* items eaten by them either with a main course or on its own as a snack, these are fried dumplings made with gram flour mixed with water and spices. Vegetables like potatoes, spinach, stuffed green chillies, and onions are commonly coated with the *besan* batter, while eggplant and cauliflower are also occasionally used. Conversely, vegetables could be chopped and mixed in the batter. The coated vegetables or vegetable batter is then spooned into hot crackling oil and deep fried to a golden colour. Pakoray are very popular as a snack at tea-time, at *iftar* during Ramazan, and are also regarded as the go-to snack in rainy weather. In the Sikh community, these are served as appetisers on special occasions, especially at weddings.

SHAHA TARIQ

Pakwan. There are several dishes that are, in particular, prepared for special occasions by Hindkowans. Among them is *pakwan*, a post-wedding dessert. When a Hindkowan bride returns to her maternal home the first time after marriage, the entire family gets together to make a sweet flour preparation with eggs and milk, thoroughly kneaded and deep fried. The bride takes these with her for all her in-laws when she returns to her new home. It is taken with tea in the evenings.

Palak paneer. Originating in Persia, *palak paneer* is a spinach dish introduced to the region by the Mughals. This lightly cooked vegetarian platter has chunks of fried cottage cheese in it.

Palapu. Traditionally, buckwheat pasta with a rich nutty sauce of walnuts and almonds, *palapu* is a Baltistani dish that is being substituted more and more by wheat pasta as the younger generation of Baltis are finding it increasingly difficult to consume buckwheat.

Palav/osh/pulao. Although *palav*, *pilau* or *pulao* is regarded as one of the oldest preparations of rice with Persian or Arab roots, there is evidence that this term existed much earlier in Sanskrit (in the *Yajnavalkya Smriti*) and Tamil. However, another school of thought holds that there is no evidence that rice was cooked by this technique in India before the Muslim invasions. Indians themselves associate *pulao/pilaf*-making with Muslim cities such as Hyderabad, Lucknow, and Delhi. According to one belief, during their stay in Bactria, Alexander the Great's army became hooked on what is regarded as the Bactrians' greatest gift to the world, the ancient *pilaf* or *pilau*, a rice dish cooked with meat, and took the recipe with them when they went back to Greece. *Pilaf's* arrival in Greece initiated its spread to Eastern Europe and it entrenched itself permanently into most cuisines of the ancient world.

Traditionally, the Persian version of *pilau* was a dish of barley or wheat with no spices, cooked with meat and infused with saffron, over coal campfires, historically cooked by nomadic Persian shepherds. The Persians substituted barley and wheat with rice, upon their discovery of this grain during their invasion of India.

Cooked with spices, meat, and vegetables by the absorption method, *pilau's* quality was always judged by how the rice was cooked, always fluffy, not sticky or forming clumps—a criterion that is considered vital in the methods of cooking *biryani* as well. In fact, this style of cooking has been the inspiration for many Pakistani rice dishes.

Panch phoron. A combination of five spices (*panch* means five), the key ingredients used in equal portion are onion seeds, fenugreek seeds, fennel seeds, cumin seeds, and mustard seeds (collectively known as *panch phoron*). The combination gives a distinctive aroma and flavour to pulse and vegetable dishes. The spice mixture comes from the eastern coastal state of Bengal and, therefore, one finds its usage more common in Karachi, where Bengalis have left their mark more vividly than anywhere else in Pakistan. The spices, which are usually left whole, are fried in hot oil or *ghee*, to which they impart their perfume, before the other ingredients are added.

Paneer. The Persian, Turkish, and Urdu word for cheese, *paneer* is generally used to denote cottage cheese specifically—the only kind of cheese used in cooking some traditional dishes. Known for combining a good supply of protein with a low-calorie count at a relatively low cost, cottage cheese has also gained popularity as a dish to be served on its own among the urban elite that is now conscious of healthful and organic foods. Otherwise, *paneer* is popularly eaten mixed with spinach in the vegetarian Punjabi dish *palak paneer*. It is also an important ingredient in many Bengali desserts.

Pani puri/gol gappa/puchka. Rolled out wheat flour dough, and deep fried into small, globular, thin, crispy and hollow shells, *pani puri/gol gappay/puchkay* are eaten as a light snack accompanied by boiled chickpeas and/or boiled and mashed potatoes and a tangy, pepper-water liquid. Originally a Gujarati snack, they are now as much a popular roadside item as a snack to be served at elitist parties, wedding occasions, etc.

Panjiri. A classic Punjabi dish made from whole wheat flour stir-fried lightly in sugar and ghee, *panjiri* is heavily laced with dry fruit—in fact, five types of finely cut dry fruits are used, thus the name *panj* meaning five—and herbal gums. It is usually eaten in winter to ward off cold, and given to mothers after delivery as it is believed to boost the production of breast milk. It is also often presented at weddings from the groom's side, to the bride's family.

Pao bhaji. A Portuguese contribution, *pao bhaji* is rather like an elastic bun, which is baked in square shape to form four sections that can be broken apart (hence the name *pao*, meaning quarter). Generally eaten with cooked vegetables (*bhaji*), mostly mixed—beans, carrots, cauliflowers, potatoes, bottle gourd, etc.—it is also a favourite staple with *daal gosht*. Today, it is more popularly consumed by the Gujarati community.

Papar (papadam). Also known as *happala*, *papar* is first mentioned in a book published in AD 1200 describing food consumed in Karnataka. Basically, *papar* is pulse flour dough rolled out very thin into discs and deep-fried or roasted to crispness, used as an accompaniment to meals. It is made from pulses like *urad*, *masoor*, *chana*, and others, and sometimes with tapioca, rice, or potato flour. Popular among the Gujaratis, it is a common accompaniment to main courses like *dahi ki karhi* and *khichri*. While the names *papar* and *papadam* are generally interchangeable, *papadam* is the more anglicised name for *papar*, used by high-end eateries or the modern younger generation. However, there is a slight difference; *papadam* is smaller, rolled out a little thicker and always fried, and puffed out more, while the *papar* is larger (about 22 cm in diameter), rolled out paper-thin, and not necessarily fried, as roasted versions are also very popular.

Papaya (*Carica papaya*). One of the best tropical fruits, papaya looks rather like a pear-shaped melon. The papaya plant is a very large, semi-woody herb, shaped like a palm tree but with huge fingered leaves. It grows quickly from seed and bears fruit within a year. The preferred type of commercial papaya is generally up to 500g in weight. It is pear shaped, pale green when unripe and blotchy yellow or orange when ripe. The pulp inside is of a creamy orange colour, soft, delicately scented, and sweet. At the centre is a mass of black seeds encased in a gelatinous coating. Although these are edible, the seeds are generally discarded. In Pakistan, the provinces of Sindh and the Punjab are rich in lavish green plantations of papaya. Seaside territories of Sindh province and Malir zone of Karachi have been developing papaya on a large scale. There are two seasons of cultivation— February to March, and July to August.

Paratha. Rich, flaky, flatbread, *paratha* is an oil-rich version of *chapati* generally made with refined flour, although whole wheat flour is also frequently used. Believed to have originated in the Punjab, *paratha* is richer both because of the oil or *ghee* it contains, and the layers of dough that are rolled out and compressed to make a single *paratha*. In fact, *parath* means layer, while *atta* is dough. The dough is divided into balls, slightly flattened, a little oil added to it, and then made into a ball again. One may just roll it out (into a square or a circle) and fry it on an iron griddle, by adding spoonful of oil to the sides of the *paratha* and fry it from both sides till done, or one could opt to flatten the ball, add more oil, and then flatten it again and fold over, repeating the process as many times as one desires to make the *paratha* richly layered and flaky, and then rolling it out and following the same process of frying.

The dough could be mixed with seasoned vegetables like potatoes, spinach, or fenugreek. Or, it could have various types of traditional fillings, such as *daal*, cooked radish, onion, chopped eggs, mince, spinach, or potatoes. Once regarded as a form of bread ideally eaten at breakfast or with barbecued food at dinner, these days *paratha* has taken on an entirely new avatar, especially in the metropolitan city of Karachi. From a food item normally shunned by the weight- and health-conscious elite of the country, it has become the most sought-after snack item to be consumed either with evening tea, or post-dinner *qehwa*/tea. From chicken *tikka paratha* to Nutella *paratha*, and from cheese and egg *paratha* to plain cheese and plain egg *paratha*, there is no dearth of choices.

SHAHA TARIQ AND SHANAZ RAMZI

Parsi. Although Persians were doing business with the subcontinent from approximately 500 BC, the exact time of the arrival of Parsis here is debatable. It is generally believed that approximately a thousand years ago, a group of Zoroastrians fled from Persia (mainly from the province of Pars) to escape religious persecution; they were given asylum in Gujarat, and settled in Surat where they eventually came to be known as Parsis or 'people of Pars'. Before Gujarat, the group had briefly inhabited the Diu region of India, but soon afterwards their dastur (leader) determined that their destiny lay elsewhere. They left Diu and after braving a life-threatening storm, reached Gujarat.

Responding to their request for asylum, King Jadav Rana, the ruler of the tiny community where they landed, sent them a bowl filled to the brim with milk (a gentle hint that his kingdom was full and couldn't accept refugees). In reply, the leader of the Persians dissolved a spoonful of sugar in the milk and sent it back to the king, suggesting that his small flock would dissolve like sugar in the milk and enrich the king's community without straining its resources. These refugees were the forefathers of the subcontinent's Parsi community. The story of their arrival and settling down in Gujarat is called the *Qea-ye Sanjān* (*The Story of Sanjān*).

King Jadav Rana's permission to the refugees to stay in his land came with a few conditions: they would have to learn and use only the local language, the women would have to wear saris, and the use of weapons and conversion of any local people were strictly prohibited. The dastur agreed to these conditions and so the Parsis settled down in the subcontinent, enriching its culture and contributing heavily towards its economy and prosperity. Although they assimilated with the local population, adopting the language and attire of their Hindu benefactors, they maintained their distinct identity. They thrived as a mercantile community with strong social and religious ethics based on 'good thought, good word and good deed.'

When the Europeans began to arrive, they adapted again, learned English, moved into shipping, and grew wealthy from the China trade. The East India Company merchants, in Bombay (now Mumbai), mixed with the Parsis during the early days of the company and later, once their rule was established, often employed Parsi butlers in their households.

By the middle of the 19th century, Parsis had settled in Karachi in substantial numbers, retaining a great deal of their ancient heritage in their religious and gastronomical habits.

In fact, despite having lived in the subcontinent for well over a thousand years, the Parsis remain a very unique minority community. Their cuisine is also very distinct; it is a blend, that reflects their Iranian ancestry and the influences of their adopted region, Gujarat. The use of spices is often complex, but moderate. Parsis like meat, and a Parsi meal normally includes a meat, fish, or chicken dish. The most famous Parsi meat dish is *dhansak*. Fish, including pomfret and Bombay duck, is much eaten and is regarded, along with coconut and rice, as a symbol of plenty. A group of curry-type sweet-and-sour fish dishes are known as *patias*.

The Iranian influence is apparent in the free use of nuts, sultanas, and raisins. Eggs are an essential part of the Parsi cuisine; they are not just eaten at breakfast but also as entree at lunch or dinner. Parsis love their eggs, which find their way on top of almost every vegetable, while there are numerous egg dishes. Parsi *pora* is a must for Sunday breakfasts, as is *akoori*. Another favourite is *salli par eeda*, regarded as a perfect Parsi breakfast, though it is just as popular at lunch or even dinner. Comprising a small heap of cooked potato shreds mixed with spiced tomatoes and onion paste, the dish is gently fried with an egg on top. Another variation is *papeta par eeda* which is baked and does not include tomatoes. However, although most Parsis adhere strictly to Zoroastrianism, they are one of the most Westernised of all Pakistani communities. As such, they have hardly any food restrictions, and their cuisine is a delicious blend of sweet and sour flavours. Although they have made quite a remarkable impact on Karachi, the size of the Parsi community in the metropolis is in decline. There are now fewer than 1,700, down from more than 7,000 several decades ago. That's just a drop in the ocean in a city that reportedly has a total population of over 14 million.

BISMA TIRMIZI

Partition. August 1947 saw the partition of the Indian subcontinent into two dominion states of India and Pakistan. The term Partition does not cover the secession of Bangladesh (1971) or the earlier one of Burma (Myanmar) from the British Administration. It also does not cover the separation of Ceylon (now Sri Lanka) from the subcontinent.

The Partition was the fulfilment of the concept agreed upon and signed in 1940 that came to be known as the Pakistan Resolution—an independent state to be carved out from within the subcontinent for the Muslims of India. Muslim majority provinces were to be selected and grouped together for the purpose. On 3 June 1947, the last Viceroy Lord Mountbatten gave his plan for the same. The boundaries were drawn, and 14 and 15 August saw the realisation of their collective dreams as Pakistan and India gained independence from the British Raj, respectively.

However, a lot of struggle, bloodshed, and massacre preceded this event, which is classified under Freedom Movement. Some territorial issues like Kashmir remain unresolved to date; it is one of the longest unresolved political disputes in the world and impacts Pakistan–India relations time and again. Kashmir was not the only province that had its heart divided; Punjab also lost its eastern part to India and a large part of Thar remained with Rajasthan on the other side.

Modern-day discussions—political, economic, social, religious, et al.—refer to Partition as a major event in changing the dynamics of the region and creating subsequent environments in which we function today.

Partition in terms of cuisine had its own impact. Provincial cuisines (Punjab, Sindh, Khyber Pakhtunkhwa, and Balochistan) gained prominence, along with Kashmiri specialities which retained their own distinction. Influences of Delhi, Lucknow, Hyderabad, Mysore, and Gujarat's flavours travelled with the migrants to make place among the essentially Pakistani dishes.

SHAHA TARIQ

Pasanda. Based on the word *pasand* meaning 'fond of', *pasanda* is a popular Pakistani dish of Mughal origin, which uses prime cuts of meat, creamy yoghurt, nuts, and screw pine. Served in the court of the Mughal emperors, *pasanda* was originally made with leg of lamb flattened into strips, marinated, and fried in yoghurt and spices. These thin steaks are now generally made of beef, especially the part known as 'undercut' in Pakistan (the meat along the edge of the spine of the cow).

Pastry. This is a collective name for items that are usually based on short, puff, or choux pastry or sponge. Pastry basically comprises flour, fat, and water made into a dough and cooked. It may incorporate other ingredients such as fruits, nuts, jam, fresh cream, chocolate, coconut and much more. Exactly what is counted among pastries depends on the country concerned. In Pakistan, the term covers all the sweet bakers' confectionaries used as selection for dessert or to serve at tea time. Although pastries are not necessarily sweet, in Pakistan the term is only used for confectionaries when referring to the prepared item. Pastry dough, however, is now sold at bakeries, and are used to prepare savoury items as well such as pie crusts and *vol-au-vent*.

Patarveliya/patra. A Gujarati speciality, *patarveliya* is a snack made with taro or *arvi* leaves, on which a spicy, sweet, and sour paste is spread. The leaves are then expertly stacked together and bound as a roll. The roll can be frozen for later consumption. Thin slices are cut to reveal elegant swirls of *patarveliya*, which are then deep-fried and eaten hot and crisp.

Pathia. A traditional Parsi dish *pathia* was brought from Persia by Parsis who settled in Tarapur, now in Gujarat. A group of curry-type sweet-and-sour seafood dishes *pathia* is made with prawns or fish (mostly pomfret) cooked in a dark vinegar sauce with spices, herbs, jaggery or palm sugar, and tamarind. Chicken or lamb versions also exist but are not originally Parsi. It is usually served on special occasions such as birthdays, weddings, or any auspicious occasion like Navroze—marking the beginning of the Persian year and the advent of spring, celebrated on 21 March—accompanied with *dhandor* which is basically made of *arhar daal* and boiled rice. The served rice is first topped with two or three tablespoons of *dhandor* and further topped with a tablespoon of *pathia*. This spicy, sweet, and sour dish can be eaten hot or cold and can be stored in the refrigerator in an air-tight jar for up to a month.

Patisa. A popular Lahori dessert, *lachchedaar patisa* is made with sugar, gram flour, flour, *ghee*, milk, and cardamom. Produced by confectioners, it has a crisp and flaky texture. Although it was traditionally sold loose, in a rolled paper cone, modern industrial production has led it to be packed as cubes or sold as flakes.

Patrani machchi. A fish dish, *patrani machchi* is a famous Parsi dish eaten on auspicious occasions and a favourite dish to be served at Parsi weddings. The fish fillets (sole, plaice, or pomfret) are cut in slices and thickly coated with a green chutney made by grinding fresh coriander, mint leaves, green chillies, desiccated coconut, lemon juice or vinegar, cumin seeds, garlic cloves, sugar, and salt. Banana leaves are singed on both sides very gently on a low flame and then the fish pieces are wrapped individually in banana leaf 'packets' with toothpicks inserted and woven through the leaf to secure them. The packets are steamed, then fried or baked till done. *Patrani machchi* is served as it is, in the parcel, and guests enjoy opening the leaves and eating the fish from it. Small whole pomfrets coated with green chutney are also often steamed in banana leaves, with slits on the fish to ensure that the masala seeps in well.

Around the world, wherever bananas grow, cooks have devised ways to use the banana leaves, wrapping them around foods, both savoury and sweet. A parcel made from banana leaves seals in moisture and flavour and infuses the contents with a subtle, grassy aroma. At Parsi weddings, food is served on large banana leaves that add to its taste and the fun in eating off it! Banana leaf also makes a beautiful background on which to serve various dishes and is also excellent for steaming, as it allows the steam to penetrate the food inside or on top of it. It is not unusual for Parsis to use banana leaves to line a steamer, or to wrap food in it and then steam it.

ZARNAK SIDHWA

Patta tikka. A favourite of the Pakhtuns living in what used to be known as the Tribal Areas, now a part of KP, *patta tikka* is a meat dish, heavily laced with fat.

Patties. Made of pastry dough rolled out thinly, the characteristic flaky texture of patties is achieved by repeatedly rolling out the dough, spreading butter on it, and folding it to produce many thin layers or folds. Patties are light, airy, and fatty, but firm enough to support the weight of the filling, which could be either mincemeat (chicken or beef) or vegetable.

Pawan matar-aloo bhaji. A Gujarati speciality, *pawan* is flattened, boiled and dried rice, hydrated with water before cooking. It is stir-fried with potatoes and peas.

Paya/paaye. Said to have originated in Persia and brought to Delhi, where it found favour among the royals and their nobles who considered it a delicacy, *paaye*—feet or trotters—of a cow, goat or sheep were the most expensive parts of the animal. Traditionally a winter breakfast dish, its preparation is a painstaking job. The *paaye* have to be first roasted over open fire to burn off the hair from the skin while taking care not to scorch the skin since that would spoil the flavour of the dish. The *paaye* are then cooked for a long time (usually overnight) in a pot of water with spices until the soupy curry acquires a sticky consistency—the prolonged cooking melts the fat in the *paaye* making the curry sticky and full of natural gelatine. The curry is generally created by sautéing onions, tomatoes, and garlic and adding a number of curry-based spices to it. There is very little meat, but the tendons, fat, connective tissues and bone marrow all contribute to producing a smoky and intense flavour. In the past, when people used wood or coal as a cooking fuel, women would cook this dish all night on low heat. *Paaye* are usually eaten with *naan* or *kulchay*. Fresh chopped coriander, ginger, green chillies, and sliced lemon are used as garnish. Recipe for this dish varies slightly from region to region. Variations of this delicacy include *kunnah paya* (a mix of the Chinioti dish *kunnah*), *bong paya* (a blend of *nihari* and *paya* with prime chunk of meat added to the trotters) and the older *siri paya* (*siri* means head, which is cooked along with the trotters). Occasionally, tongue and bone marrow are also added to the dish. *Paaye* serve as a remedy for people with joint pains and is also great for colds and coughs.

Pea. A legume which originated in western Asia, pea has been a staple food since ancient times. There are three main kinds: the first, the common cultivated garden pea, *mattar* in Urdu, is *Pisum sativum*, by far the most important. Second, and supposedly the ancestor of the garden pea, is the field or grey pea, that used to be distinguished as *P. aravense*, the small, marbled field pea still in use in the country and which has been found in Harappa sites. The third is the small, wild Mediterranean pea. Although other legumes of different genera are also popularly called 'peas'—such as chickpea, pigeon pea—this entry focuses on the popular green peas. In Pakistan, green peas are cooked as a vegetable to be eaten on their own with *chapati*, or along with rice or mince as *peas pulao* or *qeema mattar*, respectively. They are also used to make several snack items, and as an accompaniment/garnish to various meat dishes.

Peach. A fruit distinguished by its velvety skin, the peach, *Amygdalus persica*, belongs to the rose family and is classified as a drupe, i.e. fruit with a hard stone.

It is a fruit of temperate but warm climates, which will not endure either tropical heat or severe cold. Peaches are easily raised from seed. Having its origin in China, its cultivation spread westwards through areas with a suitable climate, such as Kashmir to Persia. Most of the peaches available in Pakistan come from the northern areas or from Afghanistan.

Pear. *Pyrus communis*, *P. sinensis*, and other *Pyrus* spp, the pear, or *nashpati* in Urdu, originated in the general region of the Caucasus, as did its cousin the apple. Both the fruits were spread by the Aryan tribes from that area as they migrated into Europe and the subcontinent. Both belong to the rose family, Rosaceae. Pears were brought during the time of Mughal Emperor Akbar, from Kashmir and Samarkand but were also grown in the hilly, northern areas, as they continue to do even today.

Peethi ki kachori. A Dilliwallay speciality, *peethi ki kachori* is a fried, layered *puri* stuffed with masala or a variety of fillings which include mince, vegetables, or *daal*, especially *urad daal*. It is eaten normally on special occasions or in Ramazan and on Eid.

Penhon. A Sindhi traditional dessert made of crushed rice cooked in sugared water, *penhon* is served normally at breakfast, especially the day after a wedding.

Peppercorn. The common spice, black pepper, is *Piper nigrum*. True peppers belong to the genus *Piper*, but the common name 'pepper' is applied to very different products. True peppers are only white and black pepper. The actual word 'pepper' comes from the Sanskrit *pippali* where it referred to long pepper. One of the food-related words in Tamil that entered Sanskrit is *milgu* or *miriyam* (pepper) which occurs as *maricha* (*mirchi* in Urdu). One of the oldest known spices, peppercorn is native to the subcontinent. Peppercorns are the tiny berries of a perennial vining shrub *P. nigrum* of the Piperaceae family, and one of the world's most important spice plants; they are picked when fully-developed but still unripe. They are left in heaps for a few days to ferment and then spread out on mats in the sun to dry. As they dry, the berries turn black and the skin and part of the pulp form a reticulated covering to the seed. To produce white pepper, the berries are left for longer before harvesting. They are then soaked in water so that the outer skin may be washed off to reveal the pale inner core before sun-drying. As the flavour is mostly contained in the outer skin, while the pungency lies in the inner core, white pepper is fierier than black but with a subtler flavour. Pepper is available whole or finely ground, and has become, with the exception of salt, the most used daily spice in the world. Pepper increases the metabolic rate, improves blood circulation, and stimulates bladder function. It stimulates the appetite and digestion, encourages perspiration, and has considerable antioxidant and antibacterial properties. Pepper has outstanding value in treating coughs and colds. Its main culinary function is as a preservative. It is a frequent ingredient in Pakistani cuisine, usually in the form of whole peppercorns in rice, meat, and pickles. Powdered, it is one of the main ingredients of the mixed spices that are the basis of curry powders. Pepper is also used extensively in herbal medicines.

Persian influence. Persian influences in the sub-continent (Indo-Persian) were first introduced to South Asia by the Delhi Sultanate (11–13th century Afghan kings) and then by the Mughal Empire (c.1526). Aspects of the language and culture were brought to the subcontinent by various 'Persianised' Central Asian, Turkic and Afghan rulers and conquerors, the most notable among them being Mahmud of Ghazni in the 11th century AD. Many of the sultans and noblemen in the Sultanate period were Turks from Central Asia who spoke the Turkic language, but Persian became the preferred language of the Delhi Sultanate, the Mughal Empire, and their successor states and was also the cultured language of poetry and literature. As a result of this strong Persian culture on the royal courts of the Mughals, a cuisine developed that was strongly influenced by Persian food and cooking techniques. Owing to his fondness for Persian culture, the court kitchens of the second Mughal emperor, Humayun (1506–1556), experienced an influx of a large number of Persian cooks. These cooks brought Persian cuisine to the subcontinent, and further enhanced the already established Persian cooking techniques introduced by the Abbasid caliph of Baghdad, about five centuries earlier. The *pièce de résistance* of Persian cuisine at this time was *pilau*—rice was imported from the subcontinent and was relatively expensive, therefore a rice dish was always prepared as the centrepiece rather than a side dish, leading to the development of lavish Persian rice-based recipes. These appealed to the Mughals, during their time spent in Persia, and inspired them to bring these recipes back with them, where they were developed further in combination with local spices by Persian chefs. The most significant

fusion of the subcontinental and Persian food happened when the Persian *pilau* evolved into the classic Mughlai *biryani*. Persian techniques of marinating meat with yoghurt, spices, onion, garlic and nuts were used, with the rice infused using the *dum* method with saffron and nuts. Other 'imports' from Persian cuisine were *haleem*, sherbets of crushed ice mixed with fruit juices, and stewed meat dishes with butter and rich spices, such as *roghan josh*. The use of fruits, both fresh and dried, and nuts with savoury food was popular in the royal kitchens as were rich milk- and saffron-based desserts. Also originating in Persia, *kulfi* is believed to have been introduced in the subcontinent to please the palate of the great Mughal Emperor Akbar and developed further by later Mughals who brought ice to Delhi from a mountain near Kasauli called Chur-Dhar (also known as Churi-Chandni Dhar which means mountain dressed in the moonlight) which is perennially covered with snow. The method of making *kulfi* has remained unchanged to the present day. Many subsequent nawabi, Kashmiri and other Pakistani/North Indian recipes have taken on Persian names and to this day, many of Pakistan's festive dishes are based on Persian cooking techniques.

SUMMAYA USMANI

Peshawar. Close to the Khyber Pass, at the head of the fertile Indus Valley lies verdant Peshawar, the provincial capital of Khyber Pakhtunkhwa. Peshawar represents a city of Pakistan where people still closely adhere to their local customs and traditions. It is a city where residents have not incorporated changes in lifestyle at the same rate as residents of the larger cities of Pakistan, and consequently follow a slower pace of life. Interestingly enough, the largest urban population of Pakhtuns is not concentrated in Peshawar but in Karachi. A number of Sikhs, on the other hand, are settled here, as in other parts of Khyber Pakhtunkhwa, though their largest concentration is in the Punjab. The language of the original families living in the walled city of Peshawar was Hindko which has now been replaced by Urdu and Pushto.

Phaturay/kachori. Regarded as a classic Punjabi dish, *cholay phaturay*, surprisingly enough, originated in Delhi (where it is known as *chana bhatura*) and its surrounding areas. *Phaturay* are soft and fluffy fried *puris* with *maash daal* mixed into the dough. They are popularly eaten with chickpea curry, *achar*, and salad. Although eaten at any meal, they are preferred at breakfast or tea.

Pheni. The origin of the exceedingly thin, strand-like *pheni* can be traced to AD 1129–30 as the book *Manasollasa*, from that period, contains its recipe under the name *phenaka*. Wheat vermicelli from hard wheat doughs, extruded really fine and vended in bundles, *pheni* was usually eaten with sugared milk in Karnataka, where a vast variety of sweet items were consumed, and have changed little over a millennium. It figures in Gujarati historical literature as *sutar-pheni* as well as *khajla-pheni*, terms that are still used by Gujaratis. In Mughal times, the humbler Muslims ate desserts of *pheni*. Soaked in sugared milk, *pheni* is popular especially in Ramazan, when in many households it is partaken of both at *sehri* and *iftar*.

Phitti. Probably the most famous of all Hunza breads, *phitti*, a whole wheat flour bread is a common breakfast food. Thick and nutritious, though its preparation is time consuming, it is crusty from the outside and soft from the inside. The dough is put into a sealed metal container and the *phitti* is baked overnight over the hearth's embers.

Phoshpaki. A variation of the yeast bread, *phoshpaki* is popular with the Khows of Khyber Pakhtunkhwa.

Pickle. This refers to preserved foods, especially vegetables and fruits, and occasionally prawns, in a preserving medium with a strong salt or acid content. In Pakistan, the concept of pickled foods is limited to *achars*, which are relishes that usually accompany a main course. Immersing foods in vinegar or brine, or a mixture of the two, is a long-established way of preserving foods. Highly acidic solutions and strong salt solutions prevent micro-organisms from growing and enzymes from working. The acetic acid in vinegar has a disinfectant effect; hence, vinegar is a better preservative than other acidic liquids of the same strength. While most pickled foods use vinegars, a few recipes use lime juice. Sometimes sugar plays an important part as a preservative, as in chutneys. Mustard, ground or as whole seeds, is another common addition which helps to preserve the pickle, but almost any spice may be used in pickling.

Pineapple (*Ananas comosus*). Pineapple is a tropical fruit of impressive appearance and attractive flavour and is now grown in hot regions around the world. This is a composite fruit formed of 100–200 berry-like fruitlets fused together, giving its outside a tessellated appearance. It grows on a short stem springing from a low plant with large, sword-like leaves, small versions of which form the crown of the fruit. Although the pineapple was being grown in the subcontinent by the middle of the 16th century, it was not till after 1971, when Pakistan lost its eastern wing where pineapples were being produced, that it started to be cultivated in what is now Pakistan. But, even today, pineapple cultivation in Pakistan is limited to just a few areas in Sindh because of a number of constraints.

Po cha. A typical Tibetan drink, *po cha* is butter tea which is consumed all day long by Baltis living in Gilgit–Baltistan, to sustain them and keep them warm. It is made with cooked, specific tea leaves churned with salt, baking soda (optional), yak butter and goat milk.

Pomegranate. Rich in polyphenols and vitamins C and K, pomegranate is considered one of the heavenly fruits and a gift from God. Pomegranate (*Punica granatum*) belongs to the Punicaceae family, growing well in semi-arid, mild temperatures and naturally adapted to regions with cool winters and hot summers. The fruit of a small tree which is native to Iran and still grows wild there, it came to this region very early—excavations at Harappa in the Indus Valley (*c*.2000 BC) yielded 'two polychrome earthenware vases, the former shaped like a pomegranate and the latter shaped like a coconut.' The tree is bushy with thorny branches and brilliant orange flowers, and grows to a height of five metres. Good quality pomegranates, that are worth eating, have plenty of juicy pulp with a sweet, sharp flavour which is only slightly astringent. Inferior quality pomegranates, especially those from wild trees, contain mostly seeds and membranes, and whatever pulp they have is very sour and astringent. But sour pomegranates have their uses in Pakistan, where the seeds are used as a sour condiment, *anardana*. The province of Balochistan is the main producer of pomegranates in Pakistan, while pomegranates are also being cultivated in isolated areas in Khyber Pakhtunkhwa and the Punjab on a small scale. Pomegranates are popularly consumed both on their own and as a refreshing juice extracted from the pulp. This delectable fruit boosts the immune system and helps purify the blood.

LAL MAJID

Pomfret. The name pomfret is mainly used for two deep-bodied narrow fish of Asian coastal waters. These have many characteristics in common but belong to different families. The white pomfret, *Pampus argenteus* belongs to the family Stromateidae, whereas the so-called black (brown grey in reality) pomfret, *Parastromateus niger*, is a member of the family Carangidae. The pomfrets, when adult, have no pelvic fins. The white pomfret is the larger of the two, more expensive and more esteemed. Its firm white flesh divides readily into fillets. The black pomfret is also delicious, but notorious for its fine bones. It is mostly found in Karachi's coastal waters.

Poori. A spicy version of omelette, *poori* is a Parsi breakfast dish and is a popular item with *roti* at picnics as well. Raw chopped mango is added when in season.

Poppy seed (*Papaver somniferum*; khashkhash). Tiny dried seeds of the opium poppy, poppy seeds are an ancient spice and have no narcotic properties, because the fluid in the bud that becomes opium is present only before the seeds are fully formed. The delicious nutty flavour of poppy seeds is always better when the seeds have first been roasted. The Pakistani poppy seeds (usually of the cultivar White Persian) is much smaller and off-white as compared to the more common blue-seeded ones used in most countries. They are used, often whole, to flavour curries and coat savoury items, as well as combined with jaggery syrup to make a popular sweet meat—*laddu*. Ground to a paste with water, poppy seeds are sometimes used as a thickening agent. Poppy seeds are also crushed to give an oil of fine flavour. They are recommended in many prescriptions for tonics as they contain minerals such as calcium and phosphorus.

Portuguese culinary influence. The Portuguese came to the subcontinent in large numbers in the 16th century and ruled for 150 years. They intermarried with the locals (Goans) and introduced a variety of new dishes, ingredients, tastes and produce that came to be regarded as part of the local fare in time. When Sir Charles Napier occupied Sindh in 1843, many Goans who did not want to continue living under the Portuguese rule moved to Karachi—which was then being developed as the future hub of trade and commerce—bringing with them their cuisine.

Chilli pepper was introduced to the subcontinent by the Portuguese. No south Asian had seen it, let alone used it for cooking before the Portuguese arrived in the region at the beginning of the 15th century. Three different species of chilli plants had been introduced thirty years after Vasco da Gama set foot on the subcontinent, and that in itself is the greatest impact of Portuguese culinary influence on the subcontinent spice.

Although South Asians are often slow to accept new foodstuff, a few years after chilli had been introduced it was declared the 'saviour of the poor' for it became a cheap and easy way to give taste to the simple meal of rice and lentils.

Another ingredient introduced by the Portuguese to the subcontinent is vinegar, as it is an essential component of their cuisine. *Vindaloo*, normally regarded as subcontinental curry, is a Goan adaptation of the Portuguese dish *Carne Vinha d'alhos* (Garlic Wine Marinated Pork), or meat soaked and cooked in wine vinegar and garlic—the term *vindaloo* being a local distortion of the original name. When the Portuguese arrived in the subcontinent and found that the natives did not make vinegar, they got Franciscan priests to solve the problem by manufacturing vinegar from coconut toddy. The cooks combined this with *garam masala*, tamarind, black pepper, plenty of garlic, cinnamon, and cloves. But the key ingredient, which gave bite to the granular sauce of the *vindaloo* curry, as indeed all Portuguese dishes, was the chilli.

Although the Portuguese almost certainly also introduced tomatoes and potatoes to the subcontinent, these foods were not integrated into the subcontinental culinary world until the British showed their own cooks how to use them.

It is safe to assume that on their arrival in the northern part of the subcontinent, the Goanese worked together with the native cooks, and new flavours were born. The province of the Punjab also developed a liking for the taste of the spicy curry, and the Punjabi, Lucknawi, and Delhi cooks introduced our modern-day vegetable and meat curries. The comfort food of the subcontinent, and greatly enjoyed in Pakistan—*aaloo gosht, lauki gosht, tinda gosht, arvi gosht, bhindi* curry—are all a twist on the Goanese *vindaloo* sans the wine vinegar but rich in spice, chilli, and flavour.

They baked bread for use by the English or Dutch factories, ships, and private homes, and so added a variety of European breads to the subcontinental cuisine—crusty white rolls, soft croissant-like breads, and the sweet milk bread *massa sovada*. The leavened bread enjoyed in the subcontinent is an evolution of the toddy bread (since yeast was unavailable then) made in Goa in the 17th century for the Portuguese in the subcontinent. Their other speciality was fragrant egg custard, a style of dessert entirely new to the subcontinent at that time, where sweets were *halwa*, or *kheer*, spiced with cardamom and bound by clarified butter. The modern-day caramel custard and *crème brulee* are all sophisticated versions of the egg pudding/custard of yore.

The Portuguese successfully introduced New World fruits to the subcontinent as well—papayas, custard apples, and guavas from the Americas—all of which have been incorporated into the Pakistani diet. But the most popular was the pineapple which has become a familiar sight in Pakistan today. New crops like tobacco and cashew nut were also introduced by them to the region.

BISMA TIRMIZI

Potato. The potato (*Solanum tuberosum*) was introduced to the subcontinent probably as early as 1615, where it had a slow start; it was first accepted only by the Europeans and then by the Muslims. Later, with rapid general acceptance, the potato began to be grown all over the country, though at first it grew especially well in elevated terrain. Used in cooking in many different ways, it is popular as a dry *sabzi*, cooked either on its own or in accompaniment with other veggies, and eaten in accompaniment with the *chapati*, *paratha* or *puri*. It is also commonly used as a dry stuffing in *paratha*, *samosa* and *kachori*. It is frequently incorporated in the ubiquitous *gosht ka salan*, is an integral part of *aaloo salan*—a Dilliwalla version of it—and is a popular deep-fried snack or meal item, served as finger chips or french fries, or as cutlets—with or without a filling—or as a boiled ingredient in many *chaat* varieties.

Prabhu. A Balti speciality, *prabhu* is a highly popular dish in Gilgit–Baltistan. These are boiled dumplings made from whole wheat or barley and eaten with mint and coriander chutney.

Pulse. A collective term for the edible seeds of leguminous plants like grams, beans, lentils, and peas, the name may be used for either fresh or dried seeds. They have been a major staple food in human diet since earliest times. The word derives from the Latin *puls*, meaning pottage.

Drying, the simplest way of preserving all food, is a technique particularly suited to pulses; their protein and fat content remains largely intact, while the flavour, although altered, remains good. Several pulses are in use in Pakistan, many from remote antiquity, and are especially important. A distinction is made between gram, which are whole, unpeeled pulses, and *daal*, split, skinned pulses. Legume seeds are always double in form and split easily when the skin is rubbed off.

Pulses in general are sweet, except for horse gram which is considered pungent. Numerous pulse-based dishes abound in the country, many of which are used in combination with other key ingredients such as wheat and rice.

Pumpkin. A large vegetable fruit, typically orange in colour, round, and ribbed, pumpkin is borne by varieties of the plant *Cucurbita pepo*, one of four major species in the genus *Cucurbita*. Fruits of the species *C. pepo* and its hybrids may have other common names, such as squash. Pumpkins are eaten when fully ripe. They often grow to a large size. Pumpkin flesh is rather fibrous and has an earthy taste which is not universally liked. It is used for both savoury and sweet dishes.

Punch. A blend of arrack, distilled from palm juice, spices, sugar, lime-juice and water, punch was first noted in 1638 by Mandelslo as *palepuntz*, and became a popular drink in all the British colonies. It is a classic example of unique Anglo-Indian terms that arose in the area of food, after British colonisation of the subcontinent, and the arrival of the *memsahibs* (British ladies). Punch was from *panch*, and denoted the five components used in making the drink. In the course of time, numerous recipes for the drink developed, including one with milk.

Punjab. In sharp contrast to the rugged terrain of Khyber Pakhtunkhwa are the rich and fertile plains of the Punjab. The region has derived its name from five rivers that have influenced the lifestyle of the people of the province in much the same way as the mountains have affected the culture of the people of Khyber Pakhtunkhwa. These are the tributaries of the Indus River through which the Punjab is irrigated.

Rising in Tibet, the Indus flows down through the Karakoram Mountains that form a part of the northern borders of Pakistan and continues its journey southwards and westwards through the heart of the country, carrying and depositing rich alluvium that accounts for the Punjab's highly fertile soil. Though not the largest in area, the Punjab is the most developed province, and the nerve-centre of Pakistan, with over 60 per cent of Pakistan's population comprising Punjabis. It is also the most progressive part of Pakistan in terms of administration, trade, and learning.

Home to numerous villages, small, ancient towns and large cities, the province boasts the ruins of Harappa, a city belonging to the Indus Valley Civilisation that flourished about 5,000 years ago, and Multan, a city that was born only a few hundred years after the demise of the ancient civilisation. It also has the twin cities of Rawalpindi and Islamabad, the latter the modern federal capital of the country, situated on the Potohar Plateau; as well as Lahore, the cultural, architectural, and artistic centre of Pakistan, and the country's second largest city.

Lying in the pathway of many of the invasions to which the subcontinent has been subjected through the centuries, one can see the stamp of Persian, Greek, Turkish, Sikh, Afghan, and Mughal influence on the culture and cuisine of this region. The Punjab's population comprises basically indigenous Punjabis who trace their ancestry to pre-Islamic Jat and Rajput castes that arrived from Rajputana and Jaisalmer, later inter-marrying with other ethnic groups, which came to the area. Other Punjabis trace their heritage to Arabia, Persia, Balochistan, Afghanistan, and Kashmir.

Thus, in contrast to many other areas of the country where people often remained isolated, Punjabis have very diverse origins. This diversity facilitated their coalescence into a coherent ethnic community that has historically placed great emphasis both on farming and fighting. Interaction with one another has resulted in most Punjabis developing similar eating habits, although there are certain delicacies that are associated more with one or the other of the numerous tribes. Perhaps, that is why, in spite of the Punjab being famous for its cuisine, and Lahoris in particular being known for loving their manna, there are only specific indigenous dishes that the community is famous for.

Another large group of people living in the Punjab—south Punjab to be precise—is Saraikis but they are more a linguistic group than an ethnic one, and, hence, their cuisine is not distinct. Ethnically they are the same as the natives of Sindh and the rest of the Punjab and trace their ancestry to Jat and Rajput castes. In certain parts of the Punjab Khojas form a notable minority community as do the Baloch, Pakhtuns, Afghan refugees, and Sikhs.

Among the minority groups living in the Punjab are the Sikhs, who must be mentioned here, as unlike the other communities, who reside in greater numbers in other parts of the country, the Sikhs are mostly concentrated in the Punjab. According to the 2008 population census, they roughly number 20,000.

Rich in agricultural land, the Punjab grows wheat, barley, corn, and rice among other food grains. Wheat is the staple food grain in affluent Punjabi families, while millet, barley and maize are the staple food of the people in the rural areas. Rural Punjabis also partake of meals comprising thick *chapati* made of rice of inferior quality, accompanied by *lassi*, onions and chillies. The farmers in the rural areas consume green grams and vegetables along with the staples. *Sattu*, made of barley seeds is a popular drink in some villages, especially in summer, and is often taken at lunch, along with *missi roti* made of mixed wheat and gram, flavoured with salt and chillies. In other rural areas of the province, breakfast simply comprises wheat bread or bun taken with *lassi* (incorporating dried whole milk known as *khoya*) or yoghurt mixed with sugar in summer; and with milk in winter. *Paratha* made of wheat flour is also popular for breakfast in many homes, often eaten with the previous evening's leftovers or yoghurt, along with *lassi*, or fresh cream. The bread is mostly baked in *tandoors*. Often, it is the previous night's leftover bread that is fried in oil and eaten at breakfast.

Another item commonly consumed by the common man in summer, is *achar* made of raw mangoes. It is taken as a substitute for *daal* or curry and is eaten with bread. In winter, the food usually consists of rice, maize, *saag* and *daal*, while okra is a popular vegetable in summer. Other than *saag*, the vegetables in season and popular in winter are turnips, carrots and radish. *Ghee* is an integral part of the diet. Dates also form a major part of the staple diet in some parts of the province.

In southern Punjab which is dominated by Saraikis, the cuisine is much the same as in the rest of the province. Generally, two meals are consumed—breakfast, comprising *paratha* and tea topped with cream—and supper, eaten around four in the evening. While there isn't much difference in the food, there are certain greens, such as *sohanjna*, that are grown only in the southern belt which are consumed here. Its roots and *phallian* (green beans) are used to make *achar*. *Tandoori roti* is generally made with whole wheat flour without any refined flour and baking soda added to it, and so is healthier than the *roti* in the rest of the province.

In the hilly areas, smoked meat and *kak* (baked balls of wheat flour) are served to guests. In Mianwali, meat fried on burning coal is a speciality. In other towns, families of average income normally take wheat *chapati*, meat (mostly beef) curry, cooked pulses, and vegetables. Boiled rice is occasionally eaten as well, in accompaniment with curry, and is not taken in the form of *chapati* as in the rural areas. *Lassi* and milk are universally popular accompaniments and the former is also popular at breakfast. Fish, though rarely eaten in summer, is consumed in winter.

In the Punjab, at weddings especially, guests are usually served rice or wheat *chapati*. Sweet dishes include *firni* made from cream of rice and milk, *halwa*, *sewain* (vermicelli) and milk or *malai* (double cream), and *jalebi*.

In Lahore, breakfast tends to be a bit more elaborate in affluent homes, particularly on weekends and public holidays. *Bakarkhani*, *paya*, and yoghurt with sugar or *lassi* are popular holiday breakfast items, while toast/rusk with tea is consumed on weekdays. At lunch, *phatura*, which is a large *puri* made of a flour dough mixed with either a pulse or ground meat, is often eaten with *daal*.

Although the fragrant spices used in the north such as saffron, cardamoms and cloves are also used in cooking here, emphasis is placed more on the usage of plants that grow better in the Punjab such as mustard, black pepper, asafoetida and *kari* leaf (which some say is the source of the Indo-British word, 'curry'). The main ingredients used in Punjabi cuisine, though, are basic: onions, ginger, garlic, and *ghee*.

Pura. Similar to a pancake, *pura* is a Punjabi dessert made of whole wheat flour.

Puri. Whole wheat or refined flour dough kneaded with little oil or *ghee*, and warm water into a stiff dough, rolled out into a disc, about ten centimetres across, and then deep-fried in a wok to puff up, makes a *puri*. It is either eaten hot, as part of a meal, or as a snack with dry vegetable preparations like potato *bhaji*. While this is a popular breakfast item in many parts of the country eaten with chickpea curry and potato curry, some variations are also popular in certain communities. For instance, the Bengalis settled in Pakistan make their *puri* thick and not as fully puffed as the normal *puri* since some fat is kneaded into the dough. They also stuff the centre of the ball of dough with a mash of cooked *urad daal* before rolling it out and deep frying it into one of their popular snack items—the *daal puri*.

Qabargah. A Kashmiri speciality, *qabargah* is lamb rib chops cooked in a spice mixture. The ribs are then coated in a *besan* batter and fried.

Qadeet/landhi. A Balochi food item, *qadeet* is basically mutton with its fat dried in the sun with salt. It became popular because of the nomadic nature of the Baloch tribes which required meat to be preserved for consumption during travel, particularly in the winter months. It is made by skinning the whole goat, cleaning, and cutting the meat, seasoning it with rock salt, red chillies, and asafoetida and leaving it to dry for two months. Providing warmth and nutrition, *qadeet* was and still is the perfect anathema to the severe winters of Balochistan. It is normally eaten with turnips. *Landhi* or *qadeet* made with meat that had been sacrificed on Eid-ul-Azha is known as *tabahiq*, and a number of dishes are made using this meat, including *tabahiq daal*.

Qeema/qeema aaloo. The basis of the Pakistani popular main course, *qeema* comes from the Mughals' love of minced meat, cooked with spices. Basically, a dry curry of minced lamb or beef, it is especially popular as a breakfast item, eaten with *naan* or *paratha*. The meat could be put through a mincing machine in which case the mince is fine, or it could be prepared by hand, in which case the mince is a little coarser.

A version with gravy is also popular, frequently eaten with rice. A variation of this dish is *qeema aaloo*, which as the name indicates (*aaloo* is potatoes in Urdu) has peeled and diced potatoes added to the mince.

Qeema bhara karelay. Bitter gourd filled with *qeema* and *chana daal* and cooked on *dum* for three to four hours, *qeema bharay karelay* is a Dilliwalla speciality. It is a tricky dish to make as the bitterness of the gourd has to be removed in the cooking process, but if made well, it is regarded as a dish to set before a king!

Qeema sewain. An interesting combination of ingredients, *qeema sewain/sewaiyan* is a Hyderabadi speciality consisting of minced meat (mutton) cooked in various masalas, fried onions, tomatoes and yoghurt. Roasted vermicelli and lemon juice are added to the cooked mince before it is put on *dum*.

Qehwa. This is an aromatic black tea. Most Kashmiris believe—even though its exact origins are still unclear—that *qehwa* dates back to time immemorial and has been a part of local consumption for centuries. Certain sources trace the origins of the drink to the Yarkand valley in Xinjian district. Some areas of Kashmir and Xinjiang were part of the Kushan Empire during the first and second century AD, and it is likely that the use of *qehwa* and the spread of its popularity in these regions was facilitated during the Kushan rule. In fact, its fame spread to Khyber Pakhtunkhwa to the extent that it is usually served after every meal in these areas. It is flavoured with saffron, cardamom, and almonds and served from a samovar (a large metal kettle originating in the Russian steppes).

Qorma. In Pakistan, the term *qorma* refers to a dish in the category of braise (i.e. a dish in which the main ingredient is cooked slowly with a minimum of added liquid) or of stew (a dish in which the main ingredient is cooked slowly in a relatively large amount of liquid). In the latter case it would normally be the sort of stew which finishes up with a thick rather than thin sauce. A creamy or aromatic curry, *qorma* is based on the Persian technique of marinating with yoghurt, and probably spread to the subcontinent with the Mughals through Afghanistan. It is mildly hot, and the curry is rich with nuts and has a creamy finish.

Qurutob. A Tajik speciality, the name *qurutob* connotes its preparatory method: *qurut* means dried balls of salty cheese while *ob* means water. The balls are dissolved in water and the liquid is poured over strips of thin, flaky flatbread made with butter or tallow for flakiness. Before serving, the dish is topped with onions fried in oil until golden-brown, and other fried vegetables. It is popular with the Tajiks living in Khyber Pakhtunkhwa.

Rabri. A Dilliwalla dessert comprising clotted cream flakes, *rabri's* origin can be traced to around AD 1000 when it was part of the royal fare. This calorie-laden sweet dish is made by evaporating milk over low heat till it becomes dense and changes colour. Although the addition of fresh cream, butter and sugar gives the *rabri* a curdled-milk texture, it tastes divine. Popular especially in winter, it also has a pistachio variety.

Raisin. To make raisins, bunches of black or green grapes are hung in a darkened room to dry slowly. In Pakistan, grapes are grown in Balochistan and Sindh. Raisins are used to dress food items such as *pulao, halwa* and other local desserts, as well as served on their own or mixed with other dry fruits like almonds, pistachios, and walnuts. They are particularly popular in winter.

Raita. This is a class of relishes with a spiced, lightly beaten yoghurt base, to which with added salt, often ground mint and coriander leaves, raw onions and chillies are added, while sometimes raw, diced cucumber and tomatoes may also be folded in. *Raita* is an invariable accompaniment to *pulao* and *biryani*. The more watery version of it, which is often drunk as much as it is used to dress *pulao* or *biryani*, is known as *raita*, while the Gujarati *kachumar* or *kachumber* though similar, is a more solid version, and can only be eaten as an accompaniment.

Rajput. The Punjab's population comprises basically indigenous Punjabis who trace their ancestry to pre-Islamic Jat and Rajput castes that arrived from Rajputana and Jaisalmer, later marrying in other ethnic groups, which came to the area. Almost 60 per cent of the population of the Punjab comprises Rajputs and Jats and the various branches of their race.

In Pakistan, Rajput and Jat tribes are so mixed up that often it is difficult to distinguish one from the other. It is possible that some of the Rajput tribes are probably of Jat origin and vice versa. Even tribes which bear well-known Rajput names are often classified as Jats in the Punjab. The main Muslim Rajput tribes of the Punjab are: Bhatti, Punwar, Chauhan, Minhas, Tiwana, Noon, Ranghar, Khokhar, Ghakkar, Meo, Chib, Gheba, Jodhra, Janjua, Sial and Wattu.

Ramazan. The ninth month of the Islamic calendar, Ramazan is a month of fasting and abstinence from eating and drinking from dawn to dusk, from one new moon to the next. It is compulsory for all healthy Muslims to fast, and is meant to cleanse the body and soul. Travellers, the very old, the sick, who may include pregnant women and nursing mothers, and women during menstruation are exempt from fasting but are expected to fast after Ramazan, whenever they can, in lieu of the fasts they missed.

Two meals are normally eaten daily throughout the month: one before dawn—which is known as *sehri*—and the other at sunset, known as *iftar*. While personal choices prevail as to what one eats at the two meals, there are certain dishes that are traditionally linked to each of these meals, and a large number of households partake of them. A tradition of the Prophet (PBUH) favours breaking the fast with dates, and this is widely observed in many Muslim countries, including Pakistan. Salt is a close second favourite for breaking fasts among those who don't have a taste for dates. Typically, *pakoray, samosay, jalebiyan*, and different kinds of *chaats*, not to mention fruits, are part of an *iftar* spread, while *parathay*, tea, eggs, *qeema* and leftover food items from *iftar* generally constitute the *sehri* fare.

Rasgulla. One of the most favourite Bengali sweets, *rasgulla* comprises spongy balls basically made of milk powder (or of *chhena* [an Indian cottage cheese] and semolina dough), soaked in lightly sweet sugar syrup. They are eaten cold and can be served 'wet'—with syrup. Supposedly a predecessor of *rasgulla*, *sandesh* is a lot less sweet, and has not gained as much favour with the general populace as *rasgulla*, although, it is available at certain sweet meat shops here. In fact, it was because of *sandesh's* limited popularity, that according to a legend, Nobin Chandra Das, a late 19th century sweet-maker/confectioner, not content with serving his patrons the traditional plain sweet, experimented with boiling a *sandesh* in syrup, and invented the spongy *rasgulla*.

Rasmalai. Some fifty years after the 22-year-old Nobin Chandra Das, a late 19th century sweet-maker/confectioner, came up with the recipe of *rasgulla*, his son Krishna Chandra Das invented the *rasmalai*—flattened milk powder (or *chhena*) patties floating in thickened milk flavoured with screw pine. While it is counted among the most favourite Bengali sweets, it is also extremely popular as a dessert among all communities residing in Karachi.

Rava. Eaten by Parsis generally at breakfast on festive occasions as an alternate to *sheer khurma*, *rava* is a sweet dish made with semolina, milk, sugar, butter and eggs, and flavoured with rosewater or essence and garnished with rose petals, almonds and raisins.

ZARNAK SIDHWA

Raway ka paratha. Made of *suji* (semolina) and eaten with sweet and savoury dishes by the Dilliwalla community, *raway ka paratha* is a type of bread that is also cooked in a *tandoor* and is particularly popular on Eid. It is often eaten with mangoes during the mango season.

Razmah goagji. This is a simple Kashmiri vegetarian speciality, made with boiled turnips and dried beans, stir-fried in mustard oil.

Red chilli. A major crop of Pakistan, it is not only an important food ingredient but is also used for essence production. It is used in foods for pungency and red colour. Kunri located in Sindh province, is called the red chilli capital of Asia and produces 85 per cent of all red chilli cultivated in Pakistan, generating 1.5 per cent of the country's GDP.

Dried red chillies constitute an important ingredient in Pakistani cuisine. They can be used either whole or crushed, or as chilli powder. Whole dried chillies are usually fried in oil before use and are popular ingredient of *tarka* for various dishes such as *karhi* and *daal*. They are extremely fiery and break easily once cooked, spewing their seeds into the broth. The crushed and powdered chillies, however, tend not to have the potency and flavour of the whole pods. ·

Red chillies are healthy as they are low in sodium and very low in saturated fat and cholesterol. They are also said to be good for digestive ailments and are an excellent source of vitamins A, B, C, E and P.

Relish. Relish as a noun and in a culinary context, refers to a condiment or highly-flavoured food item taken with plainer food to add flavour and interest to it. In the Pakistani food context, *achars* and chutneys are relishes that usually accompany the main course, and if one cannot afford to eat a main course then the relish often doubles as one, eaten with a staple which is either a *roti* or rice.

Reshmi kebab. Minced meat, favoured by the Persians, made its way into Mughal cuisine as mincing was found to be a good way of preserving prime cuts of meat in a hot climate and removing any toughness in the meat. *Reshmi* (silky) *kebabs* got their name from their tender, silk-like, minced texture and the addition of tenderisers; they were usually finished with a hint of smoke.

SUMMAYA USMANI

Rewri. A sesame seed-based, winter sweet treat, the *rewri* is made with melting jaggery and glucose together and then adding clarified butter and cooking the three ingredients on low heat. The mixture is then allowed to cool and formed into bite-size balls after which they are coated with roasted sesame seeds.

Rice. A grain that is a staple food for roughly half of humanity, rice (*Oryza sativa*) has several advantages over most other staple foods. It gives higher and more reliable yields than wheat and barley. It keeps well in storage; in cool, dark, and reasonably dry conditions, and its quality declines only a little after three years, usually remaining edible even after ten years. Rice has a good flavour and texture when cooked, absorbing and setting off to advantage the flavour of any sauce or other cooking liquid.

Archaeological finds of rice date back to 6000–3500 BC in northern Thailand and central China, although in 2003, BBC reported that archaeologists in South Korea had found the world's oldest known domesticated rice, which would push back the recorded origins of Asia's staple food by thousands of years.

The terraced fields of Kashmir, so typical of rice cultivation, have been placed at 10,000 BC. The earliest finds of cultivated rice in the Deccan area date as late as 1400–1000 BC, after its domestication in the well-watered Himalayan plains. Since then, innumerable names turn up in Sanskrit literature after its first mention in the *Yajurveda*, reflecting the sustained development of rice varieties throughout the region.

Rice, rarely eaten at breakfast in Pakistan, is usually consumed in its plain boiled form in accompaniment with a main dish with gravy. Culturally, rice is eaten just tender and not overcooked, with each individual rice grain separate from the other. Overcooked rice, which clumps and becomes sticky, is generally viewed as sub-standard and unpalatable.

According to a legend, fragrant Basmati rice was brought to the Dehradun valley by Amir Dost Mohammed of Afghanistan, while he was exiled there by the British in 1840. Favoured for its long fine grains and aroma, it is considered the choicest of all varieties of rice. It grows only in the subcontinent and has a higher price tag, but is preferred, especially when menu for important dinners and special occasions is being planned. Needless to say, the quality of Basmati rice also varies—the finer and more aromatic is naturally more expensive.

On special occasions, rice can be cooked in many exotic styles, varying from the relatively simple *pulao*—rice cooked with fried flavour enhancers, spices and vegetables—to a rich meat *pulao* or *biryani* which combines rice with meat and could constitute a main meal eaten on its own. Over the years, rice has also been transformed to make a series of appetising foods such as *dosas* and *kheer*.

Rigvedic Civilisation. The Vedic period or Vedic age, is the period in the late Bronze Age and early Iron Age of the history of the subcontinent when the Vedas were composed between the end of the urban Indus Valley Civilisation and a second urbanisation which began in the central Indo-Gangetic Plain *c.*600 BCE.

Among the primary Vedic Sanskrit sources is *Rigveda* (1700–1500 BC), the oldest known compilation of hymns dedicated to various deities. While certain hymns show evidence of having been formulated in some earlier homeland of the Aryans, they appear to have been set to verse form perhaps in about 1700 BC. Therefore, references to food in the *Rigveda* should be viewed with caution, as they could mirror earlier observations.

Rista. A Kashmiri speciality, often a part of the traditional feast *Wazwan, rista* is meatballs made of mutton cooked in red gravy.

River fish. Reportedly, there are anywhere from 183 to 233 species of fresh-water fish in Pakistan and Azad Kashmir, while just Chenab boasts 81 species. River fish is popular in the province of Khyber Pakhtunkhwa, especially with the fishermen residing in the Swat region. They are also found on the banks of the Chenab and in Kunhar River.

Most abundant river fish species of Khyber Pakhtunkhwa, Balochistan, as well as River Chenab include tilapia (*Oreochromis niloticus*); rohu or carp (*Labeo rohita*); mori (*Cirrhinus mrigala*); foji khaga (*Bagarius bagarius*); sangari (*Sperata sarwari*); dola (*Channa punctate*); mahseer (*Tor microlopsis*); trout and khaga. Kunhar River is a natural habitat for other species as well, such as stone loaches or *patharchatta* (Nemacheilidae), a family of traditional bony fish; salmon (Salmonidae), ray-finned fishes which include salmon; and *Sisoridae*, catfish that live in fast-moving waters.

Roasted peanut. A winter favourite, roasted peanuts are available on street carts and sold on the wayside. Five strains are available in the market—from Chakwal, Kohat, Sukkur, and India—but the best of these is from Parachinar in terms of taste and quality. The Sukkur pods are bigger in size and contain just one or two nuts in every pod, while the Parachinar pod typically has three nuts in every pod, and though smaller in size than their counterparts, they make up in taste what they lose in size. When roasted, peanuts usually cook in their own oil, and hence the difference in taste as oils have their own flavour.

Roasting. Whole spices, seeds and nuts are often first roasted before being used in Pakistani recipes as this enhances their flavours. While this is mostly done on an iron griddle in most homes, frying pans are also used nowadays. The *tawa* or pan is placed over moderate heat and the spices, seeds or nuts are stirred continuously, or the utensil is tilted and shaken to ensure even cooking till the items being roasted are well-coloured and aromatic.

Roghan josh. *Roghan* means 'clarified butter' in Persian, while *josh* means 'hot'. *Roghan josh*, thus, means meat cooked in clarified butter, at intense heat. Adopted by the Kashmiris, this aromatic curry dish comprises lamb cooked generally with browned spices and saffron, and boiled in yoghurt. It has a deep red colour thanks to the liberal use of Kashmiri dried chillies and the dried flower of the cockscomb plant (*maval*), with red flowers, indigenous to Kashmir. In fact, some historians believe that this red colour gives the dish its name, as *roghan* in Kashmiri means 'red'. It is made without onions and garlic when prepared by Brahmins (they use fennel and asafoetida instead). However, the version of *roghan josh* eaten in Pakistan, particularly by Dilliwallay, was popularised by the Mughals who ruled the Indian subcontinent for three centuries. The unrelenting heat of the plains took the Mughals frequently to Kashmir, which is where *roghan josh* was perfected. Some preparations of *roghan josh* are very lavish, with lots of sweet spices and liberal amounts of cream.

Roghni naan. A Mughlai flat bread, it is made with all-purpose flour, egg, milk yoghurt, poppy seeds, and sesame seeds. Since it is quite rich, it is not a bread that one would partake of on a daily basis; it is more of a special-occasions staple, accompanying an equally rich curry-based main course.

Rohu paratha. A Sindhi fried flatbread, *rohu paratha* comprises layers of hand-rolled dough that is fried into a *paratha*. It is encrusted with sweet water fish rohu.

Rosh. Salted roast of lamb, *rosh* is a Balochi speciality. Variations of the dish from a dry preparation to a liquid-based one exist.

Roti (bread). A generic term for all kinds of baked, grilled, or roasted breads, mostly made with wheat flour, *roti* includes indigenous bread such as *chapati*, *rumali roti*, *tandoori roti*, *naan*, *kulcha*, *sheermal*, and *bakarkhani*, as well as the Western-style loaf-bread.

History has it that the Indus Valley Civilisation, which emerged some 5,000 years ago on the banks of the River Indus, introduced the indigenous form of bread used even today. The existence of granaries at Moenjo-Daro, Harappa and Lothal (all ancient cities) further testify that wheat was the basic commodity that played a pivotal role in the barter system prevalent in those days. At a time when people in Europe lived in caves, the Indus Valley people had a centralised granary where they would deposit wheat and barley, which might have acted as the economic equivalent of our modern-day State Bank.

A large variety of *roti* is consumed throughout Pakistan, some more exotic and richer than others, although the exotic ones are normally reserved for special occasions. Daily bread is usually cooked at home on a *tawa* (a slightly concave heavy-bottomed griddle pan made of cast iron) from unleavened basic dough made from whole wheat flour (*gehon ka atta*), water

and salt, making it resplendent with vitamins (B1, B2, B3, B6, B9), iron, calcium, phosphorus, magnesium and potassium. The result is a light, thin, flat round bread called *chapati* or *phulka*. Every household has its own stamp of *roti*—varying in size and thickness. Some prefer to cook the *roti* on an upside-down tawa, others over non-stick skillets and even in *roti*-makers. In Balochistan, *koki* is made by roasting the rolled-out dough for about one-and-a-half hours, directly in a hot-stone area made with dung patties.

Some prefer large, paper-thin *rotis*, others large, thick ones, some roll out small, round ones lathered with *ghee*, while still others opt for square ones. Hunza's equivalent to today's ubiquitous *chapati* is a thin wheat bread, the *khamali*. It is much larger in diameter than the normal *chapati*, for obvious reasons—wood is a very precious commodity and conservation is essential. By baking a large bread, they take advantage of the heat from the large cooking plate of a traditional Hunza stove.

But while *chapati* or *phulka*, no matter what the size or shape, is a regular staple at all three meals in most homes in rural areas, there is a preference for the baked bread loaf/toast at breakfast in cities such as Islamabad, Karachi and Lahore. Loaf bread was once made at home in unhygienic conditions and was called *paon roti*, meaning foot bread, as the dough was kneaded by foot; however, another school of thought believes that the word was '*pao*' meaning quarter, referring to the four squares the thick, large, square loaf would be divided into—and not '*paon*'. Proper bakeries boasting machine-made, rectangular bread loaves came up only much after Independence.

Although other urban and semi-urban centres as well as some rural areas also use the bakery bread, it is in the cities, which have had greater exposure to Western tastes in general, that one finds a strong foreign influence on the Pakistani palate. Larger cities normally mean a fast-paced lifestyle and the use of bread loaf is more convenient and less time consuming than making *chapati*. For the same reason, rusks are popular at breakfast in the larger cities.

Tandoori naan, rarely made at home other than in Peshawar, is normally bought as an alternate to homemade *chapati*. Its popularity can be traced to as far back as the ubiquitous *chapati*, as remnants of a *tandoor* have been discovered from excavation at the Indus Valley sites. However, the Persian-speaking Central Asian nations—particularly the regions around Afghanistan, Uzbekistan, Iran, and Tajikistan—have also, for centuries, been consuming *naan* the way

Pakistan knows it, and it is believed that through conquests and trade, the basic recipe of the *naan* found its way to the subcontinent. Interestingly, *tandoors* started out in the Punjab as social institutions as much as a means of cooking. Since not all homes could accommodate *tandoors*, communal *tandoors* were used by the people to cook bread from flour kneaded at home, offering them the opportunity to meet neighbours and catch up with news and gossip at the same time.

Naan is eaten at breakfast only in Peshawar but is widely consumed at other meal times all over the country. Thicker and spongier than the *chapati* and usually made out of white flour, the *naan* is made of dough containing yeast. The dough is kneaded for a few minutes, then set aside to rise for a few hours. Once risen, the dough is divided into balls, patted into shape—flat, round or tear-shaped—and pushed through a hole into a large, spherical clay/earthen oven, called a *tandoor*. About 4 feet deep, a bed of charcoal heats it. The dough, plastered to the oven wall, is removed with a pair of long metal spikes when ready.

The most common derivatives of *naan* are the Peshawari and Kashmiri *naan*. These are filled with a mixture of nuts and raisins and are much broader and thicker than the normal *naan*. By adding variations to the original recipe in the form of flavourings or fillings, the *naan* can take on exotic dimensions. There are varieties of stuffed *naans* such as those with mince meat, chicken, or potato; and flavoured *naan* such as those with garlic or butter. Popular sprinklings on *naan* include cumin, sesame and nigella seeds.

One bakery situated in Lahore's Walled City since the 1850s is Mujahid Taj Din Naan Bakery. Now being run by the third generation of the family, it is as popular today, with people flocking to it from far and wide, as it was when it first opened its doors. As the name suggests, it specialises only in *naan*, boasting one of the biggest tandoors in the country and sells a large variety from *roghni* to those with beef, chicken and mutton *qeema*, to *aaloo* and *besan*. A sweet *khashkhash naan*, that remains fresh for a month, and the *gulbahar* (made to order with dried fruit and candied fruit preserve) are also among their hot selling items.

Other bread varieties include *sheermal*; *taftan*; *Kandahari naan* (long bread); *kulcha*; *bhature*; *roghni naan* (sprinkled with sesame seeds and covered with minute amounts of oil); *bateer roti* (similar to a *chapati* made on a *tawa*, it is popular in Balochistan); and *Bumbaiya naan*. *Bakarkhani* is another favourite made with white flour and *mawa*.

Occasionally, *roti* is also made with gram flour, millet, maize (*makai*), sorghum or barley, and rice, and served with special entrees. They may be stuffed with different fillings, like onion or radish, making it a complete meal for the poor.

One of the specialities in Sindh in winters is *bossari*, a *roti* sweetened with jaggery. It is relished at breakfast. Its counterpart in lower Punjab is *doli*, which is sweet and incorporates dry fruit such as almonds, walnuts and raisins. It is eaten with *halwa* and *cholay*.

Rumaali roti. The Urdu word *rumaali* literally means 'handkerchief'; *rumaali roti* is an elaborately and dexterously prepared ultra-thin bread from finely ground wheat flour made on a huge convex metal pan. Introduced by Lucknawis, it is a treat to watch one of these being prepared with great flourish by skilled cooks. It is pressed with the fingers and tossed, never rolled, till it achieves an enormous size, after which it is roasted on the pan and then folded over many times to manageable size.

Rusk (papa). Rusks are made of bread dough incorporating sugar, eggs and butter. It is shaped into a loaf or cylinder, baked, cooled and sliced and then dried on low heat until hard. Rusks have a low water content and keep well. They are popular as an accompaniment to the morning or evening tea, when the rusk is dunked into the hot tea which is eaten rather than drunk, till the rusk lasts. A variation is cake rusk, which is dried sponge cake instead of bread.

S

Sabzi challow. A traditional Afghani New Year's Eve dish, *sabzi challow* is made with spinach (*sabzi*), rice (*challow*), and lamb. The rice is crispy at the bottom and caramel-coloured, but not burned. Depending on preference, chicken thighs may replace the lamb shank.

Saffron (*Crocus sativus*; zafran, kesar). With its origins in Western Asia, particularly Persia, saffron, along with many other culinary practices was brought to the subcontinent by the Mughals. The gently dried orange-red stigma of the narcissus flower (*nargis*), saffron is the world's most expensive spice, as it takes 75,000 flowers to yield just a pound of saffron and the flower is said to bloom only one week in a whole year. The stigmas are dried and stored in sealed containers to avoid bleaching. The final product is an aromatic, matted mass of narrow, thread-like, dark orange to reddish-brown strands about 2 cm long. It has such a spicy, pungent, bitter taste and a tenacious odour that, luckily, only a small quantity is needed to flavour and impart colour and fragrance to a dish, whether sweet or savoury.

Its powerful fragrance and orange colour are prized in Pakistani cuisine among the wealthy. To best bring out the flavour and fragrance, saffron threads must be infused in hot water or soaked in hot milk for at least half an hour before use. They could also be lightly roasted before soaking them.

The cultivation of saffron in Azad Kashmir, where some of the finest crops in the world are grown, dates back to the 3rd century or beyond. The spice and its fragrance are an integral part of the dishes included in the Kashmiri feast, *Wazwan*. It is used extensively in Mughal dishes such as *qorma* and *biryani* and in desserts such as *shahi tukra*. Saffron is high in riboflavin and vitamin B, and has long been recognised for its medicinal use. Widely regarded as an aphrodisiac, especially when dissolved in milk, saffron is also said to relieve respiratory congestion. It is used in pastes to improve complexion and is reputed to purify the mind.

Sail phulka. A favourite of the Hindu community, *sail phulka* is a small, fluffy *chapati* dipped in green chutney and then steam-cooked.

Saim ke beej ka salan. This seasonal Dilliwalla dish comprises seeds of *saim ki phali* (broad beans) cooked as regular *gosht ka salan* (mutton curry). It is cooked only in winter when the *saim ki phali* are in season.

Sajji. An Arab delicacy that also became a speciality of Baloch hill tribes, *sajji* or whole-roasted lamb is traditionally cooked on a pit fire into the ground and baked over burning wood. Marinated only in salt, it is skewered in a specific way—first the front legs, then the hind legs, followed by the back, ribs, and neck. The liver, fats and other parts are not struck into the ground but suspended from a skewer. Retaining its natural moisture and fats, the meat is fully cooked when it turns a golden-brown. It initially became popular with the nomadic Baloch who depended on hunting for their meals, and had no access to stoves or elaborate cooking utensils to prepare their food. It not only provided the much-needed nutrition, it also offered opportunity for camaraderie in a nomadic lifestyle. A convenient, hassle-free meal, *sajji* is traditionally served with *kaak*.

Nowadays, variations of the traditional *sajji* are also in vogue with the marination including green papaya paste and local herbs, and the lamb being stuffed with rice.

Today, the tradition of cooking and eating *sajji* is closely interwoven in the fabric of Baloch hospitality. Interestingly, there are certain dining etiquettes attached to *sajji* that are inviolable and scrupulously observed. For instance, the back of the animal is left entirely for the hosts to eat. If a woman from the guests' family is married into the host's family, then half the rib-cage is set aside for her. A portion from which meat is never bitten off is the scapula because it is used to foretell the future. The two scapulas complement each other and are never handed over but thrown to the person who wants to read them.

Since the Balochi *sajji* is quite bland in taste, other provinces have come up with spicier variations. In Lahore and Karachi, *sajji* is made with whole cooked chicken, using a lot of spices.

Sajna ki phalli. Appropriately called drumsticks in English, *sajna ki phalli* or *saim ki phalli*, grown on a tree called *Moringa oliefera*, is from the family of pod beans and is unique for its delectable taste. Usually added to *khatta dalcha* or other dishes of pulses and curries, the pods absorb the spicy curry and make a juicy accompaniment for rice and curry/*daal* dishes. Although the outer skin of the long pod is not edible, it makes for popular vegetable and is chewed and left aside, while the leaves are just as delectable. Recently having acquired the reputation of a miracle plant the *Moringa* is supposed to be teeming with health benefits.

Salli par eedu. This is regarded as a perfect Parsi breakfast, though it is just as popular at lunch or even dinner. Comprising a small heap of cooked, shredded potato mixed with spiced tomatoes and onion paste, the dish is gently fried with an egg on top.

Salt. Since prehistoric times, much effort has been devoted to obtaining salt for use with food. Its feature as an essential culinary and dietary building block has made it central to trade and exchange from earliest times.

One main source of salt is the existence of underground deposits from which it can be mined. The other great source, which is inexhaustible, is the sea, which is made to yield salt by a process of evaporation. Salt mined from underground is called rock salt, while many kinds of salt especially prized by connoisseurs belong to the category known as sea salt.

Pakistan is rich in both rock salt and sea salt. Table salt, as the name suggests, is mostly used at the table, and is a mass-produced, refined product which comes in very small grains, and has been treated to ensure that it pours easily even in slightly damp conditions.

Samosa. This is a fried, small, crisp, flaky triangular-shaped pastry popular as a street food, snack or even side item at a meal in Pakistan. The *samosa* is stuffed with a variety of fillings, most common being minced meat, and potato, and is usually served with a chutney.

The origin of a *samosa* can be traced to thousands of miles away in the ancient empires that rose up in the Iranian plateau at the dawn of civilisation itself. Although it is not clear when the pastry was first given the now-familiar triangular shape, it is evident that the origins of its name are Persian—*sanbosag*.

The *samosa* is first mentioned in literature by the Persian historian Abul-Fazl Bayhaqi. He describes a dainty delicacy, served as a snack in the great courts of the mighty Ghaznavid Empire. The fine pastry made from refined flour was filled with minced meats, nuts and dry fruits and then fried till the pastry was crisp.

But the *samosa*, like many other dishes in Pakistani cuisine, was to be transformed as it followed the epic journey made by successive waves of migrants into the subcontinent. It was brought into the region along the route the Aryans had taken more than 2,000 years earlier—through Central Asia and then over the great mountains in what is now Afghanistan, before descending down to the fertile plains of the Indus.

Initially, it metamorphosed into something much less refined. By the time it reached what is now Tajikistan and Uzbekistan it had become what Professor Pushpesh Pant, one of the world's experts on the subcontinental food, describes as 'a crude peasant dish'. The courtly titbit was now a high-calorie staple, a much bigger and heartier dish—the sort of thing a shepherd would take out into the pastures with him. It retained its distinctive shape and was still fried, but the exotic nuts and fruits were gone—the savoury pastry was now filled with coarsely chopped goat or lamb mince with onions and flavoured simply with salt.

Over the following centuries the *samosa* made its way over the icy passes of the Hindu Kush and into the subcontinent. What happened along the way explains why Prof. Pant regards the *samosa* as the ultimate 'syncretic dish'—the ultimate fusion of cultures. Once in the subcontinent, the *samosa* was adopted and tailored to local tastes, becoming the world's first fast food. Local spices such as coriander, pepper, cumin, ginger and more were added. The filling changed, too, with vegetables often replacing meat.

Later still, it was to become the vehicle for other much more novel foodstuffs, because the modern *samosa* is the product of yet another great historical upheaval—the discovery of the New World.

These days most *samosay* are filled with potato and flavoured with green chillies, ingredients only introduced from the New World by Portuguese traders in the 16th century. And the *samosa* has continued to evolve since then. Everywhere you go in Pakistan, it is different. *Samosa* varies from region to region, and even from shop to shop as *samosa*-makers compete for customers. Sometimes they are monsters, an entire meal in a single crisp pastry casing. Elsewhere, they have re-emerged as a courtly treat—they are served as cocktail canapés at weddings and modish Karachi parties.

While it is still generally fried, baked versions also exist. The traditional minced meat filling remains popular but now other than potato, mixed vegetables, cheese or corn fillings are also in vogue. Although, the *samosa* is extremely popular as snack item all over the country, in the Gujarati community it is common to serve it as an accompaniment to an entrée at lunch or dinner.

Samosa cholay. Peculiar to the Punjab, *samosa cholay* is a *chaat* dish that is an amalgamation of a potato *samosa* broken down into bite-sized pieces and topped with *chana chaat*. For some reason, it has not picked up in popularity anywhere else, although it is the rage in the Punjab, especially in Lahore.

Sandesh. The name *sandesh* originally meant 'news' in Bengali, referring to the custom of sending sweets by messenger to one's friends and relatives when enquiring for their news, with which the messenger would return. Sandesh, supposedly a predecessor of *rasgulla*, one of the most favourite Bengali sweets, is soft and dry, spongy balls basically made of milk powder soaked in lightly sweet sugar syrup, although some recipes of *sandesh* call for the use of *chhena* or *paneer* (which is made by curdling the milk and separating the whey from it) instead of milk itself. *Sandesh* is a lot less sweet, and has not gained as much favour with the general populace as *rasgulla*, although it is available at certain Bengali sweet meat shops in Karachi. In fact, it was because of *sandesh*'s limited popularity that, according to a legend, Nobin Chandra Das, a late 19th century sweet-maker, not content with serving his patrons the traditional plain sweet, experimented with boiling a *sandesh* in sweetened syrup, and invented the spongy *rasgulla*.

Sanna. A popular Goan dish similar to *idli*, *sanna* is a spongy steamed cake made with a batter of ground rice and grated fresh coconut. The batter is fermented with yeast. In Goa, *sanna* is usually made with Goan red rice that has a special taste and is milled to leave distinctive red streaks. However, in Pakistan, and particularly among the Goans still living in Karachi, boiled rice

is substituted for Goan rice. *Sanna* is absolutely moist steamed morsel of rice cake that soaks up whatever curry it is dunked into. It complements most Goan dishes. This fluffy rice cake goes amazingly well with spicy Goan meat curries like *sorpotel*, *vindaloo* or *shakuti*. *Sanna* is prepared at festivals or on special occasions.

DEBORAH SANTAMARIA

Saraiki. The Saraikis are an ethnolinguistic group from central and south-eastern Pakistan, primarily southern Punjab. Their language is Saraiki also. The Saraiki people follow many religions, though most are predominantly followers of Islam. A small minority of Saraikis follow Hinduism, Christianity, and Sikhism. The Saraiki cuisine is much the same as that of other Punjabis. Generally, they consume two meals a day: breakfast—comprising *paratha* and tea topped with cream—and supper, eaten around four in the evening. While there is not much difference in the food, there are certain greens, such as *sohanjna*, that are grown only in the southern belt which are consumed by Saraikis. Its roots and *phallian* (green beans) are used to make *achar*. They generally make *tandoori roti* with whole wheat flour without any refined flour and baking soda added to it, and so it is healthier than the *roti* eaten in the rest of the province.

Sarson ka saag aur makai ki roti. Mustard greens, primarily *Brassica juncea*, come from a wide range of wild and cultivated mustard plants, almost all belonging to the genus *Brassica*, that of the cabbage family. They are used to make a popular vegetable dish called *sarson ka saag*, is normally eaten with maize bread called *makai ki roti*—a combo meal regarded to be very nutritious. *Sarson ka saag* and *makai ki roti* is generally eaten in winter in the Punjab, though it has now become popular in other provinces as well. The mustard green leaves and aromatics and spices such as green chillies, ginger, garlic, coriander and mixed spices powder are cooked on low heat and mashed to a porridge-like consistency. The maize flour bread is shaped by hand. The bread is yellow in colour when ready, and has much less adhesive strength than normal bread, which makes it difficult to handle. Owing to this, making *makai ki roti* is more difficult than making *roti* from wheat flour. Often *lassi* and butter form the accompaniments to this vegetarian meal.

Sattu. A cooling drink, *sattu* is made with dry roasted barley grains ground into coarse powder, mixed with cold water and brown sugar. Honey or white sugar could also substitute for brown sugar. Lemon juice could also be added to it, as also fruit pieces. *Sattu* is a natural energiser and a traditional Pakistani drink. It prevents heat stroke, hydrates the body and skin, improves the digestive system and helps keep the heart healthy. A glass full of dietary fibre, *sattu* could also be made with milk. *Namkeen sattu* (saltish *sattu*) is prepared with yoghurt, water, and salt. *Sattu* may also be used to thicken gravy and soups.

NAYYER RUBAB

Scythian. Also called Scyth, Saka and Sacae, Scythians were a group of ancient tribes of nomadic warriors originally of Iranian stock, who initially lived in what is now southern Siberia. Their culture flourished from around 900 BC to around 200 BC, by which time they had extended their influence all over Central Asia—from China to the northern Black Sea. The Indo-Greeks ultimately disappeared as a political entity in the subcontinent around AD 10 following the invasions of the Indo-Scythians. However, pockets of Greek populations probably remained, for several centuries longer, under the subsequent rule of the Indo-Parthians and Kushans under whom the country became a centre of Buddhism, leaving its mark on the culture and cuisine of the country, wherever its influence was felt. Some think that the Pakhtuns may be related to the Bactrians, Scythians and/or Kushans. Over the years, the Greeks, Persians, Scythians, Arabs, Mughals, and Rajputs also left their imprints on the ancient culture of Sindh.

Seafood. Pakistan, with an 814-km coastal line, is rich in sea fish resources and a vast variety of sea fish are exported in significant volumes worldwide. However, although Karachi is its port city, sea fish did not become popular as a main course with most Karachiites—barring the fishermen and village communities living along the coast—till perhaps a little over two decades ago. A meat-eating populace, fish did not rank as meat in the eyes of most city-dwellers, other than Gujaratis settled in Karachi. In fact, they too, avoided eating any form of seafood in months that did not have an 'r' in them, simply because their forefathers had advised them that it was not healthy to eat fish in those months. Though it is an old wives' tale, time has proved that it bears some truth because those months are the breeding season, during which the toxins produced in the fish flesh make them unsavoury.

With greater awareness, exposure to various kinds of cuisines, and willingness to experiment, fish dishes began to be slowly but steadily incorporated in the menus of various restaurants and private parties and depending on the kind of fish available, a host of dishes are now being offered. Among the sea fish available and most popularly used in Pakistan are pomfret—both white and black—pink salmon, red snapper, king mackerel, sole, Bombay duck and croaker. Pomfret is only served fried whole, as it has a lot of tiny, fine bones and is not suitable for cutting and serving in a curry, rice dish, or soup. Popular sea food here also includes prawns, crabs, lobsters, and calamari.

Seekh kebab. According to Turkish tradition, *seekh kebab* was invented by medieval Turkic soldiers who used their swords to grill meat over open-field fires. Minced beef mixed with herbs and seasonings, grilled over charcoals on skewers called *seekhs*, hence its name, *seekh kebab* was introduced in this region by Emperor Babar. It became a *pièce de résistance* on the Lucknawi *dastarkhwan*, originally prepared from beef mince wrapped around iron skewers and cooked on charcoal fire. Later influences and innovations led to the use of lamb mince, which was preferred for its soft texture. Besides, serving it on the *dastarkhwan* did not offend the sensibilities of the Hindu guests. Gradually, the *seekh kebab* found its way into other communities as well.

Seekh kebab aur malai. A quintessentially Pindi favourite, *seekh kebab aur malai* is a combination of beef kebabs and full cream. It is rarely eaten in other parts of the country.

Seena khwakha. A meat dish of Khyber Pakhtunkhwa, popular in the erstwhile FATA, *seena khwakha* is first boiled and then cooked in *ghee* using minimum spices.

Sehri. Fasting is enjoined on all faithfuls during Ramazan, the ninth month of the Muslim lunar year, and *sehri*, the daily meal before sunrise, marks the beginning of the fast. *Paratha*, eggs, minced meat, *jalebi* soaked in milk, *pheni* (vermicelli) soaked in milk, *khaja/khajla* (crisp wafers) and tea are among the items most likely to grace a table set for *sehri*. In recent years *sehri* parties have become popular amongst the elite, and on such occasions a lavish spread is laid out for the guests that may include *nihari*, *maghaz*, *paya*, and a lot more.

Semolina (suji). Semolina is usually made from the very hard durum wheat, a variety of Mediterranean origin. 'Semolina' is an Italian word, derived from the Latin *simila*, denoting fine flour. The main characteristic of semolina is that it is tough and will not turn into a starchy paste when cooked. This causes it to produce a light texture, of an interestingly granular nature. Fried golden brown and mixed with large amounts of sugar, semolina is transformed into the popular *suji ka halwa*, often a breakfast item in Pakistan, eaten with *puri*. Semolina is also used as an important ingredient in many desserts.

Sesame seed (*Sesamum indicum*; til). Both archaeological and literary evidence support the antiquity of the sesame in the subcontinent. Sesame is an upright annual herb, up to 2 m tall that bears its seeds in small, sausage-shaped pods about 3 cm long. The pods of primitive strains tend to abruptly split open when ripe, allowing the seeds to scatter. The seeds are numerous, flat, pear-shaped, and no more than 3 mm in length. They may be white, yellow, brown, or black, according to the variety, with a white inside which is revealed when they are hulled. Their full nutty flavour is best developed by roasting and they are used to flavour some curries. In fact, the seeds have many roles in Pakistani cookery—they are sprinkled on breads, pastries and biscuits; fried and sweetened to make *chikkis*, or used in *achars* and chutneys. The seeds are also cultivated all over the country for their abundant oil. The oil produced from them, in the unrefined state, also tastes slightly nutty. Thus, both the seeds and oil have a role in flavouring.

Sev. Gujarati savoury fried snacks that can be kept for days in air-tight containers, *sev* are essentially made of *besan* and fried crisp in long, thin or thick strings, or as wafers extruded from a batter through dyes into very hot fat. A special press, a *sev*-maker, is used to make them. Among the many ancient snacks called *nasto* prepared by Gujaratis, *sev* is now one of the many items eaten practically all over Pakistan and known by the new generic name of *nimco*. It is also used to garnish many *chaats*, particularly *sev puri*.

Sewain. Vermicelli or sewain (also called *sewaiyan*) are thin long strings of hard wheat that look very much like spaghetti but are processed differently. *Sewain* in Pakistan are synonymous with Eid, especially Eid-ul-Fitr, when it is typically prepared and served to celebrate the end of Ramazan, the month of fasting. Eid-ul-Fitr

is, in fact, commonly described as *meethi* Eid, because of the desserts served early in the morning to all family members after the offering of prayers. While *sewain* are used in a number of other popular desserts as well, they are delicious on their own, when fried and cooked dry in sugar syrup, with cardamoms and raisins thrown in for added flavour, if desired.

LAL MAJID

Sha balep. Tibetan in origin, *sha balep* is a bread stuffed with beef. It has been adopted by the Baltis living in Khyber Pakhtunkhwa and is regarded as one of their specialities.

Shab degh. A Kashmiri speciality, *shab degh* is a beautiful blend of whole or halved turnips, tender mutton pieces or minced mutton shaped into meatballs, *ghee* and little sugar cooked over low heat all night long (the word *shab* means 'night' in Persian) in *deghs* sealed with dough. This results in an incredibly rich and flavourful gravy laced with gentle spices, saffron and seasoning. In the early 18th century, when the Mughal Empire was on the decline, the glory of Awadh lured Kashmiri families to move to Lucknow, the capital of Awadh, in search of alternate sources of employment. They brought with them the scent of saffron and their celestial cuisine. The cooking of *shab degh* in winter for the nawab of Awadh became not only a celebration of winter, but a reminder of the bond of the migrant families with their motherland. It was then adopted by Delhi, but with a slight difference. Today, both kinds of *shab degh* are popular in Pakistan—the one made by Kashmiris which incorporates turnips and also has sugar as one of the ingredients, and the other introduced by Dilliwallay who moved to Pakistan after Partition, which incorporates carrots instead of turnips.

These days, many people have begun to incorporate both turnips and carrots in the dish. The culinary skill of a cook in preparing this dish lies in the deftness with which all the meatballs and carrots are made to look like one another and cooked to perfection. It is usually garnished with fresh green chillies and coriander.

Shab-e-Barat. Also written as *Shab-e-Brat* (night of forgiveness), *Shab-e-Barat* is celebrated culturally in Pakistan on the night between 14 and 15 Sha'ban, the eighth month of the Islamic calendar, by preparing *halwa* of any kind—of pulses like gram lentils, vegetables such as bottle gourd, dates, or semolina—and sharing it with family, friends, and neighbours.

It is regarded to be a major event in the Islamic calendar when Muslims worship through the night and ask for forgiveness for their wrongdoings—an act that they believe will reward them with fortune for the whole year and cleanse them of their sins.

Traditionally, *fateha* (verses from the Holy Quran recited at the passing away of a Muslim) is prayed before distributing the *halwa* in the hope that God will forgive the sins of all the dearly departed as well.

Shahi tukra. Literally, the name means royal pieces— *shahi* means royal in Persian, and *tukray* is an Urdu word that means pieces. It is popularly believed that *shahi tukray* was a favourite of Mughal emperors to break the fast with, in the month of Ramazan. The practice continues even today, making it a very desirable dish at *iftar*, and a dessert popularly served at the festive occasions of Eid-ul-Fitr and Eid-ul-Azha.

Saffron, cream, cardamom, pistachios, sultanas and butter-soaked bread adorn this typical Mughal dessert made with fried or baked bread slices cooked in milk with sugar and saffron, and garnished with slivers of almonds and pistachios.

Double ka meetha is another similar dessert popular among the Hyderabadi community, made with fried *double roti* (slices of a loaf of bread)—thus its name. It is served on special occasions such as weddings.

LAL MAJID

Shakhurba. A combination of minced chicken, onions and local herbs mixed with delicate spices and stuffed in *chapati*, *shakhurba* is a Baltistani speciality that tastes delicious served with mint chutney.

Shami kebab. *Shami kebabs* were made in Mughal courts with twice-minced meat and spices, chickpeas, lentils, and legumes. Introduced to the subcontinent during Babar's time in the Mughal era, *shami kebab* is a small patty of minced beef, mutton or chicken, and ground chickpeas and spices, originally cooked in earthen pots. According to one legend they were made of soft, fine, lamb mince (ideally like velvet) so that the toothless Nawab Asaf-ud-Daulah could eat this refined version of the Central Asian and Afghani kebab.

Traditionally, the preparation of *shami kebabs* required no frying, and the meat used to be tenderised by cooking it in its own steam by sealing the lid of the pot tightly with flour paste. Today, it is prepared in many different ways depending on personal and familial tastes and convenience.

The origin of the name of the dish is a mystery though. One belief is that 'Sham' refers to either Syria specifically, or the Levant in general and these kebabs literally mean Syrian kebabs or Levantine kebabs in Arabic. The other belief is that *sham* (meaning 'evening' in Urdu) refers to Sham-e-Awadh—evening in Lucknow—as it was a popular evening snack there. A parochial perfumer from Kannauj offered yet another explanation, linking the spices used in it with the seductive whiff of an *itr* (non-alcoholic perfume) called *Shamama*.

Shawarma. This Lebanese speciality, *shawarma* is made by roasting a cone of pressed lamb, chicken, or beef on a vertical spit. The meat is shaved off from the outside as the spit keeps turning, and is then sandwiched within *khubz* (Arabic bread) along with fresh and pickled vegetables, hot sauce and *tahina* (tahini). It has become as much a wayside favourite in cities as a high-end party/ wedding menu item.

Sheedi. Like the Makranis, Sheedis are of African descent. It is probable that they were an ethnic group of Sidama origin from southern Ethiopia from which many were sold into slavery mainly by local traders. However, there are linguistic indications that show that they were predominantly Swahili speaking people. Recurring famine brought them liberty and, today, the largest community of Sheedis exists in Sindh. The Sheedi cuisine is similar to that of the Makranis. Those settled in Karachi prefer to eat *roti* for lunch and rice at night. They are fond of eating dried fish which they marinate with salt, dry, boil and then scramble and cook like curry.

Sheer khurma. *Sheer* means milk while *khurma* is dates in Arabic, so literally, the name of this dessert means 'milk with dates'. Interestingly enough, nowadays many people prefer not to have dates in their *sheer khurma*.

A hot, sweet delicacy of the Hyderabadi cuisine— *sheer khurma* is a popular part of Pakistani festivals, especially Eid. Made with fried vermicelli, pistachios and almonds cooked in sweet milk, and garnished with cardamom and cloves, it is delicious when served hot, though it is also eaten cold.

The amount of vermicelli used decides the texture. Some like its consistency to be soup-like while others prefer it to be thicker, almost custard-like.

SHAHA TARIQ

Sheermal. Originating in Iran, *sheermal* is believed to have been introduced to the nawabs of Awadh by Persian tradesmen, who frequented North India and eventually settled there, thus establishing its aristocratic origins. What differentiated it from the 'plebian' bread at the time was the fact that it was prepared on an iron griddle rather than in a *tandoor*. However, according to one legend, the *sheermal* was introduced to Lucknow by a cook named Muhamdoo during the period of Nawab Nasir-ud-din Haider.

It is prepared with sweetened warm milk—thus its name: *sheer* means milk in Persian—flour, clarified butter, and eggs. The bread's soft, smooth, rich in texture, and appealing look—its crust is full of holes—not to mention its unique taste, makes it the ideal accoutrement for heavy, gravy-infused curries such as *qorma* served at marriages.

Sheermal is usually not prepared at home, and each city has its go-to places for acquiring it. The choice of outlet depends on the variant that is preferred—the Hyderabadi *bakarkhani* versus the Dilliwalla version, etc.

Sheesha. Originating from Arabia, *sheesha* has, in recent years, become a hot favourite with everybody, regardless of their age or gender. Similar to the *huqqa* that has been part of the Pakistani village culture for centuries, *sheesha* is also essentially a pipe with a water-filter for smoking tobacco leaves or dry fruit.

Sherbet. A sherbet, basically and historically, is a cold, sweetened, non-alcoholic drink, usually based on the juice of a fruit. Recipes for the traditional Middle Eastern sherbets have not changed much over the centuries. There are two main categories of ingredients: a fruit or vegetable juice, and a sweetening agent—originally honey. An optional third category would be spices.

Muslim advent in the second millennium AD introduced new beverages in the subcontinent in the form of these sherbets, often coloured and flavoured with essences like rose, *kevra* (screw pine), and herbs. Traditionally served on auspicious occasions, at *iftar* during Ramazan, at engagement parties, and as a standard offering to guests, sherbets have been replaced to a large extent by fresh juices or soft drinks among modern-day city dwellers, although it is still popular among traditionalists, and is an essential item at *iftar* at most tables in the country.

Shetu. A Khow speciality, *shetu* is a thin, watery yoghurt-like drink popular in Khyber Pakhtunkhwa.

Shikanjbeen. A great favourite in summer, *shikanjbeen* is an ice-cold drink whose origin can be traced to the Punjab but which has grown in popularity in Sindh as well. It is made with lime juice, mint leaves, sugar, salt, and black pepper.

Shikarpur ka achar. A Sindhi pickle, *Shikarpur ka achar* forms an accompaniment to the main courses. It may be sweet or sour, and based in oil or water.

Shola. The name is given to a number of dishes all over the Middle East, Iran and Afghanistan in which short-grain rice is cooked until soft and thick, with other ingredients chosen according to whether the *shola* is to be savoury or sweet. In Khyber Pakhtunkhwa, the Pakhtuns make it with sticky rice, green *mung* pulses, spices, tomatoes, onions and chunks of beef or mutton. It is cooked in pure butter fat till it becomes a thick paste. It is served on special occasions, in accompaniment with brown onions and clarified butter. On the other hand, Dilliwallay make *shola* in a very different way. Their dish is basically a local version of shepherd's pie. It is made with rice and lentils cooked with leftover food such as *qeema*, *saag*, and chillies.

Shorba. In most Islamic countries, the word for 'soup' is *shorba*. A Persian word—derived from *shor* (salty, brackish) and *ba* (stew, dish cooked with water)—in all probability, it got its name from boiling meat in salted water to yield broth, a recipe that goes back to the sixth century. *Shorba* is also the most common and popular Baloch dish made of meat stock or of *khurood*. It is similar to *shorwa* made in Afghanistan and thinner in consistency than *gosht ka salan* made in Sindh and the Punjab.

Shoshp. A simple sweet dish, *shoshp* is a Khow dessert made with wheat flour, water and germinated wheat powder cooked in *ghee*, walnut, or apricot oil. It is especially prepared on Navroze, a festival to mark the advent of spring.

Shupinak. A delicious thick, creamy cheese, *shupinak* is a Khow speciality made from yoghurt.

Shurdee. This is a sweet bread usually shaped like a pancake, which is served at the birth of a Baloch child in a colourful ceremony called *chatti*.

Sigri. A small, portable, iron-stove with a detachable, slatted iron plate to hold embers in place below the cooking vessel, *sigri* has been in use in the region as one of the two main forms of the stove—the other being the clay *chulha*—all through its history. In fact, while the usage of the clay stove is now only confined to rural areas, the *sigri* continues to be a popular item in urban areas where it is specifically used for barbecuing meat.

Sikh. The largest concentration of Sikhs in Pakistan is in the Punjab, though a substantial number is also settled in Peshawar and other areas in Khyber Pakhtunkhwa. According to the 2008 population census, they roughly number twenty thousand. Although Sikhs are permitted to eat meat—only if it is slaughtered through the *jhatka* process (a technique that allows one to kill an animal by beheading it with a single blow to the backbone side of the neck to cause sudden death)—most Sikhs in Pakistan are vegetarian since meat is slaughtered here in the *halal* manner. Their basic cuisine comprises vegetables and *chapati*. They often eat *paneer tarkari* as it is a good source of protein. Smoking is prohibited in Sikhism.

Sil batta. *Sil* is a heavy, grooved, flat stone on which ingredients are ground either dry or with a sprinkling of water by rolling them with the *batta*, a heavy, cylindrical rolling stone. Evidence of its usage dates back to Meher Garh Civilisation. The texture of the items crushed with it remains coarser than if they were ground in a blender, and the cooks who are particular about the taste of their food, especially about certain *masala*-based dishes, insist on using this ancient method to preserve the actual taste of the cuisine. It is commonly found in Pakistani kitchens especially in the rural and semi-urban areas and more specifically in taste-conscious households where electric appliances are regarded as marauders of authentic taste. However, in many urban households where quick and easy fixes are preferred to long-winded and laborious methods of grinding ingredients, the *sil batta* has been relegated to a utensil of the past.

Sindh. Sindh's topography, in vivid contrast to the Punjab's rich, fertile plains, comprises vast deserts, forests which are clean of underbrush, and stark, sculptured hills older than the Himalayas. It is also one of the two provinces—the other being Balochistan—that is not landlocked and has a coastline overlooking the Arabian Sea. The coastal fishing waters of Sindh stretch for about 120 miles with sea inlets and many picturesque creeks.

Owing to its geographical position Sindh has imbibed Iranian, Arab, Central Asian and Indian influences, which, over the years, have been assimilated in the culture of the land. With the Indus Valley Civilisation representing the mature phase of the earlier village cultures of Sindh, its chequered history dates back to about five thousand years. In fact, indigenous Sindhis trace their roots as far back as the Indus Valley Civilisation. Over the years, the Greeks, Persians, Scythians, Arabs, Mughals, and Rajputs left their imprints on the ancient culture of Sindh. Even today, one can see the remnants of the various dynasties that have left their marks on the province, be it in the ancient ruins of Mohenjo-Daro (Mound of the Dead); the Mughal architecture of its older towns, such as Thatta and Hyderabad; or in the colonial buildings of its largest city, Karachi.

During the British Raj, Sindh, situated in the south of Punjab, was the neglected hinterland of the Bombay Presidency, with the population dominated by a few major landholders (*waderas*). Before the Partition, about a quarter of the population of Sindh was Hindu, but in the aftermath of the upheaval in the province following the Partition most left for India. Instead, roughly seven million *mohajirs* (immigrants) took the place of the fairly well-educated fleeing Hindus and Sikhs in the commercial life of the province, settling primarily in Karachi. Today, the cosmopolitan nature of the province is such that its inhabitants also comprise people of Baloch origin (including Makranis), Pakhtuns, Punjabis, Sheedis, Jats, Zoroastrians, Chinese, Anglo-Indians, Goans, Afghans and Hindus.

The food in interior Sindh tends to be generally simple. The agrarian classes eat the grain that is principally produced in the area to which they belong. Thus, *jowar* and *bajra* are the staple food in a large part of Sindh, eaten as *roti*, substituted with rice in areas where rice is grown, such as in Larkana, Jacobabad and Sukkur districts, while wheat is generally preferred by those who can afford it. The *roti* can take on different forms—*busri* (*roti* with clarified butter and jaggery); *patiri* (*tandoori chapati*); *dagar* (plain *roti* made on a *tawa*); *dhodho* (thick *masalaywali roti*); or *sokh*, (crisp *roti*). Depending on affordability, the staples are eaten with vegetables or curds and whey, or *ghee* or some kind of meat—fowl, fish or goat. People in coastal areas eat fish more than the people in other areas; the nomads of Tharparkar eat wild ducks and other game whenever available, while the wandering Jats subsist on milk of their camels, and the Balochis of Kohistan on that of their goats and sheep. The diet of the upper classes is, of course, more varied including meats, pulses, fruit, and sweetmeats as well as more vegetables than the poor can afford.

Sindhi kukar. A Sindhi speciality, *Sindhi kukar* is spicy blackened chicken, with a smoky flavour, achieved by adopting the *dhuan* technique of cooking.

Snack. Considered a luxury item, snacks are regularly eaten in a large number of households in the bigger cities, where the more affluent families, regardless of their ethnic backgrounds, normally partake of snacks with evening tea. They also serve as cheap, quick filler-meals for many. Popular savoury snack items include *samosay*, crisps, french fries, sandwiches, *pakoray*, *shami kebabs*, nimco, cake and biscuits. *Chaats* such as *aaloo cholay*, *dahi baray* and fruit *chaat* are also hot favourites universally. In winter, dry fruits (almonds, walnuts, pine nuts, currants and cashew nuts) are also taken as popular snack items by those who can afford them. Sweet snacks such as *mithai* and cakes are generally not as popular as the savoury ones.

Sohan halwa. A dense, brittle, and caramelised *halwa*, *sohan halwa* is a speciality of Karachi confectioners. It is made with cornflour, sugar, *ghee*, and milk and garnished with almonds and pistachios. It is usually made into 5–6 mm thick discs, and wrapped individually in butter paper. Square, bite-size pieces have also become popular of late, while the tinned variety is normally sought to take as gifts both within Pakistan and abroad. Interestingly, while in Sindh this extremely hard *mithai* is known as *sohan halwa*, in southern Punjab *sohan halwa* refers to a dark brown, soft, sticky *mithai* made with *khoya*, flour, sprouted wheat, *ghee* and sugar. This *mithai* is known as *habshi halwa* in Sindh.

Sookha boomla nu tarapori patio. A speciality of the Parsis of Tarapore, *sookha boomla nu Tarapori patio* is made with dried Bombay duck. These are fried in *masala*, onions, and vinegar, and can be eaten hot or cold. It can be stored in an air-tight jar for up to a month in the refrigerator. When left dry, it is served as a pickle, and when cooked in slightly liquid form, it is eaten with *khichri*.

Sorghum (jowar). *Sorghum bicolor* is a cereal, related and similar to, and sometimes confused with, millet. The name sorghum is derived from the Italian word *sorgho*, meaning 'to rise' and is descriptive of the conspicuous height of the plant. The first Sanskrit names for sorghum are *yavanala* and *yavaprakara* (which means resembling barley), derived from *yava* (barley); other names are *akara* and *jurna*, from which the present term *jowar* originates. The Sanskrit terms only appear as late as the beginning of the Christian era, or perhaps a couple of centuries earlier, in the works of Charaka, Bhela, and Kashyapa. The localisation of sorghum, where its *roti* is the staple diet, may explain this late identity in Aryan consciousness.

In appearance sorghum is a typical grass with long, flat leaves and large, feathery seed heads. The main cultivated varieties vary considerably in the colour of the seeds and in the size of the plant. Among the numerous cultivars, it is generally true that those with white grains, especially white pearl, are used for food. The flavour of the better grain sorghum is robust and resembles that of buckwheat. The grains may be eaten whole or as a flour. Such flour is coarse and lacks gluten and is, therefore, not suitable for making bread, yet it is used in the subcontinent to make *chapati* and similar unleavened breads, particularly in the drier areas.

Sorpotel (sarapatel). A traditional dish of Portuguese origin, this is frequently prepared at every Goan gathering be it a christening, communion, birthday, wedding, the festive season, or even just a Sunday family get-together. Originally made with pork, blood, meat, liver and fat in vinegar and tamarind juice, in Pakistan it is made with beef. It also includes organs, such as liver and heart, that are first boiled, diced into very small pieces, sautéed and then cooked in a pungent masala. This dish tastes better as it matures. It is usually accompanied by *sanna*, a white spongy rice cake, or enjoyed with hard bread or *puri*.

DEBORAH SANTAMARIA

Souffle. A French word which literally means 'fluffed up', souffle is a culinary term in both French and English, for a light, frothy dish, just stiff enough to hold its shape, and which may be savoury or sweet, hot or cold. The British introduced the term to the region; soufflés, as popularised by them, were mostly sweet, as they are now, with seasonal fruits—such as pineapple soufflé, strawberry soufflé, and much more. Today, they are served mostly at private clubs, or private parties and weddings. Interestingly, the Bohra community is famous for its souffles which, though inspired by the traditional English souffle, are made differently from it. Using ice-cold, whipped evaporated milk, jelly, and fruits, all mixed together, this dessert is chilled for two to three hours before serving.

Soup. The most general of the terms that apply to liquid savoury dishes, soup embraces broth, consommé, bisque, potage, chowder, and the like. However, though it is a popular dish served at the beginning of a meal in most countries, it was never an item of subcontinental cuisine until the British introduced it. Since then, soups, such as cream of chicken, minestrone, French onion, and tomato have become part of the menus of clubs, restaurants, and parties. Before that *yakhni* was the only soup dish that locals in the subcontinent were familiar with, and it was not as popular as a starter to a meal as a palliative for sore throats. Later, the growing popularity of Chinese cuisine made soup an acceptable starter at meals in restaurants or even at home, with the result that today a substantial variety of soups have also made their way into the menus of restaurants serving just Pakistani cuisine.

Special occasion food. Generous hospitality is the hallmark of the traditional fabric of Pakistan. The value of guests is immense: they are offered the best, and meals served to them are a matter of honour for the host. The cost of the dish is often overlooked on these occasions, and extra time and care are devoted to cooking them. Hence, the menu for special occasions is usually not the same as for everyday meals. This trend holds true across almost all ethnic groups. A variety of dishes are cooked for a special-occasion meal, which also includes a few specialities, and is always topped with a dessert or two.

Spice. The various strongly flavoured or aromatic substances, spices, in Pakistan are always of vegetable origin and are commonly used during cooking, rather than as condiments. In fact, nothing characterises Pakistani cooking more than its vivid and imaginative use of dried spices, possibly because so many of the plants from which the spices are derived are either native to the subcontinent or grow there.

Of course, 'spicy' doesn't have to mean 'chilli'. Just as salt and pepper levels are adjusted to suit personal taste in Western cooking, the amount of salt and chillies in Pakistani cuisine may be varied without compromising the authenticity of the dish in any way.

There are many ways of using spices in local cuisine. They can be used whole, ground, roasted, fried, or mixed with yoghurt to marinate meat. Any one spice can completely alter the flavour of a dish, and combining

several in varying proportions could produce totally different colours, flavours and textures depending on the proportions.

Although packaged ground spices are now commonly used in cities, freshly ground spices are still preferred in rural areas and in homes that are not willing to compromise on the taste as there is no doubt that there is a definite difference in flavour when using freshly ground spices.

Spinach. The spinach, *palankya* in Sanskrit, and *palak* in Urdu, *Spinacia oleracea*, is native to south-west Asia and was known in the subcontinent long before it was introduced to the West. A hearty rustic vegetable, spinach is particularly an old favourite of the fertile, rural, and urban Punjab, although it is now eaten practically throughout the country.

Known for its robust mineral flavours and versatility wherever it is eaten, spinach's pungent taste was welcomed as the perfect base for the intensely spiced cuisine by the subcontinent. Abundant in flavour and nutrients, spinach is consumed in many forms—cooked on its own as a vegetable curry, mixed with cottage cheese to make the highly popular *palak paneer*, or with mutton, as *palak gosht*, or dipped in batter and deep fried to make the delectable *palak pakora*.

Spinach has a multitude of health benefits, too. People in the subcontinent eat it abundantly for this reason alone—for its age-old health benefits. It is believed to lower blood pressure and help regulate sugar levels in the body.

It is an excellent source of beta carotene, vitamin C, E, and K, potassium, iron, sulphur, sodium, folic acid, and oxalic acid. It contains more protein than most vegetables. Spinach is one of the vegetables with the highest amount of chlorophyll, a fat-soluble substance that stimulates haemoglobin and red blood cell production.

There are two varieties of spinach in Pakistan: winter spinach which is best sown in August, and summer spinach which can be sown in February. The crop is ready for harvest in six to eight weeks after sowing.

BISMA TIRMIZI

Spring roll. A Chinese snack or item of finger-food, spring roll usually consists of a wrapper of thin pastry around a savoury filling of vegetables and generally chicken. Its popularity has now gone beyond Chinese cuisine. It is often served as an *hors d'oeuvre* at dinner parties where Pakistani or continental cuisine may be on the menu, or as a snack item at tea boasting an assortment of dishes from different cuisines.

Staple. These are fundamental items of the diet that local, ethnic, regional, or national groups regard as indispensable in a meal. The traditional meal structure in an average Pakistani household comprises at least one staple and one main dish (staples are normally eaten with the main dish), with the more affluent households enjoying two staples and at least two main dishes at every meal. The staple normally eaten is grain, in the form of traditional breads, while rice constitutes either the second or the alternate staple. Interestingly, if two staples are served, there is a preference for eating rice first and *roti* later in most communities. Wheat grows more abundantly than rice in Pakistan, is cheaper and more filling, accounting for the traditionally wheat-based diet found in the country, although *roti* made with rice flour is favoured in the rice growing areas. Rice, rarely eaten at breakfast, is usually consumed in its plain boiled form with a main dish with gravy.

Stew. A Dilliwalla community speciality, onion plays a major role in the stew made by them, which is traditionally a mutton dish. It also incorporates whole spices and yoghurt.

Street food. Street food culture goes back to the 1840s when a group of Gujaratis began trading in Bombay's (now Mumbai) Fort area, starting Asia's first stock exchange a few years later. They traded mainly in cotton, and many made fortunes during 1861–65 when global supply was affected by the Civil War. These traders worked late into the night when rates were wired in and orders wired out. By the time they would be done, everyone would be hungry but it would be too late for them to eat at home as their kitchens would be closed. So, the traders began to be served by street stalls that invented a late-night special: *pao bhaji*—mashed vegetables (all the leftovers) cooked in tomato gravy and served with buttered loaves. As the city flourished, the food became more varied and snacks were included for pleasure rather than just for nourishment. Hence, among others, stalls serving *bhel* and *pani puri* came up.

However, the gentry would always consider it to be beneath them to eat from wayside stalls, and as for women, it was completely out of the question for them to be seen standing around partaking of street food or even eating while walking on the streets. In fact, eating out was once considered a social taboo. Only travellers,

labourers, and people who did not have their family in town were expected to eat at restaurants.

Today, a variety of street stalls selling anything from *bun kebab* to *gola ganda* to sweet potato to *kachori*, *haleem*, *chaat*, and a lot more have sprung up practically throughout the country, and street food culture is flourishing in all the major cities and small towns so much so that entire areas have sprung up as food streets. These are now extremely popular, serving a wide variety of fare, and people from all walks of life can be seen frequenting them—especially at night when these streets often become pedestrianised—and sitting at tables and chairs laid out on the pavements or centre of the food streets.

But it is not just these more permanent street stalls that have gained popularity in Pakistan. *Thela* food in local parlance, which is local fast food and/or snacks that is sold throughout the day on push carts of yore in busy streets and thoroughfares, has become as popular with the common man as with the elite because of the taste, freshness, reasonable price, and prompt service. The vendors generally position themselves at the same spot every day so that their regular customers know where to find them, although some prefer to push their cart from street to street in search of new customers.

From hard-boiled eggs to *kachoris* to *bun kebabs*, kebab rolls, *chaats*, *haleem*, *biryani*, corn on the cob, sweet potatoes, *challi*, roasted chickpeas and corn soup to sweets like *rabri* and *kulfi*, fresh fruits and vegetables, dry fruit, and refreshing summer and winter beverages, everything under the sun is available on the pushcart. Often, the vendors cannot even afford a pushcart, and rely on a large flat pan called *thaali* to carry the food item, which they balance on their head, while they hold a stand to rest it on, in their hands, and station it wherever they feel they can get customers.

Sufaid gosht. This is a Pakhtun community meat dish that is gently poached using the *dum* process of cooking so common in Central Asia. It is a yoghurt-based spiced curry, thus, its name which means 'white meat'.

Sugarcane (S. robustum). Sugarcane is native to the subcontinent and popular as a fruit and juice since ancient times. Buddhist literature refers to sugarcane juice being extracted with a machine (*yantra*), though in the Kushan period (AD 200), machine-extracted juice was declared inferior, presumably, to the hand-extracted product. The Sutra literature (800–300 BC), mentions the thickening of sugarcane juice to first become *phanita*, and then solid *guda* (jaggery). Later, the Persians, followed by the Greeks, discovered the famous 'reeds that produce honey without bees' in the subcontinent between the sixth and fourth centuries BC.

Sugarcane is one of the several species of tall perennial true grasses of the genus *Saccharum*, tribe Andropogoneae, native to the warm temperate to tropical regions of South Asia and Melanesia and used to produce sugar. The Persians and Greeks adopted it and then spread sugarcane agriculture. It belongs to the grass family Poaceae, an economically important seed plant family that includes maize, wheat, rice, and sorghum and many forage crops.

It has stout jointed fibrous stalks that are rich in the sugar sucrose, which accumulates in the stalk internodes. The plant is two to six metres tall. The world demand for sugar is the primary driver of sugarcane agriculture—Pakistan is one of the largest sugarcane-producing nations in the world.

Merchants began to trade in sugar from the subcontinent, which was considered a luxury and an expensive spice. Today, sugarcane juice is one of the more affordable fresh juices in Pakistan and is particularly a favourite in summer when it provides instant energy. Occasionally, it is mixed with a touch of ginger and black salt to give it a distinct added flavour.

Sukha gosht. Traditionally made with beef strips at the onset of winter, *sukha gosht* or dried beef is a variation of hunter beef and is served as an ideal accompaniment to *daal chawal*. Fat is trimmed away before seasoning for best results and preservation. The recipe is simple but tedious as it requires the meat to be strung and dried in open sunlight for four to five days. Hence, the winter season is best for its preparation, as Pakistani summers tend to be too hot to retain the freshness of the meat.

Care has to be taken as the meat must not take in any moisture; therefore, it has to be stored in a cool, dark and dry place at sunset and hung again with sunrise. Five days of this procedure will prepare the meat for storage in air-tight containers for a month-long use. The subcontinent has had a trading, hunting tradition that required men to be on the road for weeks on end and, hence, the popularity of such recipes. The only spices used in it are salt, red chilli powder, and garlic and ginger paste.

SHAHA TARIQ

Sundhera/sundheru. A dish served on *pehli raat* or the eve of Muharram in the Bohra community, *sundhera* is sweet rice made by boiling rice and mixing it with sugar and warm *ghee*. It is garnished with almonds and pistachios. It is also served as a starter in a *thaal* on special occasions, to be taken after the pinch of salt. *Sundhera* is offered in a very small plate; the objective being that each person sitting around the *thaal* gets a small bite.

Sweet potato (*Ipomoea batatas*; shakarqandi). A tropical root crop, sweet potato is the starchy tuber of a vine of the convolvulus and morning glory family. It is not related to the ordinary potato, although both plants have the same origin. There are numerous varieties. Most have tubers which are about the size of a medium ordinary potato, and generally of an elongated, slightly pointed shape, though there are also round ones.

Most sweet potatoes are used fresh: they are baked in sand and sold on pushcarts in winter in the Punjab, where they are mostly grown. They are highly nutritious and easily digested. They are believed to be good for circulation and help to eliminate toxins from the body.

T

Tabak maaz. This is a Kashmiri speciality and one of the dishes served in *Wazwan*. *Tabak maaz* are flat pieces of mutton rib chops boiled in milk or *malai* (full cream), whole spices and saffron, then fried in gravy enriched with *ghee* till they acquire a crisp crackling texture.

Taftan. A leavened rice flour bread originating from Persian cuisine and adopted by the Dilliwallay community, *taftan* incorporates sugar, milk, and lemon seeds, and is baked in a clay oven. *Taftans* are popular at weddings and are normally eaten with *shab degh*.

Tahiri. Basically, *tahiri* is plain yellow rice, with potatoes added in it. Spreading throughout the subcontinent during the Mughal rule, the *biryani*, reportedly, reached Hyderabad Deccan in Aurangzeb's time, where he had left behind Nizam-ul-Mulk as his representative in the Ara Kadu area. It is believed that the Nizam's chefs developed forty-seven varieties of *biryani*, among them was the famed *tahiri*—meatless *biryani*. This dish may have been the result of Aurangzeb's forced austerity drive.

Tajiks. These are a Persian-speaking people, with traditional homelands in present-day Afghanistan, Tajikistan, southern Uzbekistan, northern Pakistan, and western China. According to estimates there are over one million Pakistani Tajiks. They are normally considered similar to Khows and their cuisine has much in common with Persian, Afghan, and Uzbek cuisines. Traditional Tajik meals begin with a spread of dry fruits, nuts, *halwa*, and other desserts arranged in small dishes, progresses to soup and meat, and culminates in the serving of *pulao*.

Tali hui bhindi. This is a delicious dish made with okra that has been washed and dried in the sun before being finely chopped and then stir-fried with salt and red chillies till crispy.

Tamarind (*Tamarindus indica*; imli). The tamarind is a large and beautiful evergreen tree (of Caesalpiniaceae family) native to tropical Africa. However, the plant has been growing freely in the subcontinent since prehistoric times; having strong and pliant branches and an extensive root system it can be grown in places exposed to high winds; it is also resistant to drought. The tamarind is prized for its pods, which grow in clusters and contain very small beans, surrounded by an attractively sour/acidic and sticky pulp. They are harvested when fully ripe, the shells and seeds are removed, and the pulp compressed into 'cakes'. In this form tamarind provides an acidifying agent used in Pakistani cooking. However, tamarind must be soaked in hot water to extract its flavour, especially when using it in cooking. It is used especially for making chutneys, in *chaats*, and some lentil dishes, while many youngsters like to suck it raw. The pulp can also be turned into a syrup, with the addition of sugar, and then diluted to make drinks.

Tamatar kut. A unique and delicious component of Hyderabadi cuisine, *tamatar kut* is a tomato-based dish that requires tomatoes to be diced, blended and steamed with whole and ground spices, primarily curry leaves, cumin seeds, fenugreek, green chillies, ginger/garlic paste, turmeric and red chilli powder, along with tamarind paste and salt to taste. Once the tomato paste is ready, boiled eggs cut into halves are added to it. The dish is garnished with fried onions, fresh coriander and mint leaves and is normally served as an accompaniment to a main course. The term *kut* could perhaps be traced to *khatta* meaning sour as this dish has both a sweet and tangy flavour, and over time has become popular by its shorter name.

ZUBAIDA TARIQ

Tandoor. Middle Eastern clay oven, the *tandoor,* has been in use from Arab countries up to the subcontinent, while its remnants have been discovered from excavations at the Indus Valley sites. The most common *tandoors* are large, spherical clay holes/earth ovens, about four feet deep, heated by a bed of charcoals. *Tandoors* are normally used in both urban and rural areas of Pakistan to make flat bread (*roti/naan/sheermal/ taftan*) but can also be used to roast meat on vertical skewers. Though the popularity of the *tandoor* can be traced to as far back as the ubiquitous *chapati*, the Persian-speaking Central Asian nations—particularly the regions around Afghanistan, Uzbekistan, Iran, and Tajikistan—have also for centuries been consuming *naan* the way we know it. It is believed that through conquests and trade, the basic recipe of the *naan* found its way to the subcontinent. Interestingly, *tandoors* started out in the Punjab as places for socialisation as much as a means of cooking. Since not all homes could accommodate *tandoors*, communal *tandoors* were used by people to cook bread from flour kneaded at home, offering them the opportunity to meet neighbours and catch up with news and gossip at the same time.

Tandoori chicken. The origins of *tandoori chicken*, apparently, lie in Gora Bazaar in Peshawar, where nearly a hundred years ago Mokha Singh Lamba started a small restaurant. Legend suggests that the restaurant's young chef Kundan Lal Gujral decided to experiment by skewering pieces of chicken marinated in yoghurt and masala and sticking them into the *tandoor* (which was previously used only for making breads). Thus, the popular *tandoori chicken* was born.

BISMA TIRMIZI

Tas kebab. Borrowed from Irani/Turkish cuisine, *tas kebab* is now a popular dish on Pakistani tables. It is a fragrant variation of traditional, spicy, stewed meat and incorporates eggplants, carrots, and potatoes. While boneless meat (mutton/beef/chicken) is used, onions are sliced to make a base for the layer of meat. Other vegetables are added on top in layers. A cup of water helps simmer the meat and vegetables to simmer. Tomato paste, with turmeric, red chilli powder, cinnamon stick and salt is added for gravy, and dried prunes for flavour.

SHAHA TARIQ

Tash-t-nari. During a Kashmiri *Wazwan* banquet, guests sit in groups of four and the meal begins with a symbolic washing of hands with water poured from *tash-t-nari*, a vessel that looks like a kettle with a long spout, which is filled with clean warm water, and accompanied by a cauldron or a basin over which the hands are washed. Interestingly, while this is a Kashmiri custom, similar customs also exist in the Bohra and Gujarati Khoja communities where the host brings a similar vessel to wash the guests' hands before they partake of a *thaal* meal.

Tawa. A thick, flat, or slightly concave, heavy-bottomed, cast iron griddle pan on which *chapati* is cooked, *tawa* is believed to be an ancient utensil, as excavations in the Indus Valley have revealed similar clay and metal plates. *Tawa* is also used to make certain main and side dishes, such as *kata-kat* and *chapli kebab*, respectively.

Tawa tiki. This is a cake-like, thick bread made with two *shapiks*—Chitrali yeast bread—placed one on top of the other, with a filling in between, be it of vegetables, meat, or any leftovers. Deep fried, this bread is popular with the Khow community in Khyber Pakhtunkhwa. The *tikis* have different names depending on the kind of filling they have. Variations of the *tiki* include *mishtiki/ chai tiki*; *sanabach tiki* (with a paste of wheat flour); *pushur tiki* (with a meat filling); *zholai tiki* (with crushed walnuts and onions); and *phinak tiki* (with walnuts and cottage cheese).

Taway wali machli. A Punjabi speciality allegedly introduced by Darul Mahi, a restaurant in Lahore, *taway wali machli* comprises sweet water fish fried on a *tawa* and seasoned with *chaat ka masala*.

Tea-house. Traditionally, tea-houses were places frequented by the intelligentsia of the city, where they would hold conversation in which not only daily news and rumours were exchanged and discussions on politics and literature held, but cultural values were also communicated. As a rule, tea-houses were not places for conflicts; they were spaces for socialising among friends in which ethnic, social and religious boundaries were transcended. In accordance with the custom of the land, gender segregation was common so that tea-houses were traditionally a world of men and not a social locale for women. Women either sat in curtained women's section in tea houses or usually met at home for tea. The traditional tea-house more or less vanished over the years, but recently efforts are again being made to revive this practice of the literati and artists gathering together under one roof for casual chats over tea. Pak Tea House, probably the best-known tea-house in all of Pakistan, had been a literary meeting point in Lahore since the days of the British Empire. Guests included famous poets and writers such as Saadat Hasan Manto, Faiz Ahmed Faiz, Ahmad Faraz and Intezar Hussain, and the singer of classical Raga music Ustad Amanat Ali Khan, to name just a few. No other literary institution had such authority. This is where the weekly meeting of the official circle of poets was held. Some of the poets could only write here and for this they needed their daily dose of tea and tobacco. In the course of recent decades, however, the social environment of the tea-house has changed. Sadly, in 2004, the Pak Tea House had to close its doors for financial reasons.

Teetar. Basically, a winter speciality, *teetar* is a Sindhi delicacy prepared by roasting partridges (*teetar*) on a spit over a campfire. When prepared inside the home, *teetar* is normally fried.

Thaal/thaali/seni. In use since the Indus Valley Civilisation, *thaal/thaali/seni* is one of the numerous metal utensils discovered during excavations. Once a cooking pot, it is now used as an eating plate in many communities, especially Bohras, though sometimes it is also used as tray to serve desserts and fruits.

Thadal/thadai/sardai. A refreshing drink normally prepared in summer in Sindh, *thadal/thadai/sardai* is made from the extract of dried fruit seeds, such as watermelon and almonds, and aromatics.

Thar Desert. This is a large arid region in the north-western part of the subcontinent that covers an area of 200,000 sq km and forms a natural boundary between India and Pakistan. It is located partly in Rajasthan state, north-western India, and partly in Punjab and Sindh provinces, eastern Pakistan. It is the world's 17th largest desert, and the world's ninth largest subtropical desert. With 15 per cent of Thar Desert located in Pakistan, the cuisine of the area, as with the rest of Rajasthan, includes numerous types of *rotis*. Among the most common are *bhakri*—crisp *roti* made from *bajra* or *jowar* on a griddle—and *besan roti* with just a little wheat flour added to bind the dough. Also popular is *missi roti* that has spinach, green chillies and onion mixed in the dough. Their main courses comprise dishes such as *pipun*, *ker sangri* and *amaranth* made with wild herbs and vegetables indigenous to the area.

Thepla. A Gujarati dessert, *thepla* is deep fried, sweet crisp *puri*. It is basically made with whole-wheat flour, eggs, jaggery, milk, and butter. *Thepla* can be stored for days in airtight containers without going bad and is a popular tea-time snack.

Thooti wali kheer. Known as *firni* in other parts of the country, *thooti wali kheer* derives its name from *thooti*, derived in turn from *thoota*, meaning 'thumb'. In the Punjab, as indeed in Sindh, this powdered rice and milk-based dessert is served in small, earthenware bowls and often scooped out with the thumb, thus the name. It is flavoured with saffron and cardamoms, and garnished with dry fruit.

Tibet's influence on cuisine. Tibet's proximity to Pakistan's northern areas has resulted, to some extent, in the region's cuisine being influenced by Tibetan cuisine. Among the Tibetan specialities adopted in the northern areas is *momo*, steamed meat-filled dumplings that are especially popular in Gilgit–Baltistan.

Til ki chutney. A staple of Hyderabadi breakfast *til* (sesame seeds) provide a great nutty flavour to *til ki chutney* and make it an absolute favourite in many Urdu-speaking Pakistani homes. The base of this chutney is tamarind which can be either ground, if raw, or boiled, if ripe. Mixed with salt, brown sugar (optional), red chillies, ginger, diced coconut, and sesame seeds, it can be pulsed in a blender to a thick consistency. Alternatively, it may be heated and garnished with fresh curry leaves in mustard/sesame oil. Either way it is a great side item for *khichri* or *aaloo ka paratha*.

SHAHA TARIQ

Tireet. An Arab speciality that has been adopted by the Baloch community, *tireet* is a clear broth that is a cross between stock and curry. It is eaten with bits of *chapati* broken and soaked into the broth.

Tobacco. The introduction of and growth in the cultivation and trade of tobacco are some of the most interesting facts of the 17th century subcontinental economic history. A plant introduced from the new world, tobacco rapidly acclimatised itself to this region's cultivation conditions and within a few decades became a major cash crop. Until 1590, the plant and its products were entirely unknown in the subcontinent; *Ain-i-Akbari*, the great administrative compendium of Akbar's court chancellor Abul Fazl does not even mention tobacco. It was a novelty in the first decade of the 17th century. But by 1617 its use had become so widespread, not only among the nobility but also among the common people, that Jahangir issued a decree forbidding the smoking of tobacco. The decree was more well-intentioned than successful, for the habit continued to spread.

According to W.H. Moorland tobacco manufacturing barely started in the 16th century since it was unknown to the revenue officers and consequently must not have been grown to any extent at the time. It is believed that it reached the subcontinent through the agency of the Portuguese and was established first in the province of Gujarat.

Currently in Pakistan, tobacco is consumed in many forms such as manufactured cigarettes, through water pipe (*huqqa/sheesha*), *paan*, *gutka* and *naswar*. Tobacco use is growing in Pakistan as seen from the annual consumption of cigarettes which increased according to the State Bank of Pakistan report. Pakistan Demographic and Health Survey 2017–2018 reported that 23 per cent males and 5 per cent females used tobacco. Exposure to second-hand smoke is also common in Pakistan.

Keeping in view the perceived increase in the consumption of tobacco, especially among younger individuals, the government of Pakistan has taken a number of initiatives including the creation of Tobacco Control Cell at the Federal level, and the introduction of 40 per cent pictorial health warning.

BISMA TIRMIZI

Tomato. The tomato, *Solanum lycopersicum*, is an American plant which bears the familiar fruit (perceived as a vegetable because of its main culinary uses) and is now grown and consumed worldwide. Unlike several other plants from the New World, the tomato did not come directly to the subcontinent, but via England at a late but uncertain date, perhaps around 1850. By AD 1880, tomatoes had begun to be grown chiefly for the European population. However, its popularity soon grew in the region and it rapidly became an important ingredient and, indeed, the base of many Pakistani dishes. Together with onion, it is blended or cooked into a paste to form the gravy that makes up a number of Pakistani dishes. In its raw form, it is an important part of local salads and *kachumbers*.

Trami. This is a large metal platter used to serve the ultimate formal banquet in Kashmir, the royal *Wazwan*. Guests are seated in groups of four and share the meal out of it.

Trasspi bhalay. A Balti soup prepared with chicken stock, fresh mountain herbs including local coriander, hand-made wheat noodles and succulent pieces of boiled chicken, *trasspi bhalay* is delicious and typically delicately flavoured, as is the rest of Balti cuisine.

Trifle. A traditional English dessert, trifle was introduced to the subcontinent with the advent of the British Raj. The essential ingredients are sponge cake (which is soaked in fruit syrup in Pakistan as opposed to sherry or white wine in the original recipe), fruit, jelly, rich custard, and whipped cream, layered in a glass dish in that order. It soon became a people's dish, and a regular feature at weddings, and upper-class family celebrations.

Tumuro. This is a native wild thyme which is found in the mountains surrounding the Hunza valley. It is used fresh and dried, mostly by brewing in water before straining it to become Hunza's one-for-all remedy, the *tumuro chai*. This Hunzakutz drink is said to cool and clear the head, especially at high elevation.

Turai/turai gosht. *Luffa acutangla*, or ridged gourd is known as *turai* in Urdu. It is a strongly ribbed, green, tender vegetable that is either cooked and eaten as a *sabzi* on its own or incorporated in *gosht ka salan* to make *turai gosht*.

Turkish influence. The region of the subcontinent that makes up the present-day Pakistan today is a melting pot of cultures deriving from Afghan, Mongol, Arab, Turkic, and European invaders dating as far back as the 8th century. The Turkic people originally came from Central Asia and along with the Ottoman Turks created an empire which swept across Asia. The caliphs and other political leaders of Islamic countries employed Turkish prisoners of war as military slaves (*mamluk*), who were not slaves in the usual sense. *Mamluks* were allowed to carry weapons and many became powerful army generals—officials who lived lavish lifestyles and brought Turkish influence to the Islamic world. Turkish conquest of India began in about AD 1000 with Mahmud of Ghazni, a Turkish ruler of Central Asia, who originally settled in Afghanistan, and marched his armies west into Iran and east into India. His successors were the Ghaznavids, who ruled across the Indus valley, and then the Ghurids, whose armies were also led by Turkish slave generals. They successfully invaded North India, but the Ghurid king at the time was assassinated and replaced by Qutbuddin Aibak, a Turkish general, in 1206, who became the first sultan of Delhi. Thus, began a slow yet steady influence of the affluent Turkish culture that permeated into the subcontinent and ultimately allowed for a fusion of Turkish, Persian and subcontinental cuisine. One of the main Turkish culinary influences on Pakistani cuisine is the *sheesh kebab*—grilled meat on skewers. Originally, quite bland, flavoured by animal fat, salt and smoking coals, the Pakistani version is full of flavour with the addition of local spices. Other influences of Turkic cooking techniques and recipes such as barbecued meats, kebabs and the nomadic style of spit-roasting can be found in parts of Balochistan, North Pakistan and the Punjab, especially Lahore, which was an outpost of Perso-Islamic culture at the time of the Turkish Sultanate. Local dishes of breads with meat, *pulao* and yoghurt-based dips (*raita*) are also derived from the Turkish influence—which in turn had evolved through a process of exchange between different Islamic ethnic groups—on Pakistani food. Additional Turkish influences on local cuisine were also seen during the time of the Mughals, mainly in the royal kitchens of Babar (his mother was of Turkic origin). Many of the chefs in Babar's kitchens were of Turkic origin and created meals from their homeland that slowly integrated into Mughal cuisine, becoming a part of the subcontinental cuisine as well.

SUMMAYA USMANI

Turmeric (*Curcuma longa*; haldi). A spice and colouring agent obtained from the rhizomes of *C. longa* (an herbaceous perennial plant native to the subcontinent),

turmeric is now widely cultivated in the tropics, though the subcontinent remains by far the largest producer. Analyses of excavated utensils from near the eastern Punjab have uncovered residue from turmeric dating back almost 4,500 years. Vedic literature mentions the community of Nishadas, literally meaning turmeric eaters (*nisha* means turmeric, *ad* means to eat) indicative of the fact that it is being consumed since then in the subcontinent. In fact, it became an integral ingredient of the ancient practice of medicine called Ayurvedic.

The turmeric plant is related to ginger and, as with ginger, it is the rhizome or underground stem that is valued for its flavour. In Pakistan, turmeric is always used in powdered form obtained by boiling and drying the stem of the *C. longa* plant, and then grinding it, using a roller and flat slab. It is an essential ingredient in curry powder and is used in several local dishes, even as little as a pinch, enhancing their flavour and, more importantly, giving them a golden colour. It is mildly aromatic (with scents of orange or ginger) and is known to help mask fish odours. Its flavour is described as a little bitter, a little peppery like mustard or horseradish, with a slight ginger touch.

Turmeric also has numerous medicinal qualities. It helps to control blood pressure and cholesterol, treat indigestion, stomach and liver ailments (by adding it to milk) as well as to heal sores. It is also believed to be effective in combating Alzheimer's disease and is used extensively to improve complexion and as a depilatory. It is also said to cure itching, skin diseases, and conjunctivitis. It is rich in vitamin C and has anti-inflammatory and anti-carcinogenic properties.

Urad daal. *See*, **Maash daal.**

Urdong bhala. A traditional Balti soup, *bhala* is made in 18 different ways. *Urdong bhala* is prepared with a rich beef stock, crushed barley and succulent chunks of beef or mutton. It is a special favourite with the Baltis of Khaplu.

Varq/varak. A sterling silver leaf, applied in the form of very thin sheets to decorate various foods, *varq* has been in use for centuries. It is harmless, as long as it is consumed as pure metal, though many silver compounds are poisonous. It is both tasteless and odourless. Making *varq* is a very laborious process in which small, thin, coin-like pieces of silver are heated and beaten for hours until they resemble a sort of floss; a very thin layer of this floss-like substance is then compressed between two sheets of paper and transformed into wafer-like foil. It used to be highly popular garnish for Pakistani desserts and was imbibed enthusiastically in the days of the nawabs, as it enjoyed the reputation of having aphrodisiac properties. However, over the years, inflation and health concerns have reduced its use. Nonetheless, it is still used to decorate *mithai* on special occasions like weddings, and is a sign of opulence.

Vasanu. A must-have among Parsis in winter, *vasanu* is a herbal recipe that fortifies and energises the immune system. A rich recipe, a tablespoon a day is more than enough to keep the consumer warm and active in cold winter days. It is made with sugar syrup, loads of dry fruit, and *char magaz* (seeds of four types of melons: watermelon, pumpkin, cucumber, and cantaloupe), with each herb and root pounded individually and later fried in *ghee*. Although sweet, it is not classified as a dessert nor a tea-time snack. In fact, it is generally eaten at breakfast. The cumbersome and laborious preparations that go into making this dish has made it one of those almost extinct dishes that families no longer have the inclination or time to prepare. What's more, the large amounts of dry fruit that go into its preparation make *vasanu* one of the most expensive recipes in the Parsi kitchen.

ZARNAK SIDHWA

Vedic Civilisation. The Harappan Civilisation was subsumed by the Vedic Civilisation. Although it lived on in many ways in the culture that replaced it, the Harappan Civilisation was an essentially urban one, whereas the Vedic was agricultural and pastoral. Aryans set the agricultural pattern of food production that persists to date. Fields were ploughed with two oxen drawing a plough. Water was raised from rivers directly, or by deflecting them into man-made channels and building weirs across them to flood the fields. The collection of cow dung is mentioned in the *Rigveda* and the use of animal refuse as fertiliser has also been recorded in many early books. There was an early appreciation for practices such as land fallowing, crop rotation and seasonal sowing. The *Taittiriya Samhita* mentions two crops from a field in a year, the different seasons for ripening of various crops, and the proper times for harvesting them. In the *Arthashastra*, three clear crop seasons and the produce to be grown during each have been defined. Eating in public was not permitted to austere Brahmins during the Vedic era and even later times but there were no such restrictions on others.

W

Walnut (akhrot). Hailing from the Juglandaceae family, walnut is the most important species from a dozen species of the walnut tree with edible nuts, and is a very popular dry fruit in Pakistan. It can be most commonly found in Khyber Pakhtunkhwa, particularly in Dir, Mingora, and other parts of Swat District, Azad Jammu & Kashmir, and Gilgit-Baltistan. The fruit of this wild and beautiful tree is green drupe, with flesh surrounding a hard-shelled stone or nut. Inside the nut is the edible kernel. When the fruit is very young and green, the fleshy outside part can be eaten. At this time, the shell is undeveloped, so the entire fruit is edible, although sour in taste. But as the fruit ripens the fleshy part becomes thin and leathery. The shell consists of halves separated by a papery membrane, the division marked by a clear seam around the outside edge. The half-kernels within look remarkably like the brain. In Pakistan, dry fruits are mostly consumed in winter; however, roasted walnuts are vastly used all year long in preparing desserts such as biscuits, walnut cakes, and the famous *sohan halwa* of Multan along with other sweet dishes like *akhrot dhoda* of Kushab. In the Kalash Valley (Chitral District, Khyber Pakhtunkhwa) people use walnuts for making walnut bread, while in Gilgit-Baltistan the Baltis consume *kisir*, a flatbread or traditional fried pancake made from buckwheat and ground walnut, milk, and eggs paste. *Akhrot chutney* made by mixing walnut oil and yoghurt is also popular in Khyber Pakhtunkhwa, as are local tonics made by mixing walnuts with other dry fruits like pistachio and almonds in honey. Walnut oil is also used for making *zan*, a dessert popular in winter in Baltistan.

LAL MAJID

Water-buffalo (*Bubalus bubalis*). One of the most important animals of Asia, it contributes to food supplies both directly, when its milk is used, or it is eaten as meat, and indirectly because of its role as a draught animal in agriculture. There are two general types—the swamp buffalo and the river buffalo. The river buffaloes supply well over half of the subcontinent's milk and their butterfat is the major source of *ghee*. According to a 2007 article written by the faculty members of animal husbandry, University of Faisalabad, Pakistan, over 55 per cent of the national meat production was from the water buffalo. The meat of the water buffalo—at least of animals bred for the purpose—is fully comparable with beef. Its milk, too, has a higher content of both butterfat and non-fat solids than cow's milk.

Wazwan. The ultimate formal banquet in Kashmir is the royal *Wazwan* said to be brought to the region in the 14th century with the arrival of Timur Lung during the reign of the Tughlaq from Central Asia. It is a blend of the culinary styles of the Mughals and Persians who were Muslims, and the Kashmiri Pandits who were Hindu Brahmins. The Muslims introduced saffron, dry fruit, Kashmiri red chillies, butter and clarified butter, garlic, and tomatoes to the Kashmiri cuisine. *Wazwan* is served on special occasions, such as weddings or engagement ceremonies, but is also served at *taaziat* (condolences) *chaarum* or *chehlum* (forty days after death) to people who come to offer condolence. A sumptuous, multi-course meal, as many as 40 courses may be served during a formal, royal *Wazwan,* with at least 12 and up to 30 courses being non-vegetarian, cooked overnight by the *vasta waza* (master chef), and his retinue of *wazas*. 'Waz' means cook or cooking while 'wan' means shop. *Wazwan* is regarded as the pride of Kashmiri culture and identity.

The preparation of this extravagant feast requires hours of endless cooking with skill and finesse. *Wazwan* is cooked in special nickel-plated copper vessels, over simmering wood fire. Guests are seated in groups of four and share the meal out of a large metal platter called the *trami*. The meal begins with a ritual washing of hands in a basin called the *tash-t-nari*, which is taken round the guests by attendants. Then the *tramis* arrive, heaped with rice, quartered by four *seekh kebabs*, and containing four portions of *methi qorma*, two *tabak*

146

maaz, white murgh or *saffron murgh*, and much more. Yoghurt garnished with Kashmiri saffron, salads, six to eight types of Kashmiri pickles and chutneys, some of them enriched with nuts and dry fruit are served separately in small earthen pots. Every time a *trami* gets polished off, it is removed and replaced by a new one until the dinner runs its course. Just the main course runs for an hour or so.

Seven dishes that are a must in such banquets are *rista, roghan josh, tabak maaz, daniwal qorma, aab gosht, marchwangan qorma*, and *gushtaba*. The end of the main course is signalled when the *waza* brings in *gushtaba*, invariably the last entrée, and the *pièce de résistance*, as it were. Other Kashmiri specialities which could be included in the feast are *Kashmiri gobhi*—cauliflower cooked with cashew nuts and cayenne pepper, together with an aromatic tomato sauce; *Nalagarh* eggplant—eggplants served in yoghurt; *Nalagarh narangi pulao*—traditionally served with a layer of fried potatoes and yoghurt mixture sandwiched between rice, making it into a wholesome meal. *Modur pulao, matschgand, dum olav, methi maaz, dani phol*, and *muji gaad* also find their way in *Wazwan* occasionally.

The main course is followed by desserts, such as *firni, halwa*, and sweet beverages. The feast ends with an elder leading the thanksgiving to Allah, which is heard with rapt attention by everyone.

Wedding cuisine. While different regions have their own specialities which they serve at weddings, by and large *biryani* and *qorma* are regarded as standard wedding fare practically throughout the country. A barbecued or fried item often accompanies the main dishes, while for dessert, generally depending on the season, there is a choice of *gajar ka halwa, lauki ka halwa, gulab jaman, jalebi, kulfi*, trifle, or *lab-e-shireen*. At *mehendis*, the festive occasion before the wedding revolving around song-and-dance, the menu is usually barbecue—*seekh kebab* and/or *chicken boti*—and *paratha*, along with *aaloo ki bhujia* and *kachori*.

Wheat agriculture. The earliest books to mention wheat are *Yajurveda* and *Brahmanas*. The word for wheat, *godhuma*, is the same as the old Persian term *gandum*. It is contemptuously described as food for the outcasts, which could mean the vanquished Harappans who used wheat extensively. In the Vedic times, rice all but displaced wheat which then made a comeback between AD 1000 and AD 1500 when both became popular. Agriculture accounts for about one-fourth of Pakistan's gross domestic product, with wheat production accounting for just over one-fourth of agriculture's value. Wheat accounts for more than one-third of the cropped acreage. There are two main cropping seasons in most of Pakistan: *kharif* (April–November) and *rabi* (November–April). There are two basic crop-rotation systems in irrigated agriculture in Pakistan—wheat-cotton, and wheat-rice—although a number of minor crops, especially fodder, are also grown in both seasons. Wheat is a *rabi* (winter) crop, which is planted in early November and harvested in April or May.

Y

Yakhni. This is a fragrant and aromatic stock, also called *akhni*. A clear, all-purpose meat or vegetable stock, the origin of *yakhni* can be traced to ancient Persia, but it was introduced to the subcontinent by Mughal invaders, Irani travellers and merchants, and, with minor variations, is popular all over the subcontinent. Originally a yoghurt, saffron and mutton broth (*yakhni* means broth) one can find the recipe of *yakhni* in *Ain-i-Akbari*, written during the reign of Mughal emperor Akbar. *Yakhni*'s colour is pale yellow, derived from a combination of yoghurt and saffron. Tomatoes, turmeric, garlic, and onions are not used in the recipe. Only aromatic spices, such as fennel seeds, cinnamon, cardamom, cloves, and ginger, are used which collectively create its unique taste. It is often partaken of as a clear, hot, and nutritious soup, and is highly recommended for treatment of common cold and flu. Conversely, *yakhni* is also the name given to a special broth made from the mince of a lamb's tail, popular among the Pakhtuns of Landikotal in Khyber Pakhtunkhwa.

Yakhni pulao. This is a famous rice dish in the subcontinent, South Asia, and Arabia. Made by cooking rice in broth using the *dum* technique of cooking, it sits lighter on the stomach than the *biryani*. Many variations exist, depending on the community and the family it is made in, because while some use yoghurt to cook the meat, others use tomatoes. Some use green masala to cook the meat, while others don't. Variations also include the kind of meat used—chicken, mutton, fish, prawn, minced beef—while some *pulaos* only incorporate vegetables and/or pulses—potatoes, peas, mixed vegetables, chickpeas, lentils, etc.

NAYYER RUBAB

Yoghurt/Curd. One of the fermented milk foods, yoghurt's origins are probably multiple. The main role in the fermentation is always played by lactic acid-producing bacteria, and it is this acid that gives all yoghurts their characteristic sour taste. Yoghurt can be made from many different milks—cow, goat, water-buffalo, sheep, camel, and dri (female yak). These all have different characteristics in features such as texture and flavour. For millennia yoghurt used to be prepared in every household in the region using buffalo or cow milk, boiled, and cooled to room temperature, with a small quantity of yoghurt or curd from a previous run, and leaving the mass to set undisturbed overnight in a warm place. Sweetly acidic and mildly flavoured, yoghurt is now mostly bought from milk shops where it is prepared in huge clay pans, and very few homes, especially in cities, bother with the hassle of preparation. Yoghurt is normally partaken on its own as an accompaniment to a main course, or with a staple, or mixed together with chopped onions, cucumber, tomatoes, and coriander in a *kachumber*. Diluted and often with cumin added to it, it is used as *raita* served with rice dishes such as *pulao* or *biryani*. It is also used as a key ingredient in a number of dishes, both meat-based—where it serves as a marinade—and vegetarian. Yoghurt is also used throughout the country to prepare products such as the refreshing drink, *lassi*, cottage cheeses, *kashk*, and *quroot*. Yoghurt or curd carries living micro-flora, which are now recognised as regularly replenishing those in the lower intestine, thus being conducive to digestion and warding off infection.

Z

Zafran sherbet. Introduced by the Mughal Emperor Babar, *zafran ka sherbet* is a Persian drink served by the Baloch community particularly at engagements. It is made with saffron, ground cardamoms, sugar syrup, lime, and rose water.

Zafrani murgh or sufaid kukar. This is a Kashmiri speciality, often a part of the traditional feast known as *Wazwan*. *Zafrani murgh* is chicken cooked in saffron or white sauce—thus the two names it is popular by— *zafran* is saffron and *murgh* is chicken, while *sufaid kukar* is white chicken. The white sauce is prepared with refined flour and milk.

Zan. A Baltistani dessert, *zan* is a kind of *halwa* made from buckwheat. After levelling it in a pan, a hollow is made in its centre, and three types of oils, namely, almond, walnut, and coconut are mixed with sugar and placed in the hollowed centre. Especially popular in winter, it is extremely nutritious and known for its warmth-producing qualities. It is also reputed for fighting off diseases, gastric problems, and various aches and pains.

Zarda. A sweet, yellow-coloured rice dessert that has its origin in the Persian cuisine, where it is known as *sholeh zard*, *zarda* was introduced by the Mughals. *Zarda* is derived from *zard* meaning yellow in Persian, and now in Urdu as well, whereas *sholeh* means sticky rice. In the 17th century, it was known as *zard brinj* which means yellow rice served with *balai* (fresh cream) on top. It was a popular Mughal dish enriched with raisins, pistachios, sultanas, and dried apricots. During the Mughal era *zarda* was considered a Sufi dish because it was commonly distributed free among pilgrims at the shrines of Sufi saints all over the subcontinent. *Zarda* made in Pakistan consists of rice, sugar, refined butter, saffron, *khoya* and dry fruits (raisins, almonds, pistachio, cashew nuts, and walnuts). Nowadays, to give yellow colour to *zarda*, *zarday ka rang* (yellow food colour) is used. In olden days, and often even today *zarda* was/is served in combination with lamb *pulao* at weddings or other ceremonial gatherings. In the Gujarati community, it is served as an entrée and partaken of with *daal gosht*.

NAYYER RUBAB

Essays

Chulha/Zero Carbon Earthen Pakistan Chulha

YASMEEN LARI

A mud fireplace, common even today, the *chulha* is usually about 15–20 cm high, with an inlet for inserting logs of firewood or twigs, and knobs on the rim to support the cooking vessel. The device is ancient. The Vedic sacrifices prescribe the use of *chulli*. Excavations at Nageshwar (2500–2000 BC), an Indus Valley settlement, have revealed a U-shaped *chulha* with a front opening and three round knobs.

Two decades after the dawn of the 21st century, a couple of billion women in South Asia and sub-Saharan Africa are still forced to squat in front of the open-flame stoves and cook using biomass as fuel, as they know no better and find them economical, with the indigenous raw-materials easily available. The rudimentary stove is a major cause of eye and respiratory diseases among women, which remain unattended throughout their lives. In Pakistan, too, these ancient *chulhas* are still very much in use in rural areas and in impoverished areas of the cities.

However, in the last few years, a valiant effort has been made by the Heritage Foundation, Pakistan, to transform the ancient *chulha* into a specially designed, zero-carbon, earthen structure incorporating a chimney, presenting an attractive and low-cost alternative to the inefficient open-flame single stove. The double-stove *Pakistan Chulha* minimises the cooking time and reduces smoke which is, in any case, emitted at a higher level. It provides a clean, hygienic dining space for the family on a raised, lime-stabilised earthen platform. Fuelled by sawdust/cow dung briquettes, it also saves women from spending excessive time searching for fuel.

According to WHO figures, women and girls bear the largest health burden not only from domestic pollution sources, but also often from related fuel-gathering tasks. Survey data from thirteen countries shows that girls from homes with polluting cook-stoves spend about 18 hours a day collecting fuel or water, while boys spend 15 hours.

The scientifically designed Pakistan *Chulha* is women-centric making it easier and less time consuming for the housewife to cook for her family and has a number of advantages: health and hygiene, DRR-compliance, ease of cooking and environmental benefits. Moreover, advantage in social development in rural areas are sizeable and will only continue to rise as the knowledge and success of the initiative continues to spread. The utilisation of commonly found waste materials with zero biomass, such as briquettes made with sawdust and cow dung, provide a low-cost alternative to marginalised communities.

With the Pakistan *Chulha*, the easily replicable methodology enables rapid spread of construction information. Hence, women, typically the least empowered members of a household, are able to learn about the construction technique using unfired clay and lime, in order to self-build and self-decorate their double-stoves to express their own identity.

From the Pakistan *Chulha* built so far, it is clear that the rural women have been able to bring about the excitement of vernacular design and traditions to personalise what are usually seen as mundane earthen stoves. They have customised each one as a designer stove, showing the pride and ownership of the initiator. Due to the ingenuity of the rural women of the country, the Pakistan *Chulha* is not just a stove; it is akin to a work of art!

After the construction of over 60,000 Pakistan *Chulhas*, it is clear that it is a life-transforming element for women, raising their status in society that was unimaginable before this intervention. The raised earth platform has become a dining-room, where for the first time in their lives, the family members socialise with each other, and where grandmothers can now indulge in their story-telling.

In addition to the family space, it has also become a community social space, where women from neighbouring houses can sit or stand around, interacting with each other. In the absence of any working space available to women, the earthen dais has become their work platform. When they are not cooking, they use it to carry out their craft activity: embroidering, stitching, even practicing the ancient craft of glazed-tile making.

Heritage Foundation of Pakistan has trained several Barefoot Entrepreneurs (BE) as 'Chulha or Stove Sisters.' These are rural master trainers, who are mostly non-literate. They visit neighbouring villages to impart training to housewives for building the Pakistan chulha. They also provide hygiene training to encourage hand washing prior to cooking or handling food.

These Barefoot Entrepreneurs are now spreading the message on their own, at the same time earning a substantial amount for themselves. Each Chulha Adhi (Stove Sister) charges Rs 200 to provide guidance in mixing lime with mud as well as guidelines for stove construction. Take the case of one Chulha Adhi, Champa, who along with her husband, belonging to a minority community, has helped to build 30,000 stoves out of 60,000 that have been built in twenty-seven months, thereby herself earning the grand sum of Rs 6,000,000 or Rs 125,000 per month, twenty-five times her income four years ago. This reflects the popularity and potential of the product, without any promotional activity by the Foundation. The family, on the other hand, incurs a cost of Rs 800 including the fee paid to the Stove Sister for a facility that is life-changing.

Note: The reason why this article has been included in this book, although the Pakistan Chulha has a long way to go before it is adopted all across the country, and indeed across continents, is that one is hopeful that there will be a time when the chulha will have undergone complete transformation the world over and will become a source of pride, income and health to all rural women. Already, the Pakistan Chulha has been recognised by World Habitat and received an award, and is being replicated in Africa, and it is hoped that this is just the beginning.

Cooking the Pakistani Way

SHANAZ RAMZI

While it is generally easy to associate a particular food with a country, like you may link pasta with Italy, fish and chips with England and *shawarma* with Lebanon, it is difficult to link a specific food item with the whole of Pakistan as it is home to so many diverse ethnic groups. In fact, no food can be regarded as even representative of a whole province, as within each province different communities co-exist, each with its own special food, cooked in a particular way. One can, in fact, go so far as to say that in Pakistan one can learn a lot about one another's culture and ethnic background by the type of food normally cooked in their homes. Having said that, I must admit, there are certain features that are common to most types of Pakistani cuisine, which give them a distinct Pakistani flavour. For one, since Islam prohibits pork, most Pakistanis follow this diet restriction rigidly (in fact, pork is not available in the country) and even avoid packaged foods cooked in lard. Also, since alcohol is frowned upon in Islam, its usage in cooking is rare.

All meat (mutton, beef and chicken are the most popular) that is cooked is *halal* (permissible for use according to Islamic law) or kosher. Fish is also eaten, particularly in the coastal areas and near rivers and lakes. However, while the majority of Pakistanis have no religious problems eating any kind of fish, some, like the Isna Ashri Shias and the Bohras—Muslim sects that are followers of Hazrat Ali (RA)—do not eat fish without scales, while the former doesn't eat shell fish, either. Different kinds of fish are popular throughout the country. For instance, in Khyber Pakhtunkhwa, trout and silva are popular river fish. In Sindh, where fresh-water fish is available, *palla machli* (elicia) is the rage, in spite of its numerous bones. The coastal city of Karachi is traditionally known for its pomfret, as well as for sear/mackerel, grouper and silver croaker. Now, thanks to greater awareness and the growing popularity of continental dishes, fish such as red snapper and sole are also widely consumed.

Wheat being the country's staple crop, the core of all traditional Pakistani meals consists of cereals and grains consumed in the form of bread, *chapati* or *naan*, without which a meal is generally incomplete. Rice figures as a close contender, if bread is not eaten at a meal, rice takes its place as a staple.

While both rice and bread can be eaten on their own, serving as a cheap stomach-filler and energy provider, they are generally an accompaniment to a main dish, comprising a curry containing meat in one form or the other, *daal* or vegetables. The most common form of meat dishes are meat curries cooked with vegetables—*aaloo gosht* (meat with potatoes) being the most popular. Although vegetables are an integral part of the Pakistani diet, few people consume them fresh or lightly cooked. Split lentils or *daal* are traditionally considered inexpensive food items, and typically not served when guests are invited at home.

Also, no matter which community one hails from, traditional recipes and processes of cooking entail the use of fats and oils in meals, which provide the aroma, colour and taste in Pakistani cuisine. The oil/fat medium imbibes flavours, aroma and colour from spices and flavour enhancers that are fried in it and passes them on to the main body of the dish. The preparation of curries, vegetable dishes, *daal* and any other item which has gravy in it is considered to be complete only when the cooking fat surfaces to form a layer on top. In fact, without the presence of oil/fat floating on top, the dish is generally not considered to be presentable—although increasing health consciousness is changing that view somewhat in at least the larger cities.

The use of flavour enhancers is also very widespread in Pakistani cooking, regardless of the ethnic group, geographical region and the socio-economic class of the household preparing the food. The five flavour enhancers most commonly used in Pakistani cooking are onions, garlic, ginger, tomatoes and green chillies. One or more of these ingredients are found in almost every Pakistani dish, with onions topping the list.

Aromatics such as ground and whole spices including turmeric, coriander, cumin, red chillies, cinnamon and cardamom, whole grains, oil-rich nuts and seeds, however, are at the heart of Pakistani cooking, making it both immensely flavourful and healthful.

Of the large variety of spices used, many are difficult to clean and handle. Each spice can be prepared and used in many different ways in order to bring out distinctively diverse flavours. A noticeable feature about the local cuisine though, is that village food tends to be simple and uses only the very basic herbs and spices, while food preparation begins to get more elaborate, and use of ingredients increases in towns and cities.

In Pakistan, most housewives prefer to prepare their food from scratch, at the most using single packaged spices—whole or ground—rather than opting for packaged mixed spices. The main reason for this is that the combination of spices used in a dish varies so greatly from family to family that most housewives like to adhere to their own recipes, passed down to them by their mothers, mothers-in-law, and grandmothers. Thus, dishes even common to most ethnic groups become very household-specific in terms of taste and appearance and vary in identity and flavour from one family to another, preserving traditional family cooking styles. Not surprisingly, using packaged ready-made foods is an alien concept in most local households.

Also, certain traditional utensils will be found in most Pakistani kitchens, without the use of which it would be difficult to bring out the right flavour, especially in certain dishes. Since every vessel conducts heat in a different way, the flavour of the final product alters depending on the kind of pan used for cooking a particular dish, even if the ingredients in each case are the same. Therefore, many dishes are only prepared in specific kinds of pots and pans in order to acquire their authentic tastes.

The key to Pakistani cooking also lies in the understanding and practice of six fundamental techniques: frying, boiling, steaming, tempering, smoking, and tenderising as most dishes employ one or more of these techniques for their preparation.

Bread too, is prepared in a variety of ways, sometimes employing unique methods and cooking aids, some of which one may never have heard about. It is no small wonder then that in Pakistan eating constitutes the single greatest entertainment and pastime of people from all communities and classes.

Curry

IRFAN HUSAIN

Over the years, I have been asked innumerable times in Western countries if Pakistani food is like Indian food. Patiently, I explain that North Indian cuisine is almost identical to its Pakistani counterpart, the main difference being that ours is heavy on meat, while the focus is more on vegetables on the other side of the border, but the spicing is similar. However, I add that our kebabs are far superior.

The real difference lies between North and South Indian cooking: the latter is generally hotter, and makes more use of curry leaves, lentils, coconut and tamarind, as one can see in the cuisine of the migrant communities from South India now settled in Karachi. These nuances do not resonate with most foreigners for whom almost all our wonderful dishes fall under the umbrella appellation of 'curry' which does not differentiate between a *salan*, a *qorma*, *bhuna hua* or a *qeema*. All these, and more, fall under the rubric of curry.

There are many theories about the origin of this ubiquitous catch-all word, curry. *Kari* in Sanskrit meant black pepper, which was an important ingredient in meat dressing. Centuries later, the word was anglicised to curry, with the much wider connotation of any seasoned dish and was widely used during the Raj by *memsahibs* (British ladies) when discussing the day's menus with the *khansama* (cook). And when the British returned to their cold, wet island, they took their love of curries with them.

It is a little-known fact that out of the many different kinds of ethnic restaurants that flourish in foodie Britain today, more money is spent in *desi* establishments than any other. This is despite the low prices generally charged by Indian restaurants. In fact, most eateries offering food from the subcontinent are known generically as Indian, even though the vast majority of cooks at these places happen to be Bengali. This trend started in the 19th century, when some sailors from Sylhet, in present-day Bangladesh, jumped ship in London and set up *dhabas* (wayside restaurants) for other seamen from British India.

For some reason, Sylhet provided manpower for many of the merchant ships plying between Britain and its far-flung empire, and also ended up supplying cooks to most 'Indian' restaurants in Britain. This tradition lives on today. Another source of the globalised curry was the indentured labour from the subcontinent that was shipped to parts of Africa and the Caribbean to work in sugar plantations and on railway lines. Each region developed its own variation of the curry—from *coucou paka* (also spelt *kuku paka*), a chicken dish in East Africa, to *bunny chow*, a curry in a bun, popular among the Cape Malays of South Africa.

But the spread of spiced food began much earlier: there is evidence to indicate that Indian monks travelling to East Asia took their technique of grinding spices and slow-cooking vegetables in a gravy with them. This influence has produced many of the fiery dishes we see on Thai and Indonesian menus. The famous Burmese dish, *khow suey*, is basically a meat, fish, or chicken curry that is poured on to noodles and then topped with an array of garnishes.

During the Meiji era in Japan (1867–1912), when the country opened up to the outside world, British traders introduced the unsuspecting Japanese to that abomination, curry powder. The oldest curry house in Tokyo dates back to 1912, and in the district of Kanda, there are hundreds of such establishments. There is even an annual Kanda Curry Grand Prix; the winner of this event last year was the seven-seat Hinoya, and its winning entry featured a raw egg on top. Those familiar with the genuine article complain about the blandness of the Japanese version, but they can now go to Indian, Pakistani, and even African restaurants that have opened in Japan for the authentic stuff.

In fact, curry powder has a lot more to answer for: the culinary havoc it has caused in Britain has been devastating as it has given generations of Brits the completely wrong idea about what constitutes a real curry. I recall with a shudder an evening I spent in a lovely house overlooking the sea in Dorset a few years ago. The hostess considerately cooked a curry, imagining that the dish would make me feel at home. Sadly, it was so bland and insipid that I could barely swallow it. She had used curry powder, of course.

This wretched flavouring was produced in the 19th century by an enterprising businessman to cash in on the nostalgia of returning Brits for the food prepared by their Indian staff when they served the Raj. Presumably, it contains a blend of *desi* spices, but more often than not, it sits unused on shelves for months until somebody decides to make it a 'curry night' and dust a stew with the powder that has long ago lost whatever flavour it might have once contained.

Now, however, Brits are becoming more knowledge-able about *desi* food. At the top end, several Indian restaurants have won Michelin stars—the prestigious accolade every chef craves. Indeed, these upmarket establishments, apart from being very pricey, are highly innovative in their presentation and décor. Dishes that appear on no *desi* menu back home feature here and are served with a flourish. Exotica, such as game birds, venison, and oysters, are cooked in delicate sauces.

At the other end of the scale are the '*balti* joints' that are favoured by football fans after they have quaffed pints of beer. Their speciality is our popular *karhai gosht*, but with multiple variations ranging from fish to vegetarian. One Balti cookbook I flipped through, made the startling claim that the dish had originated in the mountains and valleys of Baltistan. This is quite a stretch, considering the poverty and paucity of meat in that remote region. Manchester's 'Curry Mile' features many *balti* joints, and everybody has their own favourite.

Increasingly, macho young Brits want more chilli in their *desi* food, as fiery curries need copious amounts of lager to quench the flames that light up along the mouth and throat. In Glasgow, a few years ago, an Indian restaurant ran a promotion in which the management offered a red-hot curry for free to anybody who could finish the dish. Overloaded with the Dorset *naag*—one of the hottest chillies known to man—the dish was truly a killer: one idiot who did get it down died as a result. I find it hard to sympathise.

For me, a *desi* dish is all about balance: no single spice should dominate. In a harmonious *qorma*, for instance, each spice adds to the flavour of the dish without dominating the others. For this reason, I find there is no special merit in the *chat pata*, or spicy, dish if its only claim to fame is that it is hot. Anybody can throw in a lot of chilli into a dish; knowing the right amount in relationship to the cumin, coriander, turmeric, and the other spices is the key to a successful curry.

Some scientists think that chilli is an addictive substance. It is true that after a few days without a curry, I do start missing *desi* food. But it is not the heat of chillies I miss as much as the blend of different spices that excite the taste buds without numbing them. Luckily, the popularity of *desi* food has now made our spices available in almost every supermarket in Britain. After centuries of colonising the world, it is the Brits who have been colonised by the humble curry.

Evolution of Mughal Cuisine

IRFAN HUSAIN

When considering a civilisation's achievements, we look at the art and literature it has produced, among other things, as well as the well-being of its citizens. And certainly, we take note of the level of excellence achieved by its chefs.

In this last category, the cuisines of Hyderabad Deccan and Lucknow have never been surpassed in the subcontinent. Both gastronomic traditions owe much to the Mughal presence in India, but they developed distinct flavours that were influenced as much by the local cuisines as by Central Asian, Turkish, and Persian traditions. The nawabs of both Muslim centres vied with each other to serve the most lavish meals imaginable, and *bawarchis* and *rakabdars* (chefs) were paid huge amounts to produce new dishes that became the talk of the town.

In 19th century Lucknow, a chef, famous for his *maash ki daal*, was offered a fabulous monthly salary of Rs. 1,500 to cook just his signature dish at every meal. When accepting the offer, he laid down the condition that the nawab would eat the *daal* while it was still hot. At one meal, the nawab was held up in a meeting, and the *daal* grew cold. Furious, the chef flung the dish into the garden where, as legend has it, a lovely flowering tree grew at the spot the *daal* had landed.

Another story goes that one apprentice at a Delhi nawab's kitchen began preparing a meal when his *ustad* was late. When the master chef finally appeared, he was furious to see his *shagird* at work. Throwing the pots on the floor, he shouted: 'You have only been learning for nine years, and you think you can cook for the nawab?'

With nawabs willing and able to pay fortunes in huge salaries as well as for the most expensive ingredients, the chefs were encouraged to innovate and serve new dishes to titillate the palate. Given this appreciative patronage, there was much rivalry between the two cities, with both claiming the title of India's gastronomic capital. The one thing both culinary powerhouses agreed on was that Delhi was a backwater when it came to refined dining. They charged—with some justification—that Delhi cooking lacked subtlety and balance between flavours,

and that it was heavy and over-spiced. One example of Lucknawi sophistication was the local preference for delicate *pulao* over the hefty *biryani* of Delhi.

Both Hyderabadi and Lucknawi food were often slow-cooked in pots sealed with dough, with charcoal placed on top and under the pots in the *dum* style. The Mughlai style of Delhi called for milk, cream, and lots of exotic spices. Heavy amounts of *ghee* were also a feature.

Given this preoccupation with good food, the *dastarkhwan*, or the large, elaborately embroidered covering placed on the carpet where the guests were seated, would be covered with various dishes. At an absolute minimum, there would be a *qorma*, a *salan*, and a *qeema*. These would be accompanied by a *pulao* and a variety of breads, followed by a *kheer* and a *firni*.

Of course, special occasions would see a far more impressive menu that would include several favourites. Kebabs were (and still are) popular with the Deccani and Lucknawi aristocracy: *kakori, galawat, shami, boti, patili ke kebab, seekh*, and *pasanda* featured regularly. Lucknow's *tunday ke kebab* were named after a one-armed cook of some 150 years ago and are still served at the same *dhaba* in the famous *chowk* (roundabout) in Lucknow. The recipe is a family secret and is said to contain 160 ingredients.

The breads could include any of the following: *rumali roti, tandoori roti, naan, kulcha, sheermal, bakarkhani, lachha paratha*, and *puri. Sheermals* were invented by Mamdoo Bawarchi over a century ago, and his name is still honoured in Lucknow. *Kachay gosht ki biryani, zafrani biryani*, and *pathar ka gosht*—thin slivers of meat cooked on a hot, flat stone—were all party favourites.

In those pre-refrigeration days, food was seasonal, and attention was also paid to the time of day a certain dish was supposed to be eaten. Thus, *nihari*, as its meaning in Persian implies, was served in the morning after cooking on a low heat the whole night. *Paya*, or trotters, were also cooked overnight and eaten with *naan*. The quality of a dish of *paya* is judged by how sticky one's fingers became after the meal: the glutinous tissue released from the bones thickens the dish and makes for a finger-licking experience. Certainly not a dish to enjoy with a knife and fork.

Shab degh, a Kashmiri speciality, was another winter favourite, and was prepared by cooking large turnips with meat, again overnight. *Haleem*, a dish from the Middle East, made with a mixture of grains, pulses and meat, was also slow cooked. Indeed, its name derives from the Arabic word for 'patience'.

While the Mughals, and before them the Delhi sultans from Afghanistan, introduced the relatively simple fare of Central Asia, much of the refinement in North Indian and Mughlai cuisine came from Persia. When Babar's son Humayun fled to the Persian court after being defeated by Sher Shah Suri in 1540, he remained in exile for 15 years. When he returned victoriously to the subcontinent in 1555, he did so with a large retinue of Persian nobles and soldiers. Having acquired a taste for the refined Persian cuisine, it is hardly surprising that a number of chefs accompanied him on the journey and took up residence in the royal palace in Agra. From this point on, Persian culture was dominant among the ruling elites, and filtered down to every section of educated society.

Indian foodies insist that Lucknow retains much of its early gastronomic splendour. But without the patronage the chefs received from wealthy aristocrats, it is doubtful if there is much innovation happening in Lucknawi kitchens today. The fact that, thanks to a cultured and appreciative population that takes pride in their refined cuisine, old recipes are kept alive, is a great relief.

Here in Pakistan, elements of this great tradition were brought over by migrant families from all three Muslim centres. Some restaurants, especially in Karachi's Burns Road, serve traditional fare like *nihari* very early in the morning. But it is now normal to eat this meaty dish in the evening. Families from Lucknow, Hyderabad, and Delhi take pride in serving dishes cooked according to generations-old recipes.

Sadly, a busier lifestyle prevents many from taking the time and trouble to prepare labour-intensive dishes from the past. Educated young women, preoccupied with careers and other family duties, are forced to take short cuts in the kitchen. And most Pakistani men have yet to take to cooking. Professional *khansamas* are seldom instructed in the old ways and cook whatever recipes they have picked up.

The bright spot is the appearance of TV cooking shows that highlight many techniques and recipes. Great chefs like the late Zubaida Tariq (d. 2018) have done much to popularise traditional cooking through her TV programmes and cookbook. Unfortunately, most restaurant owners are reluctant to go to the trouble of serving dishes like *shab degh* and other traditional fare. A generation of young Pakistanis is growing up thinking MacDonald's and KFC are the pinnacle of gastronomy. Unless we can popularise our culinary heritage, we are destined to lose the wonderful range of dishes our ancestors delighted in.

Karachi Cuisine

SHANAZ RAMZI

Karachiites, rich and poor alike, love to eat, and generally are more willing to experiment with their cuisine than those living in any other part of the country. This cosmopolitan city is home to not only people who have settled here from other regions of the country, but also to many different ethnic communities. Although within a given socio-economic set-up their basic meals may not have varied greatly, their specialities that are cooked on important occasions were once worlds apart. Today though, with the growing trend for assimilating cultures, one may find a dish peculiar to one community eaten by other communities as well. They are no longer as great a novelty to the rest of the Karachiites as they used to be.

Generally, breakfast in Karachi does not vary so much because of people's ethnicity as because of their income. In the middle and upper classes, bread is normally eaten with eggs, jam, or cheese. Cereals often form popular substitutes or accompaniments. Tea is an almost universal favourite, although among the more affluent classes coffee is also favoured. Over the weekends, or on public holidays, a more lavish breakfast is normally partaken, comprising *aaloo ki bhujia*, *cholay*, *suji ka halwa*, and *puri*. Breakfast for the lower income groups normally comprises *chapati* and leftover curry from the night before.

Meat consumption is heavy in the city, while prawns, shrimps, and a variety of fish including pomfret, elicia, and carp are used as substitutes for meat. The staple food at lunch and dinner in upper income groups is a meat curry with *chapati*, and some vegetable or lentil dish on the side. But usually, meals depend on the affordability of a household, and the main dish is, accordingly, either a meat or vegetable or lentils dish. Many households also serve boiled rice as staple for at least one meal. Among desserts, *shahi tukray* is a speciality, while in winter *gajar ka halwa* is a popular delicacy.

While typically, curry, and *chapati* or rice form the staple food of Karachiites, the multi-ethnic composition of the city, as stated earlier, has given rise to the adoption of a vast variety of cuisine that was once popular only in the communities of their origin. The upper strata of society, which can afford to regularly eat out or cook cuisine that involve imported ingredients or different cooking styles, has begun to frequently partake of dishes that were once alien to them. An example of a foreign cuisine that has become almost universally popular among Karachiites in particular, is Chinese. In fact, the Cantonese and Szechuan styles, patronised in Karachi, have become so localised that Chinese food has taken on a completely new dimension here.

Along with the Chinese community that settled in Karachi in large numbers after Partition—many of whom opened restaurants and were responsible for introducing their cuisine to the country—several other communities including the Urdu-speaking, commonly referred to as Mohajirs, Anglo-Indians, Goans, Khojas, Gujaratis, Bohras, Sheedis, Hindus, and Parsis also made this city their home, and not only brought their specialities along with them, but were also successful in popularising them outside their communities.

The Anglo-Indians, for instance, are a community whose impact on the cuisine has been felt not just in Karachi—the first city in Pakistan to receive their influence—but in the smaller towns and villages as well. The ubiquitous plain cake, so popular with tea even at *chai kay adday*, is one example of a food item that owes its popularity to the synthesising capability of this community.

The Urdu-speaking or Mohajir community hail from different parts of India and as such their cuisine varies, depending on their roots. In Karachi, the Urdu-speaking communities that have come to be known for their cuisine hail from Lucknow, Hyderabad Deccan, Delhi, and Bihar. Each has their own set of specialities, and over the years Karachiites, in general, have acquired a taste for them.

Other types of cuisine that have become popular in Karachi and other major cities of Pakistan owe their popularity not so much to the communities that have settled here and introduced them as to the increasing trend for embracing different cuisines and opening niche restaurants. Hence, Italian pizzas and pastas, American burgers and steaks, Arab shawarmas, Japanese sushis and tempuras and a lot more are being offered in a large number of restaurants and even cooked in many homes, today. The proliferation of cooking shows on television channels has also been responsible for the widespread popularity of, familiarity with, and adoption of, international cuisines.

Mohenjo-Daro

MICHAEL JANSEN

The Indus Civilisation or Harappan culture was, in the third millennium BC, one of the three earliest civilisations of mankind. Like the ancient Egypt and Mesopotamia, it had developed writing; people were living in large cities like Harappa, Kalibangan, Dholavira, and Mohenjo-Daro, once probably the capital, in Sindh. More than 2,000 settlements have been traced so far, spread over an area of more than one million square kilometres. Most of the settlements were located close to the River Indus and its tributaries (e.g. Harappa, Mohenjo-Daro), and the Ghaggar Hakra (Kalibangan, present-day India) or along the coast of Sutkagen Dor, Dholavira and Lothal (present-day India).

One of the riddles is: how did the people in the Indus Civilisation deal with their daily food needs and how did they cook? Taking Mohenjo-Daro with at least 40,000 inhabitants over a time span of at least 500 years and living in very close urban context, it remains unclear how the food for the inhabitants came daily to the city and how it was distributed to the people. In order to know how the residents in their quarters lived and what they consumed, more readable texts and more modern excavations of the site would be required. Unfortunately, the existing archaeological reports and also the technology of excavation are almost 100 years old. Today, there would be new facilities to read the archaeological remains, especially to identify deposits in drains, old garbage and spoils, which are the best indicators for the remains of their food. The excavation reports of those days therefore hardly help in this respect. Additional information comes from more recent excavations like the one in Mehrgarh. Experts, such as Lorenzo Costantini and Richard Meadows, analysed for years the floral and faunal remains of the site which dates from the eighth millennium till the late Harappan times. We could assume that cereals such as barley, einkorn, emmer, and wheat, known already in Mehrgarh, were also later known in Mohenjo-Daro. The same accounts for dates, vegetable, lentils, and fruits. In the early periods of Mehrgarh sheep, goat, cow, and fowl were already domesticated. Bones of such animals

were also found in the excavations in Mohenjo-Daro. In addition, a wide palette of animals, partly wild and partly domesticated, were depicted on the Indus seals. This early period, showing the change from hunter and food gatherer to farmer and cattle breeder, proved in Mehrgarh 3, was once called the 'Neolithic Revolution' by Vere Gordon Childe. Later, when in the third millennium the first civilisations developed, marked by writing and the existence of large cities, he created a second term, 'Urban Revolution'.

While the earlier sites before Mohenjo-Daro were small and primarily agricultural with mainly agricultural subsistence, the picture changed with the 'mega' city of Mohenjo-Daro. Recent calculations show that the city was much larger than anticipated, as it continues under the present surface for several hundred metres. Approximately, one million square metres visible above the recent alluvial surface, it might extend to more than three million square metres underground with an estimated population of 100,000 inhabitants. The architecture of Mohenjo-Daro, with its densely built quarters and narrow streets, clearly shows that we are not dealing with a farming society. The First Street, 10 metres wide and running for more than 1,000 metres north-south, might have served as central distribution system, but all other streets and lanes and the houses connected to them do not show 'rural' elements of agricultural subsistence. The question that needs to be answered is whether Mohenjo-Daro, as was the imperial Rome 2,500 years later, a 'spider in the net'? Was it a centre of a gigantic food supply system with regular imports from other food production areas? And if so, how did they pay, for money in the form of standardised coins was invented more than 1,000 years later by the Phoenicians in the Mediterranean.

Although exchange (barter) of goods was definitely one way of trade before money was invented, and a double row of eight similar room structures with a smaller room in the back and a larger room at the front suggest a kind of souk for exchange of produce, excavators have not reported any indications to support such an assumption. No further buildings have been found so far in Mohenjo-Daro pointing towards 'market' areas or places where animals and food were exchanged.

The many weights found in houses point towards precise weighing of goods. Ernest Mackay found in his excavation, between 1927 and 1931, 220 weights made of stone, the smallest being 0.550 grams, the largest being 11467, 58 grams.

The interpretation of a structure, excavated in 1950 by Mortimer Wheeler, in the citadel area of Mohenjo-Daro, as 'granary', points towards a centralised storage system, controlled by a central power. Wheeler thought of a 'priest-king' system, a unification of sacred and elite power, as was known from Egypt. But in Mohenjo-Daro neither a palace nor temples were found that would indicate such powers. If the building would have been a granary, it would have been much too small for centralised storage and re-distribution for such a big city. Therefore, it is unclear where the famed 'granary' actually existed in Mohenjo-Daro, if indeed it did.

One of the problems with excavations at Mohenjo-Daro is that in those days, i.e. between 1922 and 1931, modern techniques were not yet known to identify organic material and food remains. In addition, with more than 700 houses identified in the lower city hardly ten kitchens could be identified (e.g. kitchen of bricks for cooking, see Mackay 1938: 105). This makes the identification of cooking areas and their utensils in Mohenjo-Daro extremely difficult.

There is no doubt that in the third millennium in the 'Era of Integration' or the 'Era of the Urban Revolution' there was a wide variety of food consisting of all types of fruits, vegetables, cereals, fish, and meat. We can assume then that the tradition of cooking in Sindh must have survived as an intangible tradition from Harappan times till today—one reason to integrate the cooking of Sindh on the world heritage list of Mohenjo-Daro.

Nihari

ASIF NOORANI

Very rarely have specialities shifted base as has been the case with *nihari*, an immensely popular curry made of beef, which originated in what is now old Delhi in the 18th century and got entrenched in Karachi soon after the Partition. Traditionally made of *bong*, the soft meat on the backside of the lower leg of a cow, this delicacy is cooked over low flame the whole night or for several hours in the day. Those who can afford it and/or are not bothered about the abundance of cholesterol in the brain and bone marrow spend extra money to add either or both to their plates of already cholesterol-laden *nihari*. Garnished with slivers of ginger, chopped green chillies and half-cut lemons to sprinkle on the broth, this meat delicacy is a hot favourite with young and old alike.

Nihari, as the name suggests (*nihar* is Arabic for early morning), was taken at breakfast with *naan* or *kulcha* (two forms of flat bread), more so in winter than summer. Legend has it that the curry was improvised by a *hakeem* to keep cold, cough and congestion at bay. Writer Shahid Ahmed Dehlvi dedicates almost an entire chapter in his classic book, *Ujra Diyar*, to the cooks who ran *nihari* joints in the early 20th century and drifted back further to the final period of the Mughals. Even today, in Delhi and other north Indian cities, *nihari* is served only in the morning, on a first-come first-serve basis, which is why customers leave their dishes with advance payments on the previous evening to avoid disappointment at daybreak.

This was also the case in Karachi in the early post-Partition days when some of the specialist makers of *nihari* migrated to Pakistan and set up outlets in areas like Ranchore Lines and Eidgah. But as the demand for the dish increased manifold and people other than immigrants from Delhi developed a taste for *nihari*, more and more eateries specialising in the dish opened in different areas of the burgeoning city. Also, its availability was no longer confined to morning; it began to be served at noon and night as well. There are, in fact, restaurants that are open round the clock and, sure enough, *nihari* continues to be on their menus 24/7.

Initially, *nihari* was spread to other towns of Sindh such as Hyderabad and Sukkur, where a large number of migrants from northern India had settled after Partition, but now it is not surprising to find eateries serving *nihari* elsewhere in the province, as well as in other provinces too. Salty Balochi *nihari* is a case in point.

Lahore, for example, is one city where there are quite a few *nihari* outlets, but they are confined only to certain localities; instead *halwa puri* is the *numero uno* choice as a breakfast meal all over the Punjab, particularly on weekends.

I have had interesting experiences of having *nihari* in at least three cities of the US. At Chicago's Devon Avenue, the main eatery serving Pakistani cuisine is known for its *nihari*, which for some time was cooked by a Mexican, who did a fine job. He had been the man Friday of a *nihari* specialist, brought from Karachi who after a couple of years, had moved to Dallas, where he had been offered a much higher salary. The second restaurant where I found *nihari* quite mouth-watering was at Manhattan in New York. It was, and I am told it still (till the writing of this piece) is, the haunt of Pakistani taxi drivers, who go there for lunch and dinner. The third place, Troy in the outskirts of Detroit, and run by a Bangladeshi, was unfortunately, no great shake.

Wherever there is a large Pakistani (and non-vegetarian North Indian) diaspora in the world there are bound to be *nihari* eateries, be they in Europe, North America or the Middle East. A cousin who introduced the delicacy to his white fiancée in Chicago was pleasantly surprised to find her developing a taste for spicy *nihari*. 'It was a case of baptism by fire,' he quipped.

A new player in the culinary field, the packaged *nihari masala* sells very well not just abroad but in Pakistan as well. The idea is to have hygienic and relatively less time- and effort-consuming *nihari*, but what doesn't please the puritans is the replacement of beef by chicken, thanks to the scare attached to red meat by members of the medical profession. 'Eating *nihari* made of chicken is like washing your hands with gloves on,' says a *nihari* buff, who like other traditionalists insists on *nihari* being made of beef.

Nearer home, in Chennai, where I spent three stints of a month in 2007, I went to a restaurant which had *nihari* printed in bold letters on its menu. It was understandable that with restrictions on slaughter of cows, oxen and buffaloes in some Indian states, beef has been replaced with mutton but what was not pleasing was the addition of coconut milk in *nihari*.

A common sight in Karachi more than in any other city is the presence of rows of poor people squatting on the pavement outside *nihari* outlets, partaking of a meal of *nihari* and *naan* paid for by some Good Samaritans.

The *hakeem* who innovated *nihari* for consumption in chilly mornings may be turning in his grave seeing this delectable dish served on hot Karachi afternoons, but must be, at the same time, pleased to see it transforming the lives of so many people in different parts of the world.

Pakistan's Iconic Eateries

SHANAZ RAMZI

While new restaurants are opening up in Pakistan practically every day, especially in Karachi, Lahore, and Islamabad, and many have rapidly made a name for themselves, there are some eateries that have remained so popular for over half a century that their names have become synonymous with the country. Though the restaurants may appear modest in their décor and even size, the food quality over the years has remained impeccable and people from far and wide flock for the singular taste of their cuisine that they have come to crave.

One such restaurant is Dilbar Hotel in Purana Qila, Rawalpindi. Housed in a 110-year-old building, the hotel is the flag-bearer of Kashmiri cuisine since Partition. Known for its delectable Kashmiri dishes such as *gushtaba, ristay, tabaq maz, maithi maz, Kashmiri kebabs, shab degh, karam fish, karam gosht, aab gosht, saag gosht*, and *razma daal* with *lobia*, the eatery also offers the grand *Wazwan* comprising at least seven of these dishes. The breads that Dilbar hotel is known for are *girda*, a small *roti* made in a *tandoor, lavasaa*, similar to a *naan*, and *bakarkhani*, a very crisp *roti*. Their Kashmiri tea, brewed in samovars with tea leaves, a dash of saffron, cardamom, and sugar, is just as popular as the cuisine itself and a must to wash down the feast.

Another famous eatery located both in Rawalpindi and Islamabad (on Kashmir Road and Blue Area, respectively) is Jahangir Balti and Bar-B-Que. A family favourite for the last five decades, it is renowned for its delectable barbecued items as much for its traditional Pakistani cuisine, especially *murgh chana*.

An eatery that has become synonymous with Karachi, if not Pakistan, is Bundu Khan. Started by Al-Haj Bundoo Khan, a street vendor selling kebabs on a pushcart in Bolton Market, in Karachi, soon after the formation of Pakistan, the eatery, Bundoo Khan, came into being in 1966 when the owner took part in an international food exhibition and became a hit. The food quality earned him a gold medal from an army officer attending the exhibition, and soon after, Khan was inspired enough to rent a small cabin on M. A. Jinnah Road, which for decades remained the only site of this eatery in the country.

Four generations down the road, the eatery, still run by the same family, has grown exponentially, with five outlets in Karachi and one each in Faisalabad and Dubai. It is a regular representative of Pakistani cuisine at Pakistan pavilion at the Global Village during Dubai Shopping Festival. Maintaining its reputation and its signature flavour, the family claims it does not share its recipe with anyone and prepares the spices themselves, and then sends them out to the various outlets to be used in the preparation of dishes. The eatery boasts a limited fare that it has been excelling in for decades—mutton *seekh kebab, Bihari boti*, chicken *tikka, reshmi kebab*, signature *paratha, halwa, kaleji* (kidney), and tamarind chutney—and people come from far and wide to partake of it. Although the décor has improved somewhat, the outlets still remain essentially simple, with minimum frills attached, so much so that there was no change even in their crockery for years on end, thus keeping their overheads low and the food affordable by one and all.

Phajjay kay paaye from Heera Mandi, inside Taxali Gate is doubtless, one of Lahore's iconic eateries, having been established by the late Fazal Deen alias Phajja, just a few days prior to Independence. He is, in fact, credited with having popularised *paaye* in Lahore. Now run by the third generation, they have introduced another outlet in the same city.

A Lahore eatery existing since 1872, is Sadiq Sweets known for its signature breakfast of *halwa puri*, potato, and chickpea curry, which people traverse long distances to partake of. Waheed Kebab House, specialising in barbecued items like kebabs, *tikkay*, and *boti* but also renowned for its *nihari*, is a much sought-after eatery in Karachi, while Super Nursery Bun Kebab and Hanifia are Karachi's answer to burgers and fast-food. The former started as a wayside kiosk and remains a modest one-window operation selling potato and *daal* patties sandwiched in soft buns along with tomatoes, onions, and chutney, while the latter, famous for its signature hunter beef and unique mustard sauce and the burgers made with them, has expanded to include at least two branches in the city.

Quetta's Naimat Kada, on Prince Road, existing since the mid-1980s is another eatery that people flock to from near and far. Opening as only a breakfast joint serving *halwa puri*, it has rapidly grown into a full-fledged eatery serving lunch and dinner as well, and is especially renowned for its *biryani*. Another popular eatery in Quetta is Mir Afzal Karrahi located on Circular Road, existing for four decades. Boasting some of the best meat in Quetta, it is renowned for its mutton and chicken *karhai* although it has now introduced other items as well, such as *kata-kat* and brain masala, and variations in the traditional *karhai*. Babu Jani Bar-B-Que, also at Circular Road in Quetta—though it now has one branch at Samungli Road as well—perhaps exists since before Partition. Although not family-oriented, it is under the current ownership since 1959 and is famous for its *namkeen tikka boti* and *chaamp*. Lehri Sajji and Pakistan Khaddi Kebab, both specialising in their own signature items—*sajji* and *khaddi kebab* respectively—are two other iconic eateries of Balochistan.

Although not strictly qualifying as an eatery, but nonetheless deserving of mention, is Hyderabad's famous The Bombay Bakery, established in 1911 by Pahlajrai Gangaram Thadani. A modest bakery in the Saddar area of Hyderabad, the present structure was designed and planned by Thadani himself, who chose to describe his operation as 'The shop in a Bungalow'. He moved into the premises with his three children; when he died in 1948, his children kept running the cake shop which had acquired a reputation for its hygienically prepared, excellent quality signature cakes—in particular the coffee, chocolate, and almond macaroon cakes.

The business was expanded by one of the sons, Kishinchand, and when he died in 2010, the bakery was taken over by its current owner, his adopted son, Salman Shaikh, who converted to Islam, and is the fourth generation of the Thadani family to own and run the iconic The Bombay Bakery.

Bibliography

Aab gosht
Ramzi, Shanaz, *Food Prints: An Epicurean Voyage through Pakistan.* (Karachi: Oxford University Press, 2012), p. 78. (Hereinafter referred to as: Ramzi, *Food Prints*).

Aaloo salan
Ramzi, *Food Prints*, p. 113.

Accompaniments
Ramzi, *Food Prints*, p. 29.

Achar
Achaya, K.T., *A Historical Dictionary of Indian Food* (New Delhi: Oxford University Press, 1998), 8th impression, p. 1. (Hereinafter referred to as: Achaya, *Hist. Dict. of Indian Food*).
Davidson, Alan, *The Oxford Companion to Food*, 2nd ed., edited by Tom Jaine (Oxford University Press, 2006), p. 2. (Hereinafter referred to as: Davidson, *Oxford Companion to Food*),
Nasir, Zahra, 'That's A Pretty Pickle,' *Dawn*, 23 February 2020.

Acho bor
Ramzi, *Food Prints*, p. 102.

Afghan refugees
Ramzi, *Food Prints*, pp. 58–9.

Akhni
Ramzi, *Food Prints*, p. 142.

Alcohol
Achaya, *Hist. Dict. of Indian Food*, p. 25.
Achaya, K.T., *Indian Food: A Historical Companion* (New Delhi: Oxford University Press, 2004), 3rd edition, p. 109. (Hereinafter referred to as: Achaya, *Indian Food*).
Chopra, P.N., *Society and Culture in Mughal India* (Agra: Shiv Lal Agrawala and Co. (Pvt.) Ltd, 1963), 2nd ed.
Das, Sukla, *Socio-Economic Life of Northern India (c. A.D. 550 to A.D. 650)* (New Delhi: Abhinav Publications, 1980), Chapter 6, p. 134.
Hassan, S. Mahdi, 'Distillation assembly of pottery in ancient India with a single item of special construction', *Vishveshvaranand Indological Journal*, 1979, Vol. 17, p. 264.
Lane-Poole, Stanley (ed.), *Mediaeval India from Contemporary Sources: Extracts from Arabic and Persian Annals and European Travels* (Bombay: K. & J. Cooper,), pp. 47, 76, 99.

Almond
Achaya, *Hist. Dict. of Indian Food*, p. 3.

Amchoor
Husain, Shehzad, *Healthy Indian Cooking* (Stewart, Tabori & Chang Inc, 1998), p. 6.

Amirti, jilebi
Achaya, *Hist. Dict. of Indian Food*, p. 114.

Anar dana
Davidson, *Oxford Companion to Food*, p. 18.
Husain, Shehzad, *Healthy Indian Cooking*, p. 8.

Anday wala khana
Ramzi, *Food Prints*, p. 135.

Anglo-Indians
Brown, Warren, *The Secret Race: Anglo-Indians* (Lulu publishing, 2010), back page.
Griffiths, Kris, 'Anglo–Indians: Is Their Culture Dying Out?' *BBC News Magazine*, 1 January 2013, p. 55.
Pearson, Dorothy, *Grand Ma's Old Anglo-Indian Cookery Book* (Enid Legra, 2009).

Anise
Achaya, *Hist. Dict. of Indian Food* (2013), 9th impression, pp. 4–5.
Davidson, *Oxford Companion to Food*, p. 23.

Apple
Achaya, *Hist. Dict. of Indian Food*, p. 6.
Saeed, Hakeem, *The New Cookery Encyclopedia*, UK; 'Phal Boltay Hain', Pakistan Agriculture Research Council (PAR), National Geographic News.

Arab rule and culinary influences
Achaya, *Indian Food*.
Trautmann, Thomas R. *India: A Brief History of a Civilization* (Oxford University Press), pp. 143–8.

Arhar
Achaya, *Indian Food*, p. 34.
Bendre, Ashok and Ashok Kumar, *A Text Book of Practical Botany vol. 2* (Rastogi Publications, 2009), revised edition, p. 221.
Cook's Thesaurus <http://www.foodsubs.com>
Davidson, *Oxford Companion to Food*, pp. 606, 624.
Fuller, Dorian Q., 'Agricultural Origins and Frontiers in South Asia: A Working Synthesis', *Journal of World Prehistory*, 2006, vol. 20, issue 1, pp. 1–86.
Fuller, Dorian Q. and Emma L. Harvey, 'The archaeobotany of Indian Pulses; identification, processing and evidence for

cultivation', *Environmental Archaeology*, vol. 11, issue 2, Oct. 2006 pp. 219–24.

Singh, Nagendra K., et al., 'The First Draft of The Pigeon pea Genome Sequence', *Journal of Plant Biochemistry and Biotechnology*, January–June 2012, vol. 21, issue 1, pp. 98–112.

Aromatic
Husain, Shehzad, *Healthy Indian Cooking*, p. 6.
Ramzi, *Food Prints*, p. 39.

Arrowroot
Davidson, *Oxford Companion to Food*, p. 36.

Aryan
Achaya, *Indian Food*, pp. 28, 33.
Davidson, *Oxford Companion to Food*, p. 399.
Kongard-Levun, G.M., *The Origin of the Aryans*, trans. H.C. Gupta (New Delhi: Arnold Heinemann, 1980).
Pargiter F.E., *Ancient Indian Historical Tradition* (1922) (Delhi: Motilal Banarsidas, repr. 1972), pp. 297–325.

Asafoetida
Achaya, *Indian Food*, p. 33.

Ashak
Ramzi, *Food Prints*, p. 59.

Ashura
Ramzi, *Food Prints*, p. 160.

Bactrian
The Editors of Encyclopedia Britannica, Encyclopedia Britannica, Inc., 22 October 2015.

Baghar or tarka (tempering)
Ramzi, *Food Prints*, p. 18.

Bajindak
Ramzi, *Food Prints*, p. 97.

Bajra (Pearl millet)
Achaya, *Indian Food*, p. 186.
Ali, M.A.M.; El Tinay A.H., Abdalla A.H. 'Effect of fermentation on the in vitro protein digestibility of pearl millet'. *Food Chemistry*, 80, 2003, pp. 51–54.
Hulse, J.H., Laing, E.M., Pearson. O.E. *Sorghum and the Millets: Their Composition and Nutritive Value* (New York: Academic Press, 1980), pp. 1–997.
Parameswaran, K. & Sadasivam, S. 1994. 'Changes in the carbohydrates and nitrogenous components during germination of proso millet (*Panicum miliaceum*),' *Plant Foods and Human Nutrition*, 45, pp. 97–102.
Ragaee S., Abdel-Aal E.M., Noaman, M. 2006. 'Antioxidant activity and nutrient composition of selected cereals for food use.' *Food Chemistry*, 98, pp. 32–38.
Saleh, A.S.M., Qing Z, Jing C, Qun S. 2013. 'Millet grains: nutritional quality, processing and potential health benefits.' *Comprehensive Reviews in Food Science and Food Safety*, 12, pp. 281–295.

Simmonds, N.W. (ed.) *Evolution of Crop Plants* (London: Longman, 1976), p. 91.

Singh, K.P., Mishra A., Mishra H.N. 2012. 'Fuzzy analysis of sensory attributes of bread prepared from millet-based composite flours,' *LWT-Food Science and Technology*, 48, pp. 276–282.

Bakarkhani
Hasan, Shazia, 'A Journey of the Senses,' *Dawn*, 16 November 2017.
Ramzi, *Food Prints*, pp. 75, 111.

Balochistan
Hoiberg, Dale; Indu Ramchandani (contributor), *Students' Britannica India*, Vols. 1–5 (India: Popular Prakashan, 2000).
Hughes-Buller, R., *Imperial Gazetteer of India: Provincial Series: Baluchistan* (Lahore: Sang-e-Meel Publications, 1991).
Poladi, Hassan, *The Hazaras* (Stockton, California: Mughal Publishing Company, 1989).
Quddus, S.A., *The Tribal Baluchistan* (Ferozsons (Pvt.) Ltd., Lahore, 1990).
Ramzi, *Food Prints*, pp. 8–9.
Sener, Bilge (ed.), *Biodiversity: Biomolecular Aspects of Biodiversity and Innovative Utilization* (New York, NY: Springer, 2002).

Balti
Chapman, Pat, *Curry Club: Balti Curry Cookbook* (Judy Piatkus Publishers Ltd, 1994), pp. 10–13 and 193–6.
Ramzi, *Food Prints*, pp. 63–4.

Balti gosht
Chapman, Pat, *Balti Bible*, pp. 10–13, 193–6.

Barfi
Davidson, *Oxford Companion to Food*, p. 61.

Barley
Briggs, D.E., *Barley* (London: Chapman and Hall, 1978).

Barley agriculture
Jain, V.K., *Prehistory and Protohistory of India: An Appraisal* (New Delhi: D.K. Printworld (Pvt) Ltd., 2006).
Prakash, Om, *Economy and Food in Ancient India* (Bhartiya Vidya Prakashan, 1987).
Sharma, B.D., 'The Origin and History of Barley in India,' chapter 9, pp. 120–5. In: V.C. Srivastava, *History of Agriculture in India (up to c. 1200 A.D.)*, vol. 5, part 1 of History of Science, Philosophy and Culture in Indian Civilization (PHISPC) (New Delhi: Centre for Studies in Civilization, 2008).

Basmati rice
Husain, Shehzad, *Healthy Indian Cooking*, p. 28.

Bay leaf (Tej patta)
Husain, Shehzad, *Healthy Indian Cooking*, p. 16.
Ramzi, *Food Prints*, p. 41.

Bengali
Ramzi, *Food Prints*, p. 147.

Bengali cuisine
Achaya, *Hist. Dict. of Indian Food*, p. 21,

Besan
Achaya, *Hist. Dict. of Indian Food*, p. 24.
Davidson, *Oxford Companion to Food*, p. 75.
Husain, Shehzad, *Healthy Indian Cooking*, p. 29.

Betel nut
Davidson, *Oxford Companion to Food*, p. 75.

Bhakri
Sen, Colleen Taylor, *Food Culture in India* (London: Greenwood Publishing Group, 2004), p. 42.

Bhel puri
Ramzi, *Food Prints*, pp. 132, 154.

Bhoona (frying)
Ramzi, *Food Prints*, p. 16.

Bihari, Bihari specialties
Ramzi, *Food Prints*, p. 119.

Biryani
Davidson, *Oxford Companion to Food*, p. 77.
Hasan, Shazia, 'A Journey of the Senses,' *Dawn*, 16 November 2017.
Tirmizi, Bisma, 'Hail, Queen Biryani,' *Dawn*, Sunday, 20 October 2019.

Biscuit
Achaya, *Hist. Dict. of Indian Food*, p. 29.
'Food Stories,' dawn.com, 22 December 2016.

Bitter gourd
Achaya, *Hist. Dict. of Indian Food*, p. 29.
Achaya, *Indian Food* (1994).
Jois, S.N. Krishna (ed.), *Supa Shastra of Mangarasa (AD 1516)* (University of Mysore, 1969), foods of Karnataka, pp. 253–308.
The Wealth of India: Raw Materials Series, vol. 6 (New Delhi: Council of Scientific and Industrial Research, 1962), p. 408.

Black cumin
Davidson, *Oxford Companion to Food*, p. 82.

Bohra cuisine
Lakda, Shamime, *Dhaal-Chaawal Palidu: A Collection of Bohra Recipes* (Book Art, 2002).
Content department at Phegency.

Ramzi, *Food Prints*, pp. 137–8.

Boiling and tenderising
Ramzi, *Food Prints*, p. 17.

Bombay duck
Collingham, Lizzie, *Curry: A Tale of Cooks and Conquerors* (New York: OUP, 2006). (Hereinafter referred to as: Collingham, *Curry*).

Bone marrow
Davidson, *Oxford Companion to Food*, p. 90.

Boondi
Davidson, *Oxford Companion to Food*, p. 75.

Bosrak
Ramzi, *Food Prints*, p. 97.

Bossari or busri
Ramzi, *Food Prints*, p. 101.

Bottle gourd
Achaya, *Hist. Dict. of Indian Food*, pp. 29–30.
Prakash, Om, *Food and Drinks in Ancient India* (Delhi: Munshiram Manoharlal, 1961), Vedic period, pp. 7–33.
Singh, Umrao; A.M. Wadhwani; and B.M. Johri, *Dictionary of Economic Plants in India* (New Delhi: Indian Council of Agricultural Research, 1983), p. 249.

Buckwheat
Davidson, *Oxford Companion to Food*, pp. 110–11.

Buddhism
Achaya, *Hist. Dict. of Indian Food.*
Prakash, Om, *Economy and Food in Ancient India*, part 1: Economy (Bharatiya Vidya Prakashan, 1987).
Prakash, Om, *Food and Drinks in Ancient India* (Delhi: Munshi Ram Manohar Lal, 1961).
Sharma, R.S., *India's Ancient Past* (New Delhi: Oxford University Press, 2005), Chapter 14, pp. 130–44.
Thapar, Romila, *Early India* (New Delhi: Penguin Books, 2001), pp. 167–73.

Buffalo
Achaya, *Hist. Dict. of Indian Food*, pp. 33–4.
Ansari, Mohammad Azhar, *European Travellers under the Mughals, 1580–1627* (Delhi: Idarah-i Adabiyat-i Delli, 1975), pp. 76–103.
Das, Sukla, *Socio-Economic Life of Northern India (c. A.D. 550 to A.D. 650)* (Abhinav Publications, New Delhi, 1980), Chapter 6, p. 134.
Gibbs, H.A.R. (trans.), *Ibn Battuta: Travels in Asia and Africa, 1325–1354* (London: Routledge and Kegan Paul Ltd, 1957), 4th impression, pp. 185–217.

Bumbaiya naan
Achaya, *Indian Food*, p. 138.

Bunda palla machli
Ramzi, *Food Prints*, p. 101.

Burus berkutz, burusshapik
Ramzi, *Food Prints*, p. 68.

Butter
Davidson, *Oxford Companion to Food*, p. 118.

Buttermilk
Davidson, *Oxford Companion to Food*, pp. 143–4.

Cabbage
Davidson, *Oxford Companion to Food*, pp. 121–2.

Caramel custard/crème caramel/egg pudding
Davidson, *Oxford Companion to Food*, p. 226.
Ramzi, *Food Prints*, p. 129.

Cardamom
Achaya, *Indian Food*, p. 33.
Davidson, *Oxford Companion to Food*, p. 138.
Heritage, 'Elaichi the queen of spices,' issue 15, p. 61.
Husain, Shehzad, *Healthy Indian Cooking*, pp. 11–12.
Ramzi, *Food Prints*, p. 33.

Carom seed/ajwain
Davidson, *Oxford Companion to Food*, pp. 9, 21.
Ramzi, *Food Prints*, p. 38.

Carrot/gajar ka halwa
da Silva Dias, J., 'Nutritional and Health Benefits of Carrots and Their Seed Extracts,' *Food and Nutrition Sciences*, 5 (2014), pp. 2147–156.
'Food Stories,' Dawn.com, 21 January 2014.

Cattle
Achaya, *Hist. Dict. of Indian Food*, p. 38.
Davidson, *Oxford Companion to Food*, p. 147.
Randhawa, M.S., *A History of Agriculture in India* (New Delhi: Indian Council of Agricultural Research, 1980), vol. 1, p. 107.

Cauliflower
Achaya, *Hist. Dict. of Indian Food*, p. 39.
Davidson, *Oxford Companion to Food*, p. 149.
Husain, Shehzad, *Healthy Indian Cooking*, p. 20.

Central Asia
Ferguson, Priscilla Parkhurst, *Accounting for Taste: The Triumph of French Cuisine Accounting for Taste*, Chapter 3: Readings in a Culinary Culture (University of Chicago Press, 2004), pp. 83–110.
Fernandez, Keith J., 'Table Talk: The Emperor's New Iftar,' Gulfnews.com, 15 June 2017.
Gier, Nicholas F., 'From Mongols to Mughals: Religious Violence in India 9th–18th centuries,' presented at the Pacific Northwest Regional Meeting American Academy of Religion, Gonzaga University, May 2006.
Mukherjee, Soma, *Royal Mughal Ladies and Their Contributions* (Gyan Books, 2001), p. 10.
Narayanan, Divya, 'What Was Mughal Cuisine? : Defining and Analysing a Culinary Culture,' Interdisziplinäre Zeitschrift für Südasienforschung, January 2016, pp. 1–30.
Sahuliyar, Arti, 'Mughlai cuisine tops popularity charts in capital,' *The Telegraph*, Calcutta, 5 July 2008

Chaakna
Ilyas, Ferya, 'Deccan Diaries,' T Magazine, *The Express Tribune*, 1–7 December 2013.

Chaas
Achaya, *Hist. Dict. of Indian Food*, p. 24.
Davidson, *Oxford Companion to Food*, pp. 118–19.

Chaat/papri chaat
Arab, L., Blumberg, J.B., 'Introduction to the Proceedings of the Fourth International Scientific Symposium on Tea and Human Health,' J Nutr. 2008 Aug; 138(8): 1526S–1528S.
Ramzi, *Food Prints*, pp. 152–3.

Chakki
Achaya, *Hist. Dict. of Indian Food*, p. 39.

Chapati
Achaya, *Hist. Dict. of Indian Food*, p. 40.

Chapli kebab
Ramzi, *Food Prints*, p. 54.
Shinwari, Sher Alam, 'Krazy about (Chapli) kebab,' On the Menu, *Dawn*, 13 October 2013.
Tirmizi, Bisma, 'Food Stories,' dawn.com, 18 March 2014.

Chapoti
Ramzi, *Food Prints*, p. 60.

Chewra
Achaya, *Indian Food*, pp. 110 and 135.

Chicken corn soup
Ramzi, *Food Prints*, p. 146.

Chicken fried rice
Ramzi, *Food Prints*, p. 146.

Chicken karhai
Tirmizi, Bisma, 'Food Stories: Karahi Gosht,' *Dawn*, 6 October 2014.

Chicken makhni
Pal, Sanchari, 'TBI Food Secrets: The Humble Origin of the Hugely Popular Butter Chicken,' 15 November 2016.

Chikki
Achaya, *Indian Food*, p. 134.

Tirmizi, Bisma, 'The Euphoria of Desi Winter Delights,' *Dawn*, 2 December 2018.

Chilli
Achaya, *Hist. Dict. of Indian Food*, pp. 42–3.
Davidson, *Oxford Companion to Food*, p. 172.
Husain, Shehzad, *Healthy Indian Cooking*, p. 19.
Lilani, Pinky, *Spice Magic, An Indian Culinary Adventure* (Development Dynamics, 2001).

Chinese cuisine/Chinese/Chinese specialties/chow mein
Davidson, *Oxford Companion to Food*, pp. 173–4.
Ramzi, *Food Prints*, pp. 145–6.

Christmas
Ramzi, *Food Prints*, p. 161.

Chulah
Achaya, *Hist. Dict. of Indian Food*, p. 45.
Archaeology Museum, M.S. University of Baroda, Vadodara.
Sen, Chitrabhanu, *Dictionary of Vedic Rituals* (Delhi: Concept Publishing Co., 1978; repr. 1982).
Vesci, Uma Marina, *Heat and Sacrifice in the Vedas* (Delhi: Motilal Banarsidass, 1985), pp. 32, 69, 315.

Churi
Dahiya, Ashish, *Foods of Haryana: The Great Desserts* (IHTM – MDU in association with Intellectual Foundation India, 2013).

Chutney
Davidson, *Oxford Companion to Food*, p. 186.
Ramzi, *Food Prints*, p. 29.

Cinnamon
Achaya, *Hist. Dict. of Indian Food*, pp. 45–6.
Gul Hasan, Saba, 'The Health Advertiser,' *Dawn*, 10 August 2014.
Ramzi, *Food Prints*, p. 34.

Clove
Achaya, *Hist. Dict. of Indian Food*, pp. 47–8.
Davidson, *Oxford Companion to Food*, p. 194.
Husain, Shehzad, *Healthy Indian Cooking*, p. 6.
Ramzi, *Food Prints*, p. 34.

Coconut
Achaya, *Hist. Dict. of Indian Food*, pp. 48–9.
Chattopadhyaya, K.P. *The Ancient Indian Culture Contacts and Migrations* (Calcutta: Firma K.L. Mukhopadhyay, 1970), pp. 9f.
Davidson, *Oxford Companion to Food*, p. 198.
Husain, Shehzad, *Healthy Indian Cooking*.

Cooking the Pakistani way
Ramzi, *Food Prints*, pp. 13–15.

Coriander/coriander seed
Achaya, *Hist. Dict. of Indian Food*, p. 55.
Davidson, *Oxford Companion to Food*, p. 216.
Husain, Shehzad, *Healthy Indian Cooking*, p. 16.
Ramzi, *Food Prints*, p. 35.

Court cuisine
Achaya, *Indian Food*, pp. 154–6.
Azeem, Sarwat Yasmeen, 'The Naked Nawab,' *Dawn*, 19 November 2017.
Ramzi, *Food Prints*, pp. 48–9.
Sahu, K.P., *Some Aspects of North Indian Social Life 1000–1526 AD* (Punthi Pusthak, Calcutta, 1973), ch. 2, pp. 29–44.

Crop rotation
Abbas, Muhammad Akhtar, *General Agriculture* (Lahore: Publisher's Emporium, 2000).
Mohler, Charles L.; and Sue Ellen Johnson (eds.), Crop Rotation on Organic Farms – A Planning Manual, NRAES 177 (NY: Plant and Life Science Publishing, July 2009).

Cucumber
Davidson, *Oxford Companion to Food*, p. 230.

Cumin
Davidson, *Oxford Companion to Food*, p. 233.
Gul Hasan, Saba, 'The Health Advertiser,' *Dawn*, 10 August 2014.
Husain, Shehzad, *Healthy Indian Cooking*, p. 13.
Ramzi, *Food Prints*, p. 35.

Curry leaf
Davidson, *Oxford Companion to Food*, p. 236.
Husain, Shehzad, *Healthy Indian Cooking*, p. 17.
Mathur, Abhishek, et al. 'Anti Inflammatory Activity of Leaves Extracts of Murraya Koenigii,' in *International Journal of Pharma and Bio Sciences*, vol. 2, issue 1, January–March 2011, pp. 541–4.

Cutlet
Davidson, *Oxford Companion to Food*, p. 238.

Daal
Achaya, *Hist. Dict. of Indian Food*, p. 60.
Davidson, *Oxford Companion to Food*, p. 242.

Daal chawal palidu
Lakda, Shamime, *Dhaal-Chaawal Palidu: A Collection of Bohra Recipes* (Book Art, 2002).
Ramzi, *Food Prints*, p. 138.

Daal gosht with meethay chawal
Ramzi, *Food Prints*, p. 135.

Daal ka hasma
Ramzi, *Food Prints*, p. 139.

Daal makhni
Ramzi, *Food Prints*, p. 70.

Dahi bara/dahi baray/vara/bhalla
Achaya, *Indian Food*, p. 136.
Ramzi, *Food Prints*, p. 153.

Darbesh
Ramzi, *Food Prints*, p. 56.

Date
Aazim, Mohiuddin, 'Bustling Dry Fruits Market,' *Dawn*, 19 November 2012.
Achaya, *Indian Food*, p. 59.
Davidson, *Oxford Companion to Food*, pp. 243–4.
Randhawa, M.S., *A History of Agriculture in India*, vol. 2 (New Delhi: Indian Council of Agricultural Research, 1982), pp. 10–12.

Delda
Ramzi, *Food Prints*, p. 97.

Delhi Sultanate
New World Encyclopedia contributors, 'Delhi Sultanate', New World Encyclopedia, 12 August 2013, <https://www.newworldencyclopedia.org/entry/Delhi_Sultanate>.
Szczepanski, Kallie, 'Delhi Sultanates,' ThoughtCo. <thoughtco.com/the-delhi-sultanates-194993>.

Dessert
Ramzi, *Food Prints*, pp. 30–31.

Dhaga kebab
Ramzi, *Food Prints*, p. 113.

Dhansak
Rau, Santha Rama, *The Cooking of India* (Time-Life Books, New York, 1969), p. 152.

Dho do
Ramzi, *Food Prints*, p. 101.

Dhokla
Achaya, *Hist. Dict. of Indian Food*, p. 61.
Achaya, *Indian Food*, pp. 134, 136.
Ramzi, *Food Prints*, p. 142.
Sankaran, Srinivasan Saradha, 'The Relation Between Karnataka and Gujarat from the 7th to the early 14th century AD,' PhD thesis (Baroda: Maharaja Sayajirao University of Baroda, 1974), 2 vols, vol. 1, ch. 4.

Dhokri wali kari
Ramzi, *Food Prints*, p. 142.

Dhuan/dhungar (smoking)
Ramzi, *Food Prints*, p. 20.

Dilliwallay
Ramzi, *Food Prints*, p. 111.

Diltar
Ramzi, *Food Prints*, p. 68.
Karakoram Series, Cooking in Hunza, More Mountain Wisdom.

Diram phitti
Flowerday, Dr Julie, 'Hunza's Past Carried into the Present,' Karakoram Series, Cooking in Hunza.
Isani, Aamna Haider, 'The Mighty Hunza Food Journey,' Instep, *The News on Sunday*, p. 35.
Ramzi, *Food Prints*, p. 67.

Do pyaza
Ramzi, *Food Prints*, p. 71.

Doodh ka sherbet
Ramzi, *Food Prints*, p. 133.

Doodh khoya
Mahindru, S.N., *Milk & Milk Products* (New Delhi: APH Publishing Corporation, 2009), p. 23.

Doodh na puff
'Food for thought: Parsi Feast,' *Dawn*, 21 August 2011.

Doodh patti
Ramzi, *Food Prints*, p. 88.

Doodh ras lamb
Ramzi, *Food Prints*, p. 78.

Doodhi falooda
Ramzi, *Food Prints*, p. 141.

Doudo
Ramzi, *Food Prints*, p. 67.

Dried red chilli/chilli (*Capsicum frutescens*)/sabuth sookhi lal mirch
Husain, Shehzad, *Healthy Indian Cooking*, p. 12.
Ramzi, *Food Prints*, p. 34.

Dry fruit
Aazim, Mohiuddin, 'Bustling Dry Fruits Market,' *Dawn*, 19 November 2012.
Inam, Moniza, 'Nature's Bounty,' All About Lifestyles, *Dawn*, 1 February 2013.

Dum (steaming)
Kalra, Jiggs and Pupesh Pant, *Classic Cooking of Punjab* (Mumbai: Allied Publishers Pvt. Ltd., 2004).
Ramzi, *Food Prints*, p. 18.
Sen, Colleen Taylor, *Feasts and Fasts: A History of Food in India* (New Delhi: Reaktion Books, 2014; Speaking Tiger Publishing Pvt. Ltd., 2016).

Dum aloo
Ramzi, *Food Prints*, pp. 77, 154.

Dumpukht
Achaya, *Hist. Dict. of Indian Food*, p. 62.

Easter/Easter foods
Davidson, *Oxford Companion to Food*, p. 266.
Ramzi, *Food Prints*, p. 161.

Eggplant/aubergine/brinjal
Achaya, *Hist. Dict. of Indian Food*, p. 31.
Davidson, *Oxford Companion to Food*, p. 42.
Husain, Shehzad, *Healthy Indian Cooking*, p. 19.

Eid ul Azha or Baqra Eid/Eid ul Fitr
Ramzi, *Food Prints*, p. 158.

Falsa/phalsa
Ahmed, M. Shafique, 'Cool and refreshing,' Food for thought, *Dawn*, 3 July 2011.
Davidson, *Oxford Companion to Food*, p. 600.

Fennel seed/saunf
Achaya, *Hist. Dict. of Indian Food*, p. 230.
Gul Hasan, Saba, 'The Health Advertiser,' *Dawn*, 10 August 2014.
Husain, Shehzad, *Healthy Indian Cooking*, p. 13.

Fenugreek/fenugreek seeds (*Trigonella foenum-graecum*)/ methi dana
Davidson, *Oxford Companion to Food*, p. 296.
Husain, Shehzad, *Healthy Indian Cooking*, pp. 13, 17.
Lilani, Pinky, *Spice Magic: An Indian Culinary Adventure* (Development Dynamics, 2001)
Ramzi, *Food Prints*, p. 36.

Flavour enhancer
Ramzi, *Food Prints*, p. 14.

Fresh coriander (*Coriandrum sativum*) hara dhania
Ramzi, *Food Prints*, p. 41.

Fruit chaat
'Let's Chaat!,' Food For Thought, *Dawn*, 17 February 2008.

Gajar ka halwa/gajar ka halwa/gajrella
Pakistan Cuisine, *Humsafar*, March–April 2000, p. 40.
Ramzi, *Food Prints*, p. 87.
Tirmizi, Bisma, 'A Tribute to William Orange,' *Dawn*, 17 November 2019.

Gajjak
Ramzi, *Food Prints*, p. 132.

Galavat kebab
Ramzi, *Food Prints*, p. 123.

Gannay ka ras
Ramzi, *Food Prints*, p. 104.

Gannay ke ras ki kheer
Ramzi, *Food Prints*, p. 89.

Garam masala
Husain, Shehzad, *Healthy Indian Cooking*, p. 13.
Ramzi, *Food Prints*, p. 34.

Garlic
Achaya, *Hist. Dict. of Indian Food*, p. 77.
Davidson, *Oxford Companion to Food*, pp. 331–2.
Husain, Shehzad, *Healthy Indian Cooking*, p. 19.
McCollum, G.D., 'Onion and allies,' in N.W. Simmonds (ed.), *Evolution of Crop Plants*, pp. 186–190 (Longman S. & T., England, 1987).

Garnishes
Ramzi, *Food Prints*, p. 41.

Gehar
Ramzi, *Food Prints*, p. 107.

Ghambaar
'Food for thought: Parsi Feast,' *Dawn*, 21 August 2011.

Ghas ka halwa
Ramzi, *Food Prints*, p. 137.

Ghatia/ghatia salan
Achaya, *Indian Food*, p. 135.
Ramzi, *Food Prints*, p. 135.

Ghee
Achaya, *Indian Food*, 2004.
Achaya, *Hist. Dict. of Indian Food*, p. 79.
Davidson, *Oxford Companion to Food*, p. 338.
Fazl, Abul, *Ain-i-Akbari*, trans. H. Blochmann (1871), (Delhi: Aadiesh Book Depot, repr. 1965), pp. 57–78.
Gul Hasan, Saba, 'The Health Advertiser,' *Dawn*, 22 March 2015.
Prakash, Om, *Food and Drinks in Ancient India (from earliest times to c. 1200 A.D.)* (Delhi: Munshi Ram Manohar Lal, 1961).

Gilgit-Baltistan
Ramzi, *Food Prints*, p. 5.

Ginger (adrak)
Achaya, *Hist. Dict. of Indian Food*, p. 81.
Fazl, Abul, *Ain-i-Akbari*, trans. H. Blochmann (1871), (Delhi: Aadiesh Book Depot, repr. 1965), pp. 57–78.
Husain, Shehzad, *Healthy Indian Cooking*, p. 19.

Girgir aaloo
Ramzi, *Food Prints*, p. 67.

Goa/Goan
Achaya, *Indian Food*, p. 136.
Davidson, *Oxford Companion to Food*, p. 343.
Fernandes, Jennifer, *100 Easy-to-Make Goan Dishes* (New Delhi: Vikas Publishing House Pvt. Ltd., 1977).
Ramzi, *Food Prints*, p. 126.

Goat
Davidson, *Oxford Companion to Food*, p. 343.

Gola ganda
Ramzi, *Food Prints*, p. 155.

Gonglu
Ramzi, *Food Prints*, p. 85.

Gosh nu saag
Ramzi, *Food Prints*, p. 139.

Gosh-i-feel
Mujtaba, Javed, 'Afghan Sweet Delights,' *Dawn*, 19 August 2018.

Gosht ki kari
Ramzi, *Food Prints*, pp. 135–6.

Gourd
Achaya, *Hist. Dict. of Indian Food*, p. 84.

Gram
Davidson, *Oxford Companion to Food*, p. 349.

Grape
Achaya, *Hist. Dict. of Indian Food*, p. 88.
Davidson, *Oxford Companion to Food*, p. 350.
Elphinstone, M.; E.B. Cowell; W.W. Hunter; and J. Talboys Wheeler (eds.), *Ancient India* (Calcutta: Sunil Gupta Ltd., 1953), 'The Chinese-Buddhist Pilgrims in India', p. 68.
Prakash, Om, *Food and Drinks in Ancient India*, Appendix vi, pp. 260–83.
Watt, George, *The Commercial Products of India* (1980) (New Delhi: Today and Tomorrow's Printers and Publishers, repr. 1966), p. 887.

Greek
Biddulph, John, *Tribes of the Hindoo Koosh* (Karachi: Indus Publications, 1977).
Caroe, Olaf, *The Pathans* (Karachi: Oxford University Press, 1958).
Lines, Maureen, *The Kalasha People of North-Western Pakistan* (Peshawar: Emjay Books International, 1996).
Qamar, R.; Qasim Ayub; Ayesha Mohyuddin, et al. 'Y-chromosomal DNA variation in Pakistan,' *Am J Hum Genet*. 2002 May; 70(5):1107–24.

Greek influence
Achaya, *Hist. Dict. of Indian Food*, p. 89.

Jettmar, K., *Beyond the Gorges of the Indus: Archaeology before Excavation* (Karachi: Oxford University Press, 2001).
Subbarayappa, B.V., 'Indus Script: The Womb of Numbers,' *Quarterly Journal of the Mythic Society*, Bangalore, vol. 78, nos1/2, 1987.
Wolpert, S., *A New History of India* (New York: Oxford University Press, 2000).

Green chillies (*Capsium frutescens*) hari mirch
Ramzi, *Food Prints*, pp. 39–40.

Green tea
Ramzi, *Food Prints*, p. 95.

Greens
Ramzi, *Food Prints*, p. 55.
Tausif, Gulrukh, 'On the Menu: Eat your Greens,' *Dawn*, Sunday Magazine, 19 January 2014.

Guava
Davidson, *Oxford Companion to Food*, p. 360.

Gujarati
Ramzi, *Food Prints*, p. 130.
Achaya, *Indian Food*, p. 134.

Gundh phera
Ramzi, *Food Prints*, p. 140.

Gundpaak, gur paapri, gur roti
Ramzi, *Food Prints*, p. 132.

Gushtaba
Achaya, *Hist. Dict. of Indian Food*, p. 123.
Shahid, Mohammad Saleem, 'Eating Out: Going Desi,' *Dawn*, 14 August 2011.
Naqvi, Mubashar, 'Cuisine: A Feast for Kings (And Queens),' *Dawn*, 9 September 2018.

Hak
Ramzi, *Food Prints*, p. 78.

Halal
Davidson, *Oxford Companion to Food*, p. 526.

Haleem
Achaya, *Hist. Dict. of Indian Food*, p. 98.
Davidson, *Oxford Companion to Food*, p. 36.
Fazl, Abul, *Ain-i-Akbari*, trans. H. Blochmann (1871), (Delhi: Aadiesh Book Depot, repr. 1965), pp. 57–78.
Ramzi, *Food Prints*, p. 139.

Half gosht
Ramzi, *Food Prints*, p. 137.

Halwa
Davidson, *Oxford Companion to Food*, p. 368.

Halwa puri
Ramzi, *Food Prints*. Punjab, Desserts, p. 86.

Handi
Ramzi, *Food Prints*, p. 15.

Harappa
Achaya, *Hist. Dict. of Indian Food*, p. 106.
Achaya, *Indian Food*, p. 21.
Basham, A.L., *The Wonder that was India* (1954), (Grove Press Inc., New York, repr.1959), p. 18.
Chakravarthy, Indira, *Saga of Indian Food* (New Delhi: Sterling Publishers Pvt. Ltd, 1972), pp. 8–9.
Davidson, *Oxford Companion to Food*, p. 399.
Dikshit, K.N., *Prehistoric Civilisation in the Indus Valley* (Sir William Meyer Lectures, 1939), (Madras: University of Madras, repr. 1973).
Lal, B.B, 'The Harappan Fallout,' Science Age, September 1985, p. 31.
Randhawa, M.S., *A History of Agriculture in India* (New Delhi: Indian Council of Agricultural Research, 1980), vol. 1, p. 169.
Sankalia, H.D., *Some Aspects of Prehistoric Technology in India* (New Delhi: Indian National Science Academy, 1970).
Vats, M.S., *Excavations at Harappa* (Delhi: Manager of Publications, 1940), vol. 1, p. 466.

Hari mirch aur qeema
Ramzi, *Food Prints*, p. 117.

Harissa
Ramzi, *Food Prints*, p. 78.

Hazara
Poladi, Hassan, *The Hazaras* (Mughal Publishing Company, 1989).
Ramzi, *Food Prints*, p. 96.

Hindkowans
Ramzi, *Food Prints*, p. 58.

Hindu cuisine
Ramzi, *Food Prints*, pp. 105–6.

Hoilo garma
Isani, Aamna Haider, 'The Mighty Hunza Food Journey,' Instep, *The News on Sunday*, p. 35.
Karakoram Series, Cooking in Hunza, Main Courses.

Hunza water
Ramzi, *Food Prints*, p. 68.

Hunzakutz
Karakoram Series, Cooking in Hunza.
Ramzi, *Food Prints*, pp. 65–6.

Huqqa
Ramzi, *Food Prints*, p. 45.

Hyderabadi cuisine
Achaya, *Indian Food*, p. 123.
Jaffrey, Madhur, *A Taste of India* (1985), (London: Pavilion Books Ltd.); 2nd impression 1986.
Latif, Bilkees, 'The Subtle Opulence of Hyderabad,' *Sunday Express*, 8 February 1987.
Ramzi, *Food Prints*, pp. 115–18.

Idli
Achaya, *Indian Food*, p. 126.
Davidson, *Oxford Companion to Food*, p. 396.
Iyengar, H. Sesha (ed.), *Lokopakara of Chavundaraya* (Madras: Oriental Manuscripts Library, 1950), chap. 8: Supasastram, pp. 120–34.
Shivakotiacharya (AD 920), *Vaddaradhane*, Appendix, pp. 225–91.

Iftari
Ramzi, *Food Prints*, p. 158.

Imli aur aaloo bukharay ka sherbet
Ramzi, *Food Prints*, p. 104.

Imli ke phool
Ramzi, *Food Prints*, p. 114.

Indus Valley Civilisation
Achaya, *Hist. Dict. of Indian Food*, p. 106.
Bag, A.K., *Science and Civilisation in India: Harappan Period (c.3000 BC–c. 1500 BC)*, (New Delhi: Navrang, 1985), p. 99.
BBC, bite size, 'Who Were The Indus People,' <http://www.bbc.co.uk/guides/z9mpsbk#zwhy34j>.
Ghurye, G.S., *Vedic India* (Bombay: Popular Prakashan, 1979), pp. 372–80.
Hassan, S. Mahdi, 'Distillation Assembly of Pottery in Ancient India with a Single Item of Special Construction,' in K.V. Sarma (ed.), *Vishveshvaranand Indological Journal*, 1979, vol. 17, pp. 264–66.
Khanna, A.N., *The Archaeology of India* (New Delhi: Clarion Books, 1981), pp. 62–9.
Lal, B.B. and S.P. Gupta (eds.), *Frontiers of the Indus Civilisation* (New Delhi: Books and Books, 1984), p. 417.
Rao, S.R., *Lothal Vol. II: A Harappan Port Town (1955–62)* (New Delhi: Archaeological Survey of India, 1979), vol. 1, pp. 125–34.
Sankalia, H.D., *Some Aspects of Prehistoric Technology in India* (New Delhi: Indian National Science Academy, 1975), p. 45f.
The Editors of Encyclopedia Britannica, Encyclopedia Britannica, Inc., 18 July 2017
Wheeler, R.E. Mortimer, 'The Civilisation of a Subcontinent,' in Stuart Piggott (ed.), *The Dawn of Civilisation: The First World Survey of Human Cultures in Early Times* (London: Thomas and Hudson, 1961), p. 229.

Irani restaurant
Noorani, Asif, 'The Vanishing Irani Restaurants,' *Dawn*, 4 September 2016.

Islam and food
Achaya, *Hist. Dict. of Indian Food*, pp. 106–7.
Davidson, *Oxford Companion to Food*, p. 526.

Jaggery
Achaya, *Hist. Dict. of Indian Food*, p. 110.
Prakash, Om, *Food and Drinks in Ancient India* (Delhi: Munshiram Manoharlal, 1961), pp. 7–57.

Jalebi/Jil-abi
Achaya, *Hist. Dict. of Indian Food*, pp. 113–14.
Achaya, *Indian Food*, pp. 121, 155.
Annaji, 'Soundarya Vilasa'.
Dasgupta, Minakshie, *Bangla Ranna: The Art of Bengali Cooking* (Calcutta: Jaya Chaliha, 1982).
Yule, Henry and A. C. Burnell, *Hobson-Jobson being a glossary of Anglo-Indian colloquial words and phrases and of kindred terms etymological, historical, geographical and discursive* (1886). New ed. edited by William Crooke (London: J. Murray, 1903). (New Delhi: Munshiram Manoharlal Publishers Pvt Ltd., 1984), 4th ed., p. 458.

Jat
Ramzi, *Food Prints*, p. 7.
Blood, Peter R. (ed.), *Pakistan: A Country Study* (Washington, D.C., Federal Research Division, Library of Congress, 1994).

Kaak
Ramzi, *Food Prints*, p. 93.

Kabuli pulao
Ramzi, *Food Prints*, p. 59.

Kacchi lassi
Ramzi, *Food Prints*, p. 56.

Kachoomar
Ramzi, *Food Prints*, p. 30.

Kachori
Achaya, *Indian Food*, p. 136.
Ramzi, *Food Prints*, p. 131.

Kakori kebab
Ramzi, *Food Prints*, pp. 124–5.

Kalash
Bruun, Ole and Arne Kalland (ed.), *Asian Perceptions of Nature: A Critical Approach*, Nordic Institute of Asian Studies, (Curzon Press, 1995; Routledge, 2013).
Lines, Maureen, 'Kalash Festival,' *Dawn*, 1 February 2013.
Lines, Maureen, Flashback: The Enchanting Kalash Valleys,' *Dawn*, 30 September 2012.
Masood, Saira, 'The Indo-Aryans of Pakistan,' *This Fortnight in Pakistan*, spring 2011, p. 10.
Ramzi, *Food Prints*, pp. 61–2.

Kaleji (liver)
Davidson, *Oxford Companion to Food*, p. 459.

Kali
Ramzi, *Food Prints*, p. 60.

Kalmi bara
Ramzi, *Food Prints*, p. 113.

Kanji
Achaya, *Hist. Dict. of Indian Food*, p. 116.
Ramzi, *Food Prints*, p. 88.

Kantra
Ramzi, *Food Prints*, p. 133.

Karachi cuisine
Ramzi, *Food Prints*, pp. 109–11.

Karhai Namak Mandi
Khan, Teepu Mahabat, *The Tribal Areas of Pakistan* (Lahore: Sang-e-Meel Publications, 2008).
Ramzi, *Food Prints*, p. 55.

Karmo
Ramzi, *Food Prints*, p. 141.

Karri
Ramzi, *Food Prints*, p. 95.

Kashmir/Azad Kashmir
Achaya, *Hist. Dict. of Indian Food*, pp. 123–4.
Davidson, *Oxford Companion to Food*, p. 431.
Ramzi, *Food Prints*, p. 6.

Kashmiri chai
Ramzi, *Food Prints*, p. 78.

Kashmiri cuisine
Achaya, *Indian Food*, pp. 137–8.
Kapur, M.L., *The History of Medieval Kashmir* (Delhi: Oriental Publishers and Distributors, 1975), p. 218.
Ramzi, *Food Prints*, pp. 73–5.
Rau, Santha Rama, *The Cooking of India* (Time-Life Books, New York, 1969),
Tirmizi, Bisma, 'A Feast from the Mountains,' *Dawn*, 7 May 2017.

Katakat
Ramzi, *Food Prints*, p. 85.

Kataway
Ramzi, *Food Prints*, p. 57.

Kebab
Achaya, *Hist. Dict. of Indian Food*, p. 115.
Fazl, Abul, *Ain-i-Akbari*, trans. H. Blochmann (1871), (Delhi: Aadiesh Book Depot, repr. 1965), pp. 57–78.

Ramzi, *Food Prints*, p. 53.

Sahu, Kishori Prasad, *Some Aspects of North Indian Social Life (1000–1526 AD)*, (Calcutta: Punthi Pustak, 1973), ch. 2, pp. 29–44.

Kebab roll
Kaleem, Amna, 'Rock 'n' Roll, Hot Seat,' *Dawn*, 2 September 2007.

Kewra (screw pine)
Davidson, *Oxford Companion to Food*, p. 705.
Husain, Shehzad, *Healthy Indian Cooking*, p. 29.

Khadda kebab
Betini, Asad Khan, 'Travel: Jinn Mountain,' *Dawn*, 8 April 2018.
Javaid, Mujtaba, 'Cuisine: Meat Up in Quetta,' *Dawn*, 16 April 2017.

Khakra
Achaya, *Indian Food*, p. 138.
Ramzi, *Food Prints*, p. 130.

Khameer roti
Ramzi, *Food Prints*, p. 92.

Khamuloot pie
Ramzi, *Food Prints*, p. 68.

Khandvi
Achaya, *Hist. Dict. of Indian Food*, p. 98.
Ramzi, *Food Prints*, p. 112.

Khara papeta ma gosht
Ramzi, *Food Prints*, p. 144.

Khara prashad
Achaya K.T., *Indian Food: A Historical Companion*, 3rd ed., p. 61.
Achaya, *Hist. Dict. of Indian Food*, p. 195.
Ramzi, *Food Prints*, p. 89.

Kharak
Ramzi, *Food Prints*, p. 141.

Khatia
Ramzi, *Food Prints*, p. 140.

Kheel
Achaya, *Hist. Dict. of Indian Food*, p. 130.

Kheer
Davidson, *Oxford Companion to Food*, p. 434.

Khichra
Ramzi, *Food Prints*, p. 134.

Khichri
Ramzi, *Food Prints*, pp. 120, 135.

Khoja/Khoja specialties
Lilani, Pinky, *Spice Magic, An Indian Culinary Adventure* (Development Dynamics, 2001), p. 22.
Ramzi, *Food Prints.*, pp. 133–7.

Khow
Ramzi, *Food Prints*, p. 60.

Khow suey
Ramzi, *Food Prints*, p. 149.

Khoya
Achaya, *Hist. Dict. of Indian Food*, p. 130.

Khurood
Ramzi, *Food Prints*, p. 93.

Khyber Pakhtunkhwa
Bruun, Ole and Arne Kalland (ed.), *Asian Perceptions of Nature: A Critical Approach*, Nordic Institute of Asian Studies, (Curzon Press, 1995; Routledge, 2013).
Nijjar, Bakhshish Singh, *Origins and History of Jats and Other Allied Nomadic Tribes of India: 900 B.C.–1947 A.D.* (New Delhi: Atlantic Publishers, 2008).
Ramzi, *Food Prints*, pp. 1–5.

Khyber Pass
ANI, *Mughalnama: changing the contours of Mughlai cuisine in India, 5 January 2018, <https://www.aninews.in/news/ lifestyle/food/mughalnama-changing-the-contours-of- mughlai-cuisine-in-india201801051517270001/>*.

Koftay
Ramzi, *Food Prints*, p. 125.

Kokum
Baliga, Manjeshwar Shrinath; Harshith P. Bhat, Ramakrishna J. Pai, Rekha Boloor, and Princy Louis Palatty. 'The chemistry and medicinal uses of the underutilized Indian fruit tree Garcinia indica Choisy (kokum): A review.' *Food research international* 44, no. 7 (2011): 1790–1799. doi: 10.1016/j. foodres.2011.01.064.
Kureel, R.S.; R. Kishor; A. Pandey; and D. Dutt, *Kokum: A Potential Tree Borne Oilseed* (National Oilseed & Vegetable Oils Development Board, 2009), pp. 1–15.
Shiva, Vandana and Maya Goburdhun, 'Kokum: The Malabar Tamarind,' *The Hindu*, 21 November 2014.

Koonday ki niaz
Ramzi, *Food Prints*, p. 160.

Kulcha
Hasan, Shazia, 'A Journey of the Senses,' *Dawn*, 16 November 2017.
Achaya, *Indian Food*, p. 138.

Javaid, Mujtaba, 'Cuisine: Afghan Sweet Delights,' *Dawn*, 19 August 2018.

Kulfi
Achaya, *Hist. Dict. of Indian Food*, p. 132.
Ramzi, *Food Prints*, pp. 114–15.

Kunna
Ramzi, *Food Prints*, p. 85.

Kurutz
Ramzi, *Food Prints*, p. 68.
Karakoram Series, Cooking in Hunza, More Mountain Wisdom, A Different Kind of Cheese.

Labsi
Ramzi, *Food Prints*, p. 132.

Laddu
Achaya, *Hist. Dict. of Indian Food*, p. 132.
Achaya, *Indian Food*, p. 121.

Lagan seekh
Ramzi, *Food Prints*, p. 139.

Lahori fried fish
Ramzi, *Food Prints*, p. 84.

Lai
Ramzi, *Food Prints*, p. 107.

Langar
Ramzi, *Food Prints*, p. 103.

Lassan
Ramzi, *Food Prints*, p. 136.

Lassi
Achaya, *Hist. Dict. of Indian Food*, p. 24.

Lazhek
Ramzi, *Food Prints*, p. 61.

Lentil
Davidson, *Oxford Companion to Food*, p. 452.

Lettuce
Davidson, *Oxford Companion to Food*, pp. 453–4.

Lime
Davidson, *Oxford Companion to Food*, p. 455.

Loganu
Ramzi, *Food Prints*, p. 61.

Long cheray
Ramzi, *Food Prints*, p. 113.

Luknawi
Ramzi, *Food Prints*, p. 122.

Luknawi cuisine
Collingham, *Curry*.

Lychee
Achaya, *Hist. Dict. of Indian Food*, p. 135.
Singh, Sham; Krishnamurthy S.; and Katyal, S. L., *Fruit Culture in India* (New Delhi: Indian Council of Agricultural Research, 1963).
Davidson, *Oxford Companion to Food*, p. 467.

Maash daal
Achaya, *Indian Food*, p. 188.
Bendre, Ashok and Ashok Kumar, *Economic Botany*, 4th ed. (Meerut: Rastogi Publications, 1980), pp. 21–5.

Mace
Achaya, *Hist. Dict. of Indian Food*, p. 136.
Davidson, *Oxford Companion to Food*, p. 470.

Machli ka kebab
Ramzi, *Food Prints*, p. 102.

Machli kofta
Ramzi, *Food Prints*, p. 103.

Maggio
Ramzi, *Food Prints*, p. 139.

Maghaz (brain)
Davidson, *Oxford Companion to Food*, p. 94

Main dish
Ramzi, *Food Prints*, pp. 27–9.
Southworth, Franklin C., *Linguistic Archaeology of South Asia* (RoutledgeCurzon, 2005).

Maize/makki
Achaya, *Hist. Dict. of Indian Food*, p. 139.
BR Research, 'Maize in a post-sugarcane Pakistan,' *Business Recorder*, 7 December 2018.
Davidson, *Oxford Companion to Food*, p. 472.
Pakistan's Most "A-Maize-Ing" Crop,' *The Nation*, 18 May 2018.

Makrani
Ramzi, *Food Prints*, p. 9.

Malai khaja
Ramzi, *Food Prints*, p. 140.

Malido
Ramzi, *Food Prints*, pp. 141, 145.

Malpura
Achaya, *Indian Food*.
Ramzi, *Food Prints*, p. 137.

Maltashta
Karakoram Series, Cooking in Hunza, More Mountain
    Wisdom.
Ramzi, *Food Prints*, pp. 67, 96.

Mamtu
Ramzi, *Food Prints*, p. 97.

Mandazi
Ramzi, *Food Prints*, p. 131.

Mango
Paracha, Nadeem F., 'Smokers' Corner: 'Mango Diplomacy,'
    Dawn, 21 July 2019.

Mangro qeema
Ramzi, *Food Prints*, p. 103.

Mantou
Davidson, *Oxford Companion to Food*, p. 480.

Marzan
Ramzi, *Food Prints*, p. 65.

Masala
Davidson, *Oxford Companion to Food*, p. 485.

Masala dosa
Achaya, *Hist. Dict. of Indian Food*, p. 61.
Achaya, *Indian Food*, p. 46.
Ramzi, *Food Prints*, p. 106.

Masalaydar gur
Ramzi, *Food Prints*, p. 55.

Masoor
Achaya, *Hist. Dict. of Indian Food*, p. 142.

Masoor pulao
Ramzi, *Food Prints*, p. 131.

Meethay chawal
Ramzi, *Food Prints*, p. 56.

Meethi dahi
Ramzi, *Food Prints*, p. 147.

Meetha paratha
Ramzi, *Food Prints*, p. 92.

Mehrgarh
Gangal, K.; G.R. Sarson; A. Shukurov, 'The near-eastern roots
    of the Neolithic in South Asia.' PLoS One. 2014;9(5):e95714.
Jarrige, J.F. et al., 'The Early Architectural Traditions of the
    Greater Indus as Seen from Mehrgarh, Baluchistan,' *Studies
    in the History of Art* 31: pp. 25–33, 2013.
Jarrige, J.F., *Mehrgarh: Neolithic Period Seasons 1997-2000,
    Pakistan* (Editions de Boccard, 2013).

Khan, A. and C. Lemmen, 'Bricks and urbanism in the Indus
    Valley rise and decline,' History and Philosophy of Physics
    (physicshist ph), arXiv:1303.1426v1, 2013.
Moulherat. C.; M. Tengberg; J.F. Haquet; and B. Mille, 'First
    Evidence of Cotton at Neolithic Mehrgarh, Pakistan:
    Analysis of Mineralized Fibres from a Copper Bead,'
    Journal of Archaeological Science 29(12), 2002: pp. 1393–
    1401.
Possehl, G., 'Mehrgarh,' *Oxford Companion to Archaeology*,
    edited by Brian Fagan (Oxford: Oxford University Press,
    1996).
Possehl, G., 'Revolution in the Urban Revolution: The
    Emergence of Indus Urbanization'. *Annual Review of
    Anthropology* 19, 1990: pp. 261–82.
Sellier, Pascal, 'Hypotheses and Estimators for the
    Demographic Interpretation of the Chalcolithic Population
    from Mehrgarh, Pakistan', *East and West* 39(1/4), 1989:
    pp. 11–42.

Melmastia
Ramzi, *Food Prints*, pp. 52–3.

Melon
Whitaker, T.W. and W.P. Bemis, 'Cucurbits'. In: Simmonds,
    N.W. (ed.) *Evolution of Crop Plants* (London: Longman,
    1976), pp. 64–9.

Memon
Ramzi, *Food Prints*. Karachi Cuisine, p. 141.

Methi anda
Ramzi, *Food Prints*, p. 135.

Methi maaz
Ramzi, *Food Prints*, p. 78.

Mewawalla gur
Ramzi, *Food Prints*, p. 87.

Milk
Achaya, *Hist. Dict. of Indian Food*, pp. 154–7.
Davidson, *Oxford Companion to Food*, p. 504.
Rangappa, K.S. and Achaya, K.T., *Indian Dairy Products*
    (Bombay: Asia Publishing House, 1974), p. 109.

Millet
Habib, Nusrat; M. Zubair Anwer; and Ikram Saeed,
    'Forecasting of Millet Area and Production in Pakistan,'
    Journal of Social Welfare and Human Rights 1(1); June 2013
    pp. 47–52.

Mint
Husain, Shehzad, *Healthy Indian Cooking*, p. 17.

Mohenjo-Daro
Costantini, L. (1990). 'Harappan Agriculture in Pakistan: The
    Evidence of Nausharo.' In: M. Taddei (ed.), *South Asian
    Archaeology 1987*, pp. 321–32.

Costantini, L., 'Phase 4: Palaeobotany'. In Jarrige, Catherine, Jean-François Jarrige, Richard H. Meadow, & Gonzague Quivron, *Mehrgarh: Field Reports, 1974–1985, From Neolithic Times to the Indus Civilization: The Reports of Eleven Seasons of Excavations in Kachi District, Balochistan by the French Archaeological Mission to Pakistan*. Published by Department of Culture and Tourism, Government of Sindh, in collaboration with the French Ministry of Foreign Affairs, 1995, p. 218.

Dales, George Franklin and Jonathan Mark Kenoyer, *Excavations at Mohenjo Daro, Pakistan: The Pottery* (UPenn Museum of Archaeology, 1986).

Hemmy, A.S., 'Systems of Weights.' In: *Further Excavations at Mohenjo-Daro: Being an official account of Archaeological Excavations at Mohenjo-daro carried out by the Government of India between the years 1927 and 1931*, pp. 601–606 (New Delhi: Government of India Press, 1938).

Jansen, M. (ed.), *Report on Field Work Carried Out at Mohenjo-Daro Interim Reports, Vol. 2: Pakistan 1983–84 by the ISMEO-Aachen-University Mission*.

Jansen, Michael & Günter Urban (eds.), *Mohenjo-Daro Report of the Aachen University Mission 1979–1985: Section one: Data Collection Volume 1: Catalogue and Concordance of the Field Registers 1924–1938. Part 1: The HR-Area Field Register 1925–1927: X–XV* (Leiden: E. J. Brill, 1985).

Jansen, Michael; Máire Mulloy, and Günter Urban, *Forgotten Cities on the Indus: Early Civilization in Pakistan from the 8th to the 2nd Millennium BC* (Verlag Philipp von Zabern, 1991).

Jarrige, Catherine; Jean-François Jarrige; Richard H. Meadow, & Gonzague Quivron, *Mehrgarh: Field Reports, 1974–1985, From Neolithic Times to the Indus Civilization: The Reports of Eleven Seasons of Excavations in Kachi District, Balochistan by the French Archaeological Mission to Pakistan.* Published by Department of Culture and Tourism, Government of Sindh, in collaboration with the French Ministry of Foreign Affairs, 1995.

Mackay, E.J.H., *Further Excavations at Mohenjo-Daro: Being an Official Account of Archaeological Excavations at Mohenjo-daro Carried Out by the Government of India Between the Years 1927 and 1931*. 2 vols. (Delhi, 1938).

Mark Kenoyer, J. 'Measuring the Harappan world: Insights into the Indus order and cosmology.' In I. Morley & C. Renfrew (eds.), *The Archaeology of Measurement: Comprehending Heaven, Earth and Time in Ancient Societies*, pp. 106–122 (Cambridge: Cambridge University Press, 2010).

Marshall, J. *Mohenjo-daro and the Indus civilization, being an official account of archaeological excavations at Mohenjo-daro carried out by the government of India between the years 1922 and 1927*. 3 Vols. (London: Arthur Probsthain, 1931).

Meadow, R. 'Animal Exploitation During the Harappan Period.' In: *South Asian Archaeology 1989: Papers from the Tenth International Conference of South Asian Archaeologists in Western Europe*. Edited by Catharine Jarrige, John P. Gerry, Richard H. Meadow (Musée national des arts asiatiques Guimet, Paris, France, 3–7 July 1989).

Meadow, R., 'Notes on the Faunal Remains from Mehrgarh, with a Focus on Cattle (*Bos*)'. In: *South Asian Archaeology 1981: Proceedings of the Sixth Conference of the Association of South Asian Archaeologists in Western Europe*. Edited by Bridget Allchin. University of Cambridge Oriental Publications No. 34 (Cambridge: Cambridge University Press, 1984).

Murgh sajji
Ramzi, *Food Prints*, p. 103.

Muri
Achaya, *Indian Food*, p. 110.

Mushroom
Davidson, *Oxford Companion to Food*, pp. 521–3.

Mustard/mustard seed
Achaya, *Hist. Dict. of Indian Food*, pp. 168–9.
Davidson, *Oxford Companion to Food*, p. 526.
Husain Shehzad, *Healthy Indian Cooking*, p. 13.
Vishnu-Mittre, 'The beginnings of agriculture: Palaeobotanical evidence in India.' In J. Hutchinson (ed.), *Evolutionary Studies in World Crops: Diversity and Change in the Indian Subcontinent*, pp. 3–30 (Cambridge: Cambridge University Press, 1974).

Mutanjan
Ramzi, *Food Prints*, p. 77.

Muthia
Achaya, *Hist. Dict. of Indian Food*, p. 98.
Ramzi, *Food Prints*, p. 130.

Naan
Babbar, Purobi, 'Breads of India,' *Namaskar*, Air India, vol. 6, no. 1, 1986, p. 19.
Ramzi, *Food Prints*, pp. 25–6.

Naan chaap
Ramzi, *Food Prints*, p. 136

Nadur palak, nadur yakhni
Ramzi, *Food Prints*, p. 78.

Namkeen gosht
Bisma Tirmizi, 'Food Stories: Namkeen gosht', *Dawn*, 2 June 2015.

Namkeen tikka
Ramzi, *Food Prints*, p. 54.

Nargisi koftay
Achaya, *Indian Food*, p. 123.
Achaya, *Hist. Dict. of Indian Food*, p. 63.

Nashasta ka meetha
Ramzi, *Food Prints*, p. 55.

Navroze
Ramzi, *Food Prints*, p. 159.

Nimco
Ramzi, *Food Prints*, p. 155.

Nutmeg
Husain, Shehzad, *Healthy Indian Cooking*, p. 14.

Offal
Davidson, *Oxford Companion to Food*, p. 551.

Ogra
Ramzi, *Food Prints*, p. 93.

Okra
Davidson, *Oxford Companion to Food*, p. 553.
Husain, Shehzad, *Healthy Indian Cooking*, p. 20.

Onion
McCollum, G.D., 'Onion and allies,' in N.W. Simmonds (ed.), *Evolution of Crop Plants*, pp. 186–190 (Longman S. & T., England, 1987).
Achaya, K.T., *A Historical Dictionary of Indian Food*, pp. 172–3.
Shrigondekar, K.L., *Manasollasa of King Someshwara*, Gaekwad's Oriental Series (Baroda, 1939), vol. 84, pt 2, Vimsati 3, Annabhoga, pp. 21–3.
Sahu, Kishori Prasad, *Some Aspects of North Indian Social Life (1000–1526 AD)*, (Calcutta: Punthi Pustak, 1973), ch. 2, pp. 29–44.
Davidson, *Oxford Companion to Food*, p. 558.
Paan
Achaya, *Indian Food*, p. 48.

Pakhtunwali
Mehsud, Rafiuddin, 'Pashtunwali,' *Dawn*, 6 December 2015.

Pakistan's iconic eateries
Jamal, Nasir, 'Eating Out: Going Desi,' *Dawn*, 13 August 2011.
Mise en Place, edition 1, Restaurant Trail, Bundoo Khan, 2017.
Shahid, Mohammad Saleem, 'Eating Out: Going Desi,' *Dawn*, 14 August 2011.

Pakora
Achaya, *Indian Food*, p. 136.

Pakwan
Ramzi, *Food Prints*, p. 58.

Palak paneer
Ramzi, *Food Prints*, p. 126.

Panch phoron
Davidson, *Oxford Companion to Food*, p. 574.

Paneer (cottage cheese)
Davidson, *Oxford Companion to Food*, p. 219.

Panjiri
Ramzi, *Food Prints*, p. 86.

Pao
Achaya, *Indian Food*, p. 140.
Achaya, *Hist. Dict. of Indian Food*, p. 176.

Pao bhaji
Ramzi, *Food Prints*, p. 131.

Papar/papadam
Achaya, *Hist. Dict. of Indian Food*, p. 176.
Davidson, *Oxford Companion to Food*, p. 623.
Papaya
Davidson, *Oxford Companion to Food*, p. 575.

Parsi, Parsi food
Collingham, *Curry*, p. 121.
Davidson, *Oxford Companion to Food*, p. 579.
Hussain, Saima S., 'Food for Thought: Sugar and Spice,' *Dawn*, 17 February 2013.
Monier-Williams, M., *Sanskrit-English Dictionary* (Oxford: The Clarendon Press, 1899).

Pasanda
Ramzi, *Food Prints*, p. 71.

Patarveli/patra
Contractor, Zara, 'Food for Thought: Parsi Feast,' *Dawn Review*, 21 August 2011, p. 10.

Patia
Achaya, *Hist. Dict. of Indian Food*, p. 179.
Ramzi, *Food Prints*, p. 144.

Pattay tikka
Ramzi, *Food Prints*, p. 63.

Patties
Ramzi, *Food Prints*, p. 128.

Pawan matar-aloo bhaji
Ramzi, *Food Prints*, p. 131.

Paya
Ramzi, *Food Prints*, p. 83.
Hussain, Saima S., 'On the Menu: A Winter Affair,' *Dawn*, 5 January 2014, p. 8.

Pea
Davidson, *Oxford Companion to Food*, p. 588.

Peach
Davidson, *Oxford Companion to Food*, p. 589.

Pear
Davidson, *Oxford Companion to Food*, p. 590.

Peethi ki kachori
Ramzi, *Food Prints*, p. 114.

Penhon
Ramzi, *Food Prints*, p. 104.

Peppercorn/pepper
Achaya, *Hist. Dict. of Indian Food*, p. 183.

Achaya, *Indian Food*, p. 214.
Davidson, *Oxford Companion to Food*, p. 595.
Heyn, Birgit, *Ayurvedic Medicine: The Gentle Strength of Indian Healing* (New Delhi: Indus-Harper Collins India, 1992).
Husain, Shehzad, *Healthy Indian Cooking*, p. 8.
Ramzi, *Food Prints*, p. 37.

Persian influence
Collingham, *Curry*, pp. 24–39.
Ludden, David, *India and South Asia: A Short History* (Oxford: Oneworld, 2002), pp. 84–5, 248.
Ramzi, *Food Prints*, p. 115.

Phaturay
Ramzi, *Food Prints*, p. 83.

Pheni
Achaya, *Hist. Dict. of Indian Food*, pp. 185–6.

Phitti
Karakoram Series, Cooking in Hunza, More Mountain Wisdom, the Staple Food of the Hunzakutz.
Ramzi, *Food Prints*, p. 67.

Phoshpaki
Ramzi, *Food Prints*, p. 60.

Pickle
Davidson, *Oxford Companion to Food*, p. 602.
Nasir, Zahra, 'That's A Pretty Pickle', *Dawn*, 23 February 2020.

Pineapple
Davidson, *Oxford Companion to Food*, p. 608.

Po cha
Ramzi, *Food Prints*, p. 65.

Pomegranate
Ahmed, Amena, 'Diet,' *Dawn*, 1 February 2013.
Davidson, *Oxford Companion to Food*, pp. 618–19.

Pomfret
Davidson, *Oxford Companion to Food*, p. 619.

Poppyseed
Achaya, *Hist. Dict. of Indian Food*, pp. 129–30.
Husain, Shehzad, Healthy Indian Cooking, p. 15.
Ramzi, *Food Prints*, p. 38.

Portuguese culinary influence
Achaya, *Indian Food*, p. 128.
Collingham, *Curry*.

Potato
Achaya, *Hist. Dict. of Indian Food*, pp. 194–5.

Prabhu
Ramzi, *Food Prints*, p. 64.

Pulao/pilaf
Aiyangar, P.T. Srinivasa, *Pre-Aryan Tamil Culture* (Madras: University of Madras, 1930), p. 57.
Davidson, *Oxford Companion to Food*, p. 606.
Majumdar, Girija Prasanna, *Some Aspects of Indian Civilization (in plant perspective)* (Calcutta: The author, 1938), p. 30.
Tirmizi, Bisma, 'Food Stories: Pulao,' *Dawn*, 4 March 2014.

Pulse
Achaya, *Hist. Dict. of Indian Food*, pp. 196–7.
Davidson, *Oxford Companion to Food*, pp. 640–1.
Ramprasad, Vanaja and Sudarshan S.R., 'Ahara Tattwa, An Introduction to Ayurvedic perspective of Nutrition' (Bangalore Ayurveda Academy, 1989).

Pumpkin
Davidson, *Oxford Companion to Food*, p. 641.

Punch
Achaya, *Hist. Dict. of Indian Food*, p. 201.
Achaya, *Indian Food*, p. 176.
Yule, Henry and A.C. Burnell, *Hobson-Jobson* (1886), p. 737.

Punjab
Ramzi, *Food Prints*, pp. 6–7, 81–2.
Blood, Peter R. (ed.), *Pakistan: A Country Study* (Washington, D.C., Federal Research Division, Library of Congress, 1994).

Pura
Ramzi, Food Prints, p. 87.

Puri
Achaya, *Hist. Dict. of Indian Food*, p. 201.
Achaya, *Indian Food*, p. 138.

Qabargah
Ramzi, *Food Prints*, p. 77.

Qadeet
Ramzi, *Food Prints*, p. 95.

Qeema bhara karela
Ramzi, *Food Prints*, p. 113.

Qeema sewaiyan
Ramzi, *Food Prints*, p. 117.

Qehwa
Ramzi, *Food Prints*, p. 79.

Qorma
Davidson, *Oxford Companion to Food*, p. 439.
Ramzi, *Food Prints*, p. 69.

Qurutob
Ramzi, *Food Prints*, p. 73.

Rabri
Ramzi, *Food Prints*, p. 115.

Rahu paratha
Ramzi, *Food Prints*, p. 101.

Raisin
Achaya, *Hist. Dict. of Indian Food*, p. 203.

Raita
Achaya, *Hist. Dict. of Indian Food*, p. 204.

Rajput
Blood, Peter R. (ed.), *Pakistan: A Country Study* (Washington, D.C., Federal Research Division, Library of Congress, 1994).
Ramzi, *Food Prints*, p. 7.

Ramazan
Ramzi, *Food Prints*, p. 157.

Rasgulla
Achaya, *Indian Food*, p. 132.
Ramzi, *Food Prints*, p. 147.

Rasmalai
Achaya, *Indian Food*, p. 132.

Rava/ravou
Achaya, *Indian Food*, p. 75.
'Eating in: Happy Feasting,' *Dawn*, 12 August 2012.
Manekshaw, Bhicoo J., 'Parsi bhonu: a traditional mix,' *Times of India*, 19 July 1986.
Ramzi, *Food Prints*, p. 145.

Raway ka paratha
Ramzi, *Food Prints*, p. 111.

Razmah goagji
Ramzi, *Food Prints*, p. 78.

Red chilli
Ramzi, *Food Prints*, p. 34.

Relish
Davidson, *Oxford Companion to Food*, p. 660.

Rewri
Tirmizi, Bisma, 'The Euphoria of Desi Winter Delights,' *Dawn*, 2 December 2018, p. 8.

Rice
Achaya, *Hist. Dict. of Indian Food*, p. 208.
Grist, D.H., *Rice* (Longman, 1975), 5th ed., repr. 1978, p. 3.
Mohamed, Osman S., 'The Royal Refugees,' *The Times of India*, Sunday Review, 20 August 1982.
Prakash, Om, *Food and Drinks in Ancient India* (Delhi: Munshi Ram Manohar Lal, 1961).

Ramzi, *Food Prints*, p. 27.

Rigvedic Civilisation
Achaya, *Indian Food*, p. 32.
Dowson, John, *A Classical Dictionary of Hindu Mythology and Religion* (London: Kegan Paul, Trench, Trubner and Co. Ltd, 1928), 6th edition, pp. ix–xv.

River fish
Zaman, Fahim, 'Death of a River,' *Dawn*, 29 November 2020.

Roasted peanut
Yusuf, Ahmed, 'Peanuts Parachinarvi,' *Dawn*, 1 February 2015.

Roasting
Husain, Shehzad, *Healthy Indian Cooking*, p. 8.

Rogan josh
Ramzi, *Food Prints*, p. 77.
Collingham, *Curry*.

Roti
Achaya, K.T., *Hist. Dict. of Indian Food*, p. 220.
Achaya, K.T., *Indian Food*, p. 138.
Achaya, K.T., *The Food Industries of British India* (New Delhi: Oxford University Press, 1994), pp. 169–92.
Gidwani, Bhagwan S., *Return of the Aryans* (Penguin Random House India Pvt. Ltd., 2000).
Noorani, Asif, 'More is less...,' *Dawn*, All about Lifestyles 2013.
Pruthi, R.K., *Indus Civilization* (New Delhi: Discovery Publishing House, 2014).
Ramzi, *Food Prints*, pp. 25–6.
Rizwan, Sheharyar, 'Bread, Sweat and Tears,' *Dawn*, 29 November 2020, p. 3.

Rumaali roti
Ramzi, *Food Prints*, p. 122.

Rusk
Davidson, *Oxford Companion to Food*, p. 676.

Saffron
Davidson, *Oxford Companion to Food*, p. 680.
Husain, Shehzad, *Healthy Indian Cooking*, p. 15.
Ramzi, *Food Prints*, p. 38.
Tirmizi, Bisma, 'The Golden Threads,' *Dawn*, 17 March 2019.

Sail phulka
Ramzi, *Food Prints*, p. 106.

Saim ke beej ka salan
Ramzi, *Food Prints*, p. 113.

Sajji
Ramzi, *Food Prints*, p. 94.

Salli pur eeda
Hussain, Saima S., 'Food for Thought: Sugar and Spice,' *Dawn*, 17 February 2013.

Salt
Davidson, *Oxford Companion to Food*, p. 687.

Samosa
Ramzi, *Food Prints*, p. 134.
Rowlatt, Justin, 'The Story of India as Told by a Humble Street Snack,' *BBC*, 24 June 2016.

Samosa chola
Ramzi, *Food Prints*, p. 87.

Sandesh
Achaya, *Indian Food*, p. 132.
Davidson, *Oxford Companion to Food*, p. 692.
Ramzi, *Food Prints*, p. 147.

Sarson ka saag aur makai ki roti/mustard green
Davidson, *Oxford Companion to Food*, p. 527.
Ramzi, *Food Prints*, p. 85.

Sea fish
Ali, Sajida, 'Fishing for Compliments,' *Dawn*, 24 February 2019.

Seekh kebab
Ramzi, *Food Prints*, p. 124.

Seekh kebab aur malai
Ramzi, *Food Prints*, p. 86.

Seel batta
Ramzi, *Food Prints*, pp. 16, 44.

Seena khwakha
Ramzi, *Food Prints*, p. 63.

Sehri
Ramzi, *Food Prints*, p. 157.

Semolina
Davidson, *Oxford Companion to Food*, p. 711.

Sesame
Davidson, *Oxford Companion to Food*, p. 712.
Husain, Shehzad, *Healthy Indian Cooking*, p. 15.

Sev
Achaya, *Indian Food*, p. 135.

Seviyan
Achaya, *Hist. Dict. of Indian Food*, p. 233.

Sha balep
Ramzi, *Food Prints*, p. 64.

Shab daigh
Collingham, *Curry*.
Ramzi, *Food Prints*, pp. 76, 113.

Shab-e-barat
Ramzi, *Food Prints*, p. 159.

Shami kebab
Collingham, *Curry*.
Ramzi, *Food Prints*, pp. 123–4.

Shawarma
Ramzi, *Food Prints*, p. 148.

Sheedi
Ramzi, *Food Prints*, p. 145.
Yimene, Ababu Minda, 'Transplant and Ampersand Identity: The Siddis of Diu, India,' *Journal of African Diaspora Archaeology and Heritage*, 4:1, 2015, pp. 19–33.

Sheermal
Kaleem, Sheherzad, 'Diners Delight: The Wedding Delight,' *Dawn*, 26 November 2017.
Ramzi, *Food Prints*, p. 122.

Sheesha
Ramzi, *Food Prints*, p. 149.

Sherbet
Davidson, *Oxford Companion to Food*, p. 717.

Shetu
Ramzi, *Food Prints*, p. 61.

Shikanjbeen
Ramzi, *Food Prints*, p. 88.

Shikarpur ka achar
Ramzi, *Food Prints*, p. 104.

Shola
Ramzi, *Food Prints*, pp. 54, 112.

Shorba
Ramzi, *Food Prints*, p. 93.

Shoshp
Ramzi, *Food Prints*, p. 61.

Shupinak
Ramzi, *Food Prints*, p. 61.

Shurdee
Ramzi, *Food Prints*, p. 96.

Sigri
Achaya, *Hist. Dict. of Indian Food*.

Sikh
Ramzi, *Food Prints*, p. 89.

Sindh
Ramzi, *Food Prints*, p. 10.
Gidwani, Bhagwan S., *The March of the Aryans* (India Penguin, 2012).

Sindhi kukar
Ramzi, *Food Prints*, p. 102.

Siraiki
Ramzi, *Food Prints*, pp. 81–2.

Snack
Ramzi, *Food Prints*, p. 151.

Sohan halwa
Ramzi, *Food Prints*, p. 89.

Sookha boomla nu tarapori patio
Ramzi, *Food Prints*, p. 144.

Sorghum
Davidson, *Oxford Companion to Food*, p. 735.
Doggett, H., 'Sorghum'. In: Simmonds, N.W. (ed.), *Evolution of Crop Plants* (New York: Longman, 1976), pp. 112–11.
Hulse, J.H.; E.M. Laing; and O.E. Pearson, *Sorghum and the Millets* (Academic Press, 1980), p. 33f.
Prakash, Om, *Food and Drinks in Ancient India* (1961), pp. 260–3.
Watt, George, *The Commercial Products of India* (1908), (New Delhi: Today's and Tomorrow's Printers and Publishers, repr, 1966), p. 393.

Sorpotel
Achaya, *Indian Food*, p. 136.

Souffle
Davidson, *Oxford Companion to Food*, p. 734.
Ramzi, *Food Prints*, p. 141.

Soup
Davidson, *Oxford Companion to Food*, p. 734.

Special occasion food
Ramzi, *Food Prints*, p. 157.

Spice
Husain, Shehzad, *Healthy Indian Cooking*, p. 10.

Spinach
Achaya, *Hist. Dict. of Indian Food*, p. 93.
Smith, P.M., 'Minor Crops, Spinach.' In: Simmonds, N.W. (ed.), *Evolution of Crop Plants* (New York: Longman, 1976).
'Venturing in Spinach Cultivation,' *Dawn*, 11 December 2006.

Spring roll
Davidson, *Oxford Companion to Food*, p. 750.

Staple
Ramzi, *Food Prints*, p. 24.

Stew
Ramzi, *Food Prints*, p. 114.

Street food
Ramzi, *Food Prints*, p. 49.

Sufaid gosht
Ramzi, *Food Prints*, p. 54.

Sugarcane
Achaya, *Indian Food*.
Prakash, Om, *Food and Drinks in Ancient India* (1961), pp. 7–57, 102–131.

Sundhera
Ramzi, *Food Prints*, p. 141.

Tabak maaz
Achaya, *Hist. Dict. of Indian Food*, p. 123.
Naqvi, Mubashar, 'A Feast for Kings (And Queens),' *Dawn*, 9 September 2018.
Ramzi, *Food Prints*, p. 77.
Shahid, M.S., 'Eating Out,' *Dawn*, 14 August 2011.

Taftan
Ramzi, *Food Prints*, p. 111.

Tahiri
Tirmizi, Bisma, 'Hail, Queen Biryani,' *Dawn*, 20 October 2019.

Tajik
Ramzi, *Food Prints*, p. 72.

Tali hui bhindi
Ramzi, *Food Prints*, p. 102.

Tamarind
Achaya, *Hist. Dict. of Indian Food*, p. 248.
Husain, Shehzad, *Healthy Indian Cooking*, p. 15.

Tandoor
Ramzi, *Food Prints*, pp. 25–6.

Tawa
Ramzi, *Food Prints*, p. 15.

Tawa tiki
Ramzi, *Food Prints*, p. 60.

Taway wali machli
Ramzi, *Food Prints*, p. 85.

Tea
Frembgen, Jürgen Wasim, *A Thousand Cups of Tea: Among Tea Lovers in Pakistan and Elsewhere in the Muslim World*, 'Shall we meet for tea? Literary Teahouses on the Internet'; 'Which kinds of tea,' Pettigrew, Tee (cf. Note 1), p. 74.
Hasan, Shazia, 'The Steaming Hot Tea,' *Dawn*, 12 January 2014.
Hussain, Saima, 'Going green,' *Dawn*, 20 July 2014.
Weisburger, J.H., 'Tea and Health,' Proceedings of the Society for Experimental Bio and Medicine, vol. 220, no. 4, April 1999, pp. 271–5.

Teetar
Ramzi, *Food Prints*, p. 102.

Thadal
Ramzi, *Food Prints*, p. 104.

Thepla
Ramzi, *Food Prints*, p. 132.

Thooti wali kheer
Ramzi, *Food Prints*, p. 86.

Tireet
Ramzi, *Food Prints*, p. 95.

Tobacco
Gokhale, B.G. 'Tobacco in Seventeenth-Century India.' *Agricultural History*, vol. 48, no. 4, Agricultural History Society, 1974, pp. 484–92.
Saqib, M.A.N., et al. 'Burden of Tobacco in Pakistan: Findings from Global Adult Tobacco Survey 2014.' *Nicotine & tobacco research: official journal of the Society for Research on Nicotine and Tobacco* vol. 20, 9 (2018): 1138–1143.

Tomato
Achaya, *Hist. Dict. of Indian Food*, p. 253.
Davidson, *Oxford Companion to Food*, p. 802

Trami
Ramzi, *Food Prints*, pp. 74–5.

Tumuro
Ramzi, *Food Prints*, p. 68.
Karakoram Series, Cooking in Hunza, Ingredients.

Turkish influence
Collingham, *Curry*, p. 15.
Ludden, David, *India and South Asia: A Short History* (Oneworld), p. 10.
Trautmann, Thomas R., *India: A Brief History of a Civilization* (New York: OUP, 2011), pp. 148–53.

Turmeric
Husain, Shehzad, *Healthy Indian Cooking*, p. 15.
Mukhopadhaya, Sankarananda, *The Austrics of India Their Religion and Tradition* (Calcutta: K.P. Bagchi and Co., 1975).

Ramzi, *Food Prints*, p. 36.

Tirmizi, Bisma, 'Epicurious: Sunshine in My Kitchen,' *Dawn*, 14 April 2019.

Varq

Achaya, *Hist. Dict. of Indian Food*, p. 345.

Ramzi, *Food Prints*, p. 41.

Vedic Civilisation

Achaya, *Indian Food*, pp. 29–30.

Auboyer, Jeannine, *Daily Life in Ancient India* (Bombay: Asia Publishing House, 1965), p. 63f.

Chandra, A.N., 'Survival of the prehistoric civilization of the Indus Valley,' *Memoirs of the Archaeological Survey of India*, 1929, no. 41.

Gopal, Lallanji, *Aspects of History of Agriculture in Ancient India* (Varanasi: Bharati Prakashan, 1980), p. 90.

Raychaudhuri, S.P., *Agriculture in Ancient India* (New Delhi: Indian Council of Agricultural Research, 1964), p. 81.

Shamasastry, R., *Kautilya's Arthashastra* (Mysore: Mysore Printing and Publishing House, 1967), 8th edition, pp. 129–31.

Thakur, Vijay Kumar, *Urbanisation in Ancient India* (New Delhi: Abhinav Publications, 1981), p. 202.

Vindaloo

Davidson, *Oxford Companion to Food*, p. 830.

Walnut

Davidson, *Oxford Companion to Food*, p. 836.

Water-buffalo

Davidson, *Oxford Companion to Food*, p. 839.

Wazwan

Naqvi, Mubashar, 'Cuisine: A Feast for Kings (And Queens),' *Dawn*, 9 September 2018.

Ramzi, *Food Prints*, pp. 74–5.

Wedding cuisine

Ramzi, *Food Prints*, p. 161.

Wheat agriculture

Achaya, *Indian Food*, pp. 34, 88.

Raychaudhuri, S.P., *Agriculture in Ancient India*, p. 79.

Yakhni

Ramzi, *Food Prints*, p. 54.

Yoghurt

Davidson, *Oxford Companion to Food*, p. 861.

Achaya, *Hist. Dict. of Indian Food*, pp. 57–8.

Zafran sherbet

Ramzi, *Food Prints*, p. 95.

Zerda

Ramzi, *Food Prints*, pp. 29, 78.

Santa Maria, Jack, *Indian Sweet Cookery* (Vintage/Ebury, 1979).

Index